Dementia with Lewy Bodies

Kenji Kosaka
Editor

Dementia with Lewy Bodies

Clinical and Biological Aspects

Springer

Editor
Kenji Kosaka
Emeritus Professor
Yokohama City University
Yokohama, Japan

ISBN 978-4-431-55946-7 ISBN 978-4-431-55948-1 (eBook)
DOI 10.1007/978-4-431-55948-1

Library of Congress Control Number: 2016957400

Printed on acid-free paper

This Springer imprint is published by Springer Nature
The registered company is Springer Japan KK
The registered company address is: Chiyoda First Bldg. East, 3-8-1 Nishi-Kanda, Chiyoda-ku, Tokyo 101-0065, Japan

Preface

Dementia with Lewy bodies (DLB) is now well known to be the second most frequent dementia following Alzheimer disease (AD). Of all types of dementia, AD is known to account for about 50 %, DLB about 20 %, and vascular dementia (VD) about 15 %. Thus, AD, DLB, and VD are now considered to be the three major dementias.

Although the first case of AD was reported by A. Alzheimer in 1906, the first case of DLB was reported by me and my colleagues in 1976. Following a series of our papers (1976–1990), the name "Dementia with Lewy bodies" was proposed in the first International Workshop on DLB, held in Newcastle upon Tyne, England, in 1995, with the results of the workshop reported in *Neurology* in 1996. The second workshop was held in Amsterdam in 1997, and the third was again held in Newcastle upon Tyne in 2003. The results of the third workshop were published in 2005, with the clinical diagnostic criteria then reported in *Neurology*. Those criteria have been used even up until the present. I organized the fourth International Workshop, held in Yokohama, Japan, in 2005. Since then, a fifth workshop has not been convened, for reasons not entirely clear to me; however, the International Conference on DLB was held in Washington, DC, in 2006. A similar international conference was held in Germany in 2009, and B. Boeve and D. Dickson conducted a similar international conference on DLB in Florida in 2015. I took part in all these international workshops and conferences and presented lectures on DLB in all of them.

Since 2006, I have convened the Japan DLB Research Conference in Yokohama every November. The memorial tenth Japan DLB Research Conference was held last November. In addition, since 2007 I have led the Japan DLB Family Organization, the name of which was changed to the Japan DLB Support Network in 2015. Twenty branches of that network have already been established throughout the country. I also have delivered many lectures on DLB in Japan. Consequently, DLB has become well known not only by doctors but also by care workers and the public. In addition, as the result of our clinical tests, Aricept was publicly accepted as the sole medication for DLB, having been granted the first public permission for use in the world. Furthermore, I have published books on DLB not only for doctors but also for care workers and the general public. As a result of these efforts, DLB has become well known in Japan, and my hope is that DLB will also come to be well known worldwide.

This book is published based on that deep hope.

Yokohama, Japan
September 2016

Kenji Kosaka

Contents

Part I
Introduction

Chapter 1
History and Latest Concepts of Lewy Body Disease and Dementia with Lewy Bodies

Kenji Kosaka

Abstract We proposed the term "Lewy body disease" (LBD) in 1980. Subsequently, we classified LBD into three types according to the distribution pattern of Lewy bodies: a brain stem type, a transitional type, and a diffuse type. Later, we added the cerebral type. As we have proposed since 1980, LBD has recently been used as a generic term including Parkinson's disease (PD), Parkinson's disease with dementia (PDD), and dementia with Lewy bodies (DLB).

LBD has neuropathological characteristics whereby numerous Lewy bodies are present in the central and sympathetic nervous systems, and it is a type of alpha-synucleinopathy because the main component of Lewy body is alpha-synuclein. On the other hand, the nomenclature of DLB was proposed at the first International Workshop, which was held in Newcastle upon Tyne (England) in 1995. The result of the Workshop was published in Neurology in 1996. DLB is now called the second most frequent dementia, following Alzheimer's disease (AD). In this chapter, the author explains the most recent concept of LBD and DLB from the historical viewpoint.

Keywords Dementia with Lewy bodies • Lewy body disease • Diffuse Lewy body disease • Parkinson's disease • Parkinson's disease with dementia

1.1 History of Lewy Body Disease

We [1] proposed the term "Lewy body disease (LBD)" in 1980. LBD is now understood to be the generic term including Parkinson's disease (PD), Parkinson's disease with dementia (PDD), and dementia with Lewy bodies (DLB) [2, 3]. Not a few dementia specialists, however, misunderstand how LBD and DLB are related. Therefore, we explain the concept of LBD and DLB from a historical point of view.

K. Kosaka (✉)
Department of Psychiatry, Yokohama City University School of Medicine, 65 Fukuura, Kanazawa-ku, Yokohama 256-0002, Japan
e-mail: kenji@memosync.com

K. Kosaka (ed.), *Dementia with Lewy Bodies*, DOI 10.1007/978-4-431-55948-1_1

1.1.1 From the Discovery of Lewy Bodies to the Proposal of LBD

Fritz Heinrich Lewy [4], who had studied neuropathology under the leadership of Alois Alzheimer at Munich University, reported eosinophilic intracytoplasmic and intraneuritic inclusions in the dorsal vagal nuclei and substantia innominata of PD brains in 1912. At that time, he called these inclusions "eosinophilic bodies." These inclusions were dubbed "Lewy bodies" by Tretiakoff [5] in 1919. From the 1920s to the 1950s, the differences between PD and postencephalitic parkinsonism were topical not only clinically but also neuropathologically. For example, a German neuroanatomist Hassler [6] reported the difference of distribution pattern of neuronal cell loss in the substantia nigra between these two types of parkinsonism in 1938. Greenfield and Bosanque [7], for the first time, disclosed in 1953 that Lewy bodies were always found in the brain stem nuclei in PD, while neurofibrillary tangles were present in postencephalitic parkinsonism. Bethlem and Den Haltog Jager [8] (1960) reported the detailed distribution of Lewy bodies in both the central and autonomic nervous systems.

Thus, the neuropathological base of PD, which had first been found by James Parkinson in 1817, was established. Since then, it had been widely believed that only rarely were Lewy bodies found in the cerebral cortex, although Okazaki et al. [9] reported two autopsied cases in 1960 in which numerous Lewy bodies were found in the cerebral cortex. In 1976, we [10] reported an autopsied case with progressive dementia and parkinsonism, of which I myself was the chief doctor. At that time, I clinically diagnosed the case as atypical presenile Alzheimer's disease with parkinsonism and carried out the dissection myself. As a result, I found numerous intracytoplasmic eosinophilic inclusions in small neurons at the deeper cortical layers and typical Lewy bodies in the brain stem nuclei (Figs. 1.1 and 1.2), in addition to Alzheimer pathology. I also found similar pathological findings in another older patient with depression, visual hallucinations, persecutive delusions, mild dementia, and mild parkinsonism. In 1978, I [11] reported the features of cortical Lewy bodies in comparison with brain stem type of Lewy bodies in three autopsied cases. In addition, I also found and reported two German autopsied cases [12], when I was at Max-Planck Institute for Psychiatry in Munich. These were the first autopsied cases with DLB, not only in Germany but also in Europe. In 1980, we [1] proposed the term "Lewy body disease" based on our 20 autopsied cases. Subsequently, we classified the disease into three types: type A (brain stem type), type B (transitional type), and type C (diffuse type). The brain stem type is consistent with PD, and the diffuse type was later called "diffuse Lewy body disease (DLBD)" [13]. In 1996, we [14] added a cerebral type of LBD, in which Lewy pathology was widely present in the cerebral cortex, but rare in the brain stem. In this case, no Parkinson symptoms were detected in any of the clinical stages. The presence of the cerebral type of LBD is important, since it means that Lewy bodies can develop from the upper area (cerebral cortex) to the lower (brain stem nuclei), contrary to "Braak theory"[15] in which Lewy bodies are usually developed from the lower area to the upper area.

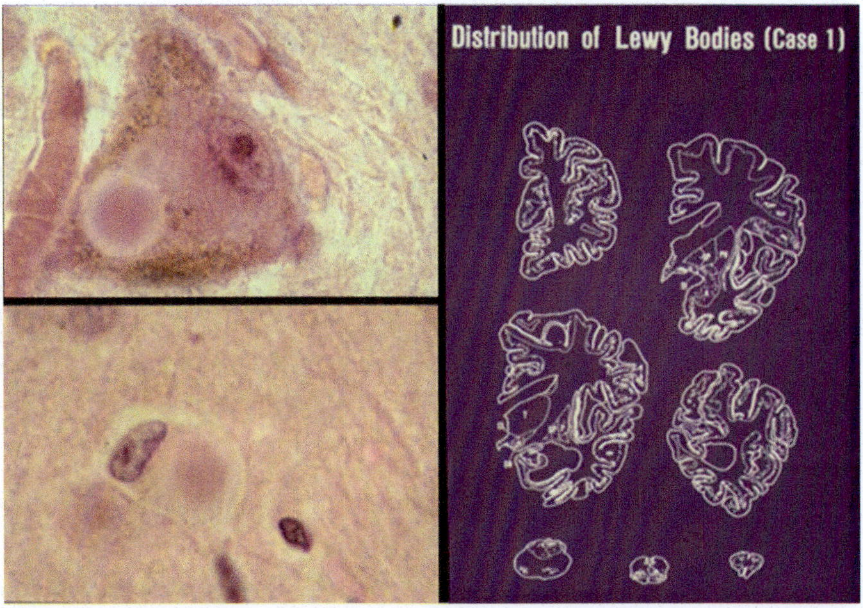

Fig. 1.1 Typical brain stem-type Lewy body (*upper*) and cortical Lewy body (*lower*) and the distribution of Lewy bodies in our first case

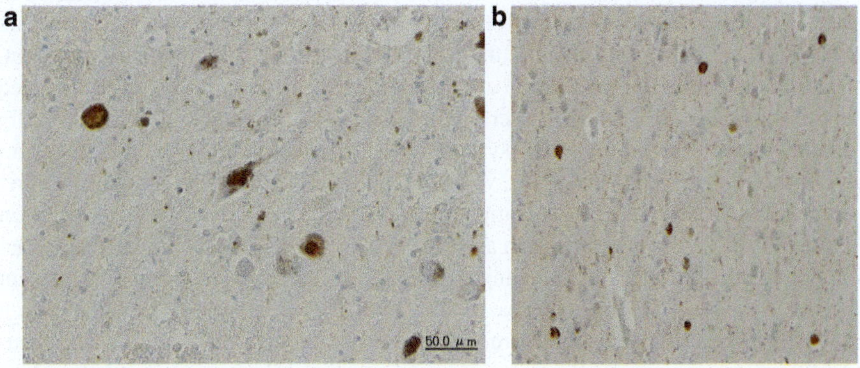

Fig. 1.2 Alpha-synuclein-immunostained Lewy bodies in the substantia nigra (**a**) and in the temporal cortex (**b**)

1.1.2 From the Proposal of Lewy Body Disease to the Proposal of Diffuse Lewy Body Disease

LBD is now defined as follows: "LBD is a chronic progressive neuropsychiatric disorder, which is clinically characterized by Parkinson symptoms of presenile or senile, or often younger onset, usually followed by dementia at the later stages.

Case by case, progressive dementia or various kinds of psychiatric symptoms including characteristic visual hallucination and delusions are the chief symptoms, frequently followed by Parkinson symptoms. It is neuropathologically characterized by numerous Lewy bodies and Lewy neurites (Lewy pathology), and neuronal cell loss in the central and autonomic nervous systems." Yoshimura [16] reconfirmed our study of LBD when he was in Vienna and proposed the term DLBD in 1983. Based on our 11 autopsied cases with the diffuse type of LBD, we [13, 17] also proposed the term "diffuse Lewy body disease (DLBD)" in 1984 and 1990.

DLBD was defined as follows: DLBD is characterized clinically by progressive dementia and Parkinson symptoms of presenile or senile, or sometimes younger onset, and neuropathologically by numerous Lewy bodies and neuronal cell loss in the central and autonomic nervous systems, frequently followed by various degrees of Alzheimer pathology."

1.1.3 From the Proposal of DLBD to the Proposal of DLB

Since we intensified in our paper of 1984 that DLBD had been overlooked in European and American countries, several autopsied cases with DLBD were also reported in those countries. Furthermore, in 1990 I indicated in my review [17] of 36 autopsied DLBD cases reported in Japan that DLBD could be classified into two forms, a common form and a pure form, and that clinical features were different in the two forms. In the common form, the onset was usually older than 65 years (presenile or senile onset), and the chief symptom was cognitive impairment, followed by parkinsonism in 70 % of the cases, while no parkinsonism was detected in 30 % of the cases. On the other hand, in the pure form, the onset was usually much younger, and the initial symptoms were usually those of parkinsonism followed by dementia. Thereafter, when I was invited to the 150th Annual Meeting of the German Psychiatry Association, on the basis of a comparative study between Japanese and European-American autopsied cases with DLBD, I reported [18] that no apparent differences of the clinical features in the common form were present between the two groups, but that in the pure form, Japanese cases had much younger onset and Parkinsonism preceded dementia, while most European-American cases were of presenile or senile onset and dementia preceded parkinsonism. Perry et al. (1990) [19] proposed "senile dementia of Lewy body type," and Hansen et al. (1990) [20] proposed the term "Lewy body variant of Alzheimer's disease." In 1995, the first International Workshop on DLB was held in Newcastle upon Tyne in England. At the workshop, the title of my lecture was "Diffuse Lewy body disease within the spectrum of Lewy body disease" [21]. It was at this International Workshop that "dementia with Lewy bodies" (DLB) was proposed [22]. The results of the Workshop were reported [23] in Neurology in 1996. Then, the clinical and pathological guidelines for DLB (CDLB guidelines) [23] were published, and the clinical diagnosis of DLB became possible. Thereafter, clinical studies were developed further.

1.1.4 From the Proposal of DLB to the Present

The Second International Workshop on DLB was held in Amsterdam in 1998, and the results of the workshop [24] were published in 1999. The Third Workshop was again held in Newcastle upon Tyne in 2003, and the CDLB guidelines-Revised [2] were published in 2005. A symposium titled "A cross-road at DLB and PDD" was held in Washington in 2005, and the results [3] were published in 2007. In 2006, I held the forth International Workshop on DLB and PDD in Yokohama, Japan. Since 2007, I have held the Japan DLB Research Meeting in Yokohama every November. In the Second Japan Annual Meeting, I organized the DLB Family Association in Japan. In 2012, we published "Front Line of DLB Research in Japan" [25].

Over the last 18 years, many important reports on DLB have been published. For example, DLB has been reported to be the second most frequent dementia following AD [26]. Some biological markers for the clinical diagnosis of DLB have also been developed, such as brain SPECT/PET, dopamine transporter imaging [27] (FP-CIT SPECT or DaT scan), and MIBG myocardial scintigraphy [28]. Alpha-synuclein gene mutations [29–31] were found in familial PD and DLB in 1997 to 2004. Alpha-synuclein was defined to be the main component of Lewy bodies in 1997 [32]. Alpha-synuclein is a 149 kDa protein encoded by the SNCA gene, and it is rich in nuclei and presynaptic areas, but its function is not yet well understood. In 2000, alpha-synuclein-positive inclusions were produced in transgenic animals [33, 34]. Braak et al. [35] hypothesized that Lewy pathology initiates in the brain stem and propagates upward to the cerebral cortex. However, in the cerebral type of LBD [14], numerous Lewy bodies were found in the cerebral cortex; in spite of their only being a few in the brain stem nuclei, Lewy pathology was thought to occur in the cerebral cortex and to propagate downward to the brain stem. Lewy pathology might also start from Auerbach's plexus of the lower esophagus [36] or the olfactory bulb [35, 37]. Recently, aggregation of alpha-synuclein might spread transcellulary throughout the brain in a prion-like way [38].

Since attempts to correlate Lewy body pathology to either neuronal cell death or severity of clinical symptoms have not been successful, the synaptic pathology [39] of alpha-synuclein aggregation in Lewy body disease has garnered more attention. For example, it was shown [39] that 90 % or even more of alpha-synuclein aggregates in DLB cases were located at the presynapses in very small deposits.

Some therapeutic trials of galantamine [40] and donepezil [41, 42] to DLB have been reported. In 2014, "Aricept" was, for the first time, recognized as the therapeutic medicine for DLB in Japan. Recently, PD, PDD, and DLB are usually called Lewy body disease [2, 3, 43] as we [1, 13] have used in 1980.

We expect that the mechanism of alpha-synuclein aggregation will be solved and that the effective therapy for LBD will be developed in the near future.

References

1. Kosaka K, Matsushita M, Ooyanagi S, et al. Clinicopathological study of Lewy body disease. Psychiat Neurol Jpn. 1980;82:292–311 (in Japanese).
2. McKeith IG, Dickson DW, Lowe J, et al. Diagnosis and management of dementia with Lewy bodies: third report of the DLB Consortium. Neurology. 2005;65:1863–72.
3. Lippa CF, Duda JE, Grossman M, et al. DLB and PDD boundary issues. Diagnosis, treatment, molecular pathology, and biomarkers. Neurology. 2007;68:812–9.
4. Lewy FH. Paralysis agitans. I. Pathologische Anatomie. In: Lewandowsky M, editor. Handbuch der Neurologie, vol. 3. Berlin: Springer; 1912. p. 920–58.
5. Tretiakoff C. Contribution a l'etude de l'Anatomie pathologique du Locus Niger de Soemmering avec quelques deductionrelatives a la pathogenie des troubles du tonus musculaire et de la maladie de Parkinson. Theses de Paris; 1919.
6. Hassler R. Zur Pathologie der Paralysis agitans und des postencephlitischcn Parkinosnismus. J Psychol Neurol. 1938;48:387–467.
7. Greenfeeld JG, Bosanque FD. The brain-stem lesions in Parkinsonism. J Neurol Neurosurg Psychiatry. 1953;10:213–6.
8. Bethlem J, Den Haltog Jager WA. The incidence and characteristics of Lewy bodies in idiopathic paralysis agitans (Parkinson's disease). J Neurol Neurosurg Psychiatry. 1960;23:74–80.
9. Okazaki H, Lipkin LE, Aronson SM. Diffuse intracytoplasmic ganglionic inclusions (Lewy type) associated with progressive dementia and quadriparesis in flexion. J Neuropathol Exp Neurol. 1961;20:237–44.
10. Kosaka K, Oyanagi S, Matsushita M, et al. Presenile dementia with Alzheimer-, Pick- and Lewy body changes. Acta Neuropathol. 1976;36:221–33.
11. Kosaka K. Lewy bodies in cerebral cortex; report of three cases. Acta Neuropathol. 1978;42:127–34.
12. Kosaka K, Mehraein P. Dementia-Parkinsonism syndrome with numerous Lewy bodies and senile plaques in cerebral cortex. Arch Psychiat Nervenkr. 1979;226:241–50.
13. Kosaka K, Yoshimura M, Ikeda K, et al. Diffuse type of Lewy body disease. A progressive dementia with numerous cortical Lewy bodies and senile changes of various degree. A new disease? Clin Neuropathol. 1984;3:185–92.
14. Kosaka K, Iseki E, Odawara T, et al. Cerebral type of Lewy body disease. Neuropathology. 1996;1:32–5.
15. Braak H, Del Tredici K. Nervous system pathology in sporadic Parkinson disease. Neurology. 2006;70:1916–25.
16. Yoshimura M. Cortical changes in the Parkinsonian brain: a contribution to the delineation of "diffuse Lewy body disease". J Neurol. 1983;229:17–32.
17. Kosaka K. Diffuse Lewy body disease in Japan. J Neurol. 1990;237:197–204.
18. Kosaka K. Diffuse Lewy-Koerperchen Krankheit:Vergleich klinisch-pathologischer Daten zwischen Japanischen und Europaeischen/Amerikanischen Faellen. 150. Jahren Psychiatrie in Deutschlnd; 1992.
19. Perry RH, Irving D, Blessed G, et al. Senile dementia of Lewy body type. A clinically and neuropathologically distinct form of Lewy body dementia in the elderly. J Neurol Sci. 1990;95:119–39.
20. Hansen L, Salmon D, Galasko D, et al. The Lewy body variant of Alzheimer's disease. A clinical and pathological entity. Neurology. 1990;40:1–8.
21. Kosaka K, Iseki E. Diffuse Lewy body disease within the spectrum of Lewy body disease. In: Perry R et al., editors. Dementia with Lewy bodies. Clinical, pathological and treatment issues. Cambridge: Cambridge University Press; 1996.
22. Perry R, McKeith I, Perry E. Dementia with Lewy bodies. Clinical, pathological, and treatment issues. Cambridge: Cambridge University Press; 1996.

23. McKeith IG, Galasko D, Kosaka K, et al. Consensus guidelines for the clinical and pathological diagnosis of dementia with Lewy bodies(DLB). Neurology. 1996;47:1113–24.
24. McKeith IG, Perry EK, Perry RH. Report of the second dementia with Lewy body international workshop. Neurology. 1999;53:902–6.
25. Japan DLB Research Association. The Front Line of Japan DLB Research, the Fifth Anniversary; 2012.
26. Aarsland D, Rongve A, Nore SP, et al. Frequency and case identification of dementia with Lewy bodies using the revised consensus criteria. Dement Geriatr Cogn Disord. 2008;26:445–52.
27. Walker Z, Jaros E, Walker RMW, et al. Dementia with Lewy bodies: a comparison of clinical diagnosis, FP-CIT single photon emission computed tomography imaging and autopsy. J Neurol Neurosurg Psychiatry. 2007;78:1176–81.
28. Yoshita M, Taki J, Yamada M. A clinical role for [(123)I]MIBG myocardial scintigraphy in the distinction between dementia of the Alzheimer's type and dementia with Lewy bodies. J Neurol Neurosurg Psychiatry. 2001;71:583–8.
29. Polymeropoulos MH, Lavedan C, Leroy E, et al. Mutation in the α-synuclein gene identified in families with Parkinson's disease. Science. 1997;276:2045–7.
30. Singleton AB, Farrer M, Johnson J, et al. α-synuclein locus triplication causes Parkinson's disease. Science. 2003;302:841.
31. Farrer M, Kachergus J, Forno L, et al. Comparison of kindreds with Parkinsonism and α-synuclein genomic multiplication. Ann Neurol. 2004;55:174–9.
32. Spillantini MG, Schmidt ML, Lee VMY, et al. α-synuclein in Lewy bodies. Nature. 1997;388:839–40.
33. Feany MB, Bender WW. A drosophila model of Parkinson's disease. Nature. 2000;404:394–8.
34. Masliah E, Rockenstein E, Veinbergs I, et al. Dopaminergic loss and inclusion body formation in α-synuclein mice implications for neurodegenerative disorders. Science. 2000;287:1265–9.
35. Braak H, Del Tredici K. Nervous system pathology in sporadic Parkinson disease. Neurology. 2008;70:1916–25.
36. Wakabayashi K, Takahashi H, Takeda S, et al. Parkinson's disease: the presence of Lewy bodies in Auerbach's and Meissner's plexuses. Acta Neuropathol. 1988;76:217–21.
37. Sengoku R, Saito Y, Ikemura M, et al. Incidence and extent of Lewy body-related alpha-synuclein in aging human olfactory bulb. J Neuropathol Exp Neurol. 2008;67:1072–83.
38. Visanji NP, Brooks PL, Hazrati LN, et al. The prion hypothesis in Parkinson's disease: Braak to the future. Acta Neuropathol Commun. 2013;1:2.
39. Schulz-Schaeffer WI. The synaptic pathology of alpha-synuclein aggregation in dementia with Lewy bodies, Parkinson's disease and Parkinson's disease dementia. Acta Neuropathol. 2013;120:131–43.
40. McKeith I, Del Ser T, Spano P, et al. Efficacy of rivastigmine in dementia with Lewy bodies: a randomized, double-blind, placebo- controlled international study. Lancet. 2000;356:2031–6.
41. Mori E, Ikeda K, Kosaka K. Donepezil for dementia with Lewy bodies: a randomized, placebo-controlled trial. Ann Neurol. 2012;72:41–52.
42. Ikeda M, Mori E, Kosaka K, et al. Long-term safety and efficacy of donepezil in patients with dementia with Lewy bodies: results from a 52-week, open-label. multi-center extension study. Dement Geriatr Cogn Disord. 2013;36:229–41.
43. Kosaka K. Diffuse Lewy body disease. Neuropathology. 2000;20(Suppl):73–8.

Chapter 2
Epidemiological Study on Dementia with Lewy Bodies

Takashi Asada

Abstract Lewy bodies are the hallmark of the brainstem pathology of Parkinson's disease. Dementia with Lewy bodies (DLB) is a common degenerative dementing illness characterized by visual hallucination, fluctuation of cognitive function and consciousness, and REM-related behavior disorder. With the spread of the disease entity of DLB, the reported prevalence has been increasing; however, its accurate prevalence and incidence remains uncertain. In this chapter, we review the previous studies which reported the prevalence and incidence for DLB using the data from community and secondary care setting. As a result, DLB accounts for more than 4 % of all dementia cases, and the incidence of DLB is around 4 % of new dementia cases. However, with more widespread recognition of the clinicopathological entity of DLB, the values of its prevalence and incidence have recently been increasing. Although the consensus clinical criteria for DLB have been revised, its sensitivity remains lower. On the other hand, the results of pathological examination from a cohort study showed much higher prevalence of DLB. In the future, effort should be indispensable to dissipate the discrepancy between clinical and pathological diagnosis of DLB.

Keywords Prevalence • Incidence • Epidemiology • Dementia with Lewy bodies

2.1 Introduction

Lewy bodies, which are the hallmark of the brainstem pathology of Parkinson's disease, were found relatively recently to occur diffusely in the cerebral cortex and to be accompanied by a dementia syndrome with characteristic clinical features. Dementia with Lewy bodies (DLB) is now used as a preferred term for a variety of clinical diagnoses including diffuse LB disease (DLBD) [1], LB dementia (LBD) [2], and senile dementia of LB type (SDLT) [3].

T. Asada (✉)
Faculty of Medicine, Tokyo Medical and Dental University, 1-5-45 Yushima, Bunkyo-ku, Tokyo 113-8510, Japan
e-mail: asada@memory-cl.jp

K. Kosaka (ed.), *Dementia with Lewy Bodies*, DOI 10.1007/978-4-431-55948-1_2

Although DLB was initially thought to be uncommon, with the spread of the disease entity of DLB, the reported prevalence has been increasing recently. Nevertheless, it is said that DLB remains underdiagnosed, with more than half cases missed [4]. Accurate diagnosis of DLB is particularly important, because it facilitates management of common associated symptoms such as hallucination, increased risk of falls, loss of consciousness, and REM-related behavior disorder. These symptoms of DLB are very burdensome for caregivers compared to those presented in other dementing illnesses. To determine the population prevalence and incidence of DLB, we review the previous studies which reported the prevalence and incidence for DLB using the data from community and secondary care setting.

2.2 Summarized Results of the Previous Studies

Thus far, two previous systematic reviews of epidemiological studies [5, 6] are available. Besides the data from studies reviewed in the reviews, we used three additional studies on the epidemiology of DLB. Hereafter, we describe the summarized results of the two reviews and show the main results of the additional studies.

2.2.1 Description of the Studies Examined

First we show the description of population-based studies reporting the prevalence or incidence of DLB listed in the above-noted systematic review 6) (Tables 2.1 and 2.2).

2.2.2 Zaccai's Review 2005 [5]

This is the first systematic review of epidemiological studies of DLB, which identified just six population prevalence studies and one incidence study [7–13]. All studies used the DSM-III-R or DSM-IV criteria to diagnose dementia. Five prevalence studies used the McKeith 1996 criteria [14] (Table 2.3), while one did a modified McKeith 1995 criteria [15]. with no restriction on duration of Parkinson's disease.

Study results are as follows. Prevalence estimates for clinical DLB ranged from 0 to 5 % (median 0.1 %) with regard to the general population and from 0 to 30.5 % (median 6.6 %) of all dementia cases. The Cache County study provides the only incidence report, estimated at 0.1 % a year for the general population and 3.2 % a year for all new dementia cases. Six studies did not report on the sex of those diagnosed, while one reported that they were all men. The authors noted that the

Table 2.1 Population-based prevalence studies

Study	No. in study	Age (years)	No. with dementia	No. of DLB	DLB/over 65 years, % (95 %CI)	DLB/all dementia, % (95 %CI)
Yamada (2001)	3715	65	142	4	0.11 (0.03–0.28)	0.28 (0.08–0.71)
Ikeda (2001)	1145	>65	60	1	0.09 (0.00–0.49)	1.67 (0.04–8.94)
Yamada (2002)	157	>70	19	0	0.00 (0.00–2.32)	0.00 (0.00–17.7)
Stevens (2002)	1085	>65	72	7	0.65 (0.26–1.32)	9.72 (4.0–19.0)
Herrera (2002)	1656	>65	118	2	0.12 (0.01–0.44)	1.69 (0.21–5.99)
de Silva (2003)	703	>65	28	1	0.14 (0.00–0.79)	3.57 (0.09–18.35)
Rahkonen (2003)	601	>75	137	30	4.99 (3.39–7.05)	21.9 (15.29–29.76)
Tognoni (2005)	1600	>65	99	3	0.19 (0.04–0.55)	3.03 (0.63–8.60)
Galasko (2007)	1984	>65	243	1	0.05 (0.00–0.28)	0.41 (0.01–2.27)
Molero (2007)	2438	>65	196	4	0.16 (0.04–0.42)	2.04 (0.56–5.14)
Fernandez Martinez (2008)	1931	>65	108	10	0.52 (0.25–0.95)	9.23 (4.53–16.37)
Gascon-Bayarri (2007)[a]	1754	>65	165	15	0.86 (0.48–1.41)	9.09 (5.18–14.55)
Jhoo (2008)	714	>65	37	2	0.28 (0.03–1.01)	5.41 (0.66–18.2)
Gurvit (2008)	1019	>65	93	9	0.88 (0.04–1.67)	9.68 (4.52–17.58)
Arslantas (2009)	3100	>55	262	0	0.00 (0.00–0.12)	0.00 (0.00–1.4)
Kim (2011)	1673	>65	351	2	0.12 (0.01–0.43)	0.57 (0.07–2.04)
Yusuf (2011)	322	>65	9	0	0.00 (0.00–1.14)	0.00 (0.00–33.63)
Dimitrov (2012)[a]	540	>65	39	2	0.37 (0.05–1.33)	5.13 (0.63–17.32)
Total	26137		2178	93	0.36 (0.29–0.44)	4.24 (3.44–5.17)

Van Jones et al. [6]
DLB dementia with Lewy bodies, *CI* confidence interval
[a]Used the revised 2005 criteria

number of available studies was too small to hypothesize on the potential effect of age, sex, and genetic background on the results.

It is of note the authors referred to the issue of the nosological relationship between DLB and Parkinson's disease dementia (PDD) which remains not yet clear. Theoretically, 1-year rule is the key to differentiate DLB from PDD;

Table 2.2 Population-based incidence studies

Study	No. in study	Age (years)	Dementia incidence (case/1000 person-years)	DLB incidence in whole population (cases/1000 person-years)	DLB incidence per dementia diagnosis (%)
Miech (2002)	5092	>65	36.3	0.57	3.2 (6/185)
Matsui (2009)[a]	887	>65	32.3	1.40	4.4 (12/275)
Perez (2010)[a]	3777	>65	26.9	1.12	4.5 (28/644)
Total				0.87	3.8 (3.39–4.15)

Van Jones et al. [6]
DLB dementia with Lewy bodies
[a]Used the revised 2005 criteria

Table 2.3 The 1996 original criteria for probable and possible DLB

1. The central feature required for a diagnosis of DLB is progressive cognitive decline of sufficient magnitude to interfere with normal social or occupational function. Prominent or persistent memory impairment may not necessarily occur in the early stages but is usually evident with progression. Deficits on tests of attention and of fronto-subcortical skills and visuospatial ability may be especially prominent
2. Two of the following core features are essential for a diagnosis of probable DLB; one is essential for possible DlB:
(a) Fluctuating cognition with pronounced variations in attention and alertness
(b) Recurrent visual hallucinations which are typically well formed and detailed
(c) Spontaneous motor features of Parkinsonism
3. Features supportive of the diagnosis are:
(a) Repeated falls
(b) Syncope
(c) Transient loss of consciousness
(d) Neuroleptic sensitivity
(e) Systematized delusions
(f) Hallucinations in other modalities
4. A diagnosis of DLB is less likely in the presence of:
(a) Stroke disease, evident as focal neurological signs or on brain imaging
(b) Evidence on physical examination and investigation of any physical illness, or other brain disorder, sufficient to account for the clinical picture

Consensus guidelines for the clinical and pathological diagnosis of dementia with Lewy bodies (DLB): report of the consortium on DLB international workshop (McKeith et al. [15])

however, the differential diagnosis is difficult in general and community survey in particular.

2.2.3 *Vann Jone's Review 2014 [6]*

This is the second review on the epidemiological studies of DLB, which identified 18 population-based prevalence study [7–12, 16–27] and two [28, 29] population-based incidence studies. Of the 18 prevalence studies, seven had been included in the review by Zaccai et al. All of the studies reviewed used the DSM-III-R or DSM-IV criteria to diagnose dementia. As to the prevalence studies of DLB, two studies used the revised 2005 criteria and the remaining 16 did the original 1996 criteria. For the incidence studies, two did the revised 2005 criteria [30] (Table 2.4) and one the 1996 one.

Table 2.4 The 2005 revised criteria for DLB

Diagnostic criteria for Dementia with Lewy Bodies 2005
Central feature:
Progressive dementia – deficits in attention and executive function are typical. Prominent memory impairment may not be evident in the early stages
Core features:
Fluctuating cognition with pronounced variations in attention and alertness
Recurrent complex visual hallucinations
Spontaneous features of Parkinsonism
Suggestive features:
REM sleep behavior disorder (RBD), which can appear years before the onset of dementia and Parkinsonism
Severe sensitivity to neuroleptics occurs in up to 50 % of LBD patients who take them
Low dopamine transporter uptake in the brain's basal ganglia as seen on SPECT and PET imaging scans
Supportive features:
Repeated falls and syncope (fainting)
Transient, unexplained loss of consciousness
Autonomic dysfunction
Hallucinations of other modalities
Visuospatial abnormalities like depth perception, object orientation, directional sense, and illusions
Other psychiatric disturbances like systematized delusions, aggression, and depression
A probable LBD diagnosis requires either:
Dementia plus two or more core features
Dementia plus one core feature and one or more suggestive features
A possible LBD diagnosis requires:
Dementia plus one core feature
Dementia plus one or more suggestive features

Synucleinopathies, with and without dementia, encompass a wide range of diseases including Parkinson's disease, multiple system atrophy, rapid eye movement (REM) sleep behavior disorder, and dementia with Lewy bodies (DLB). DLB is a neurodegenerative disorder resulting in slowly progressive and unrelenting dementia until death

Regarding population prevalence of DLB, the mean value in the whole population over 65 years old was 0.36 % or one in 270 people, with a wide range from zero to 21.9 %. Among those with dementia, 4.2 % were found to have DLB. This equates to one in 24 cases. There was a wide variation in prevalence rates across studies. Among the more recent (after 2005) studies, the prevalence of DLB in the over-65 population ranged from zero to 1.2 % and from zero to 9.7 % of those with dementia. This is a narrower range than the results from previous report by Zaccai et al. [5]. According to the 1996 consensus criteria, probable DLB can be diagnosed if any two of the three key symptoms are present, namely, fluctuation, visual hallucinations, or spontaneous motor features of Parkinsonism, and possible DLB if only one is present. Above-described mean prevalence for all included studies is a reflection of probable DLB cases only. Two studies included possible and also probable DLB cases: these reported an increase in DLB diagnoses from 9.7 to 30.5 % and from 9.1 to 12.7 % of all dementias, respectively, once possible cases were added to probable ones.

Population prevalence studies that used the 2005 criteria reported a mean prevalence of 8.2 % compared to 3.7 % among those who used the 1996 criteria, a finding that indicated statistically significant difference. Consistent with these findings, the only study [24] that directly compared and contrasted the 1996 and 2005 criteria on the same sample found a 25 % increase in probable DLB cases identified.

As to population incidence of DLB, annual incidence rates for DLB were found to be 3.8 % (range 3.2–4.5 %) of new dementia diagnoses and 0.87 (range 0.57–1.4) cases/1000 person-years. The two most recent incident studies both used the 2005 criteria [28, 29] and found a 35–40 % increase in DLB compared to the only previous incidence study (1996 criteria), although this was not statistically significant.

Of the 11 population samples that included an average age of participants, there was a positive correlation between age and the proportion of DLB compared to all dementia, although this was not found to be significant. Regarding the gender difference of DLB, the authors showed controversial results.

2.2.4 Additional Recent Reports

An additional study that has not been examined in the review by Van Jones et al. [6] came from Japan. The study [31] was conducted in a rural island of Japan using door-to-door 2-phase design. As a result, the prevalence (cases/100 persons aged 65 years and older) was 11.0 for all types of dementia and 0.53 for DLB. Thus DLB accounted 4.8 % of all diagnosed dementia in this survey. This result appears to be similar with that reported in the review by Van Jones et al. A recent Spanish study [32] showed similar result. This study was conducted in an urban region of Valladolid, Spain. The authors showed that DLB accounted 7.7 % of all diagnosed dementia.

On the other hand, an incidence study has recently been reported from the USA [33]. This study was conducted among residents of Olmsted County, Minnesota, from 1991 through 2005. The report showed that the incidence rate of DLB was 3.5 per 100,000 person-years overall, and it increased steeply with age and is markedly higher in men.

Recognition of DLB has recently become more widespread since the discovery of α-synuclein as the major constituent of Lewy bodies in 1997. Particularly, immunostaining of α-synuclein makes it easy to identify neocortical-type Lewy bodies. Consequently, with the liberal definition of the pathological criteria of DLB in 1996, no less than 60 % of Alzheimer's disease cases may be considered to meet pathological criteria for DLB. Fujimi et al. [34] first reported a community-based clinicopathological study of DLB. Using the 2005 criteria, they examined community-based consecutive autopsy cases. As a result, 10.3 % of the non-demented subjects and 31.2 % of the demented subjects showed the Lewy body pathology. Applying the revised pathological criteria to the 205 demented subjects, they determined the types of Lewy body pathology. The results are as follows: 11 cases (5.4 %) were brainstem predominant, 24 (11.7 %) were limbic type, and 24 (11.7 %) were diffuse neocortical type. Thus, 28.8 % of the demented subjects were diagnosed as having Lewy body pathology in terms of the revised pathological criteria.

2.3 Issues for the Future Studies

When we discuss the epidemiological issues of DLB, we must refer to the predictive accuracy of consensus clinical criteria for DLB. Litvan et al. [35] showed that sensitivity of case detection was variable and unacceptably low in several others but one prospective study. In contrast, specificity was generally found to be high, suggesting that the clinical criteria for probable DLB are best used for confirmation of diagnosis (few false positives), whereas those for possible DLB may be more valuable in screening but have a relatively high false-negative rate. Improved methods of identifying the core feature "fluctuation" have potential to increase diagnostic accuracy [36].

2.4 Summary

Reviewing the previous epidemiological studies, DLB accounts for more than 4 % of all dementia cases, and the incidence of DLB is around 4 % of new dementia cases. However, with more widespread recognition of the clinicopathological entity of DLB, the values of its prevalence and incidence have recently increased. Although the consensus clinical criteria for DLB have been revised, its sensitivity remains lower. On the other hand, the results of pathological examination from a cohort study showed much higher prevalence of DLB. In the future, effort should be indispensable to dissipate the discrepancy between clinical and pathological diagnosis of DLB.

References

1. Kosaka K, Yoshimura M, Ikeda K, et al. Diffuse type of Lewy body disease: progressive dementia with abundant cortical Lewy bodies and senile changes of varying degree–a new disease? Clin Neuropathol. 1984;3:185–92.
2. Gibb WR, Esiri MM, Lees AJ. Clinical and pathological features of diffuse cortical Lewy body disease (Lewy body dementia). Brain. 1987;110:1131–53.
3. Perry RH, Irving D, Blessed G, et al. Senile dementia of Lewy body type and spectrum of Lewy body disease. Lancet. 1989;1(8646):1088.
4. Palmqvist S, Hansson O, Minthon L, et al. Practical suggestions on how to differentiate dementia with Lewy bodies from Alzheimer's disease with common cognitive tests. Int J Geriatr Psychiatry. 2009;24:1405–12.
5. Zaccai J, McCracken C, Brayne C. A systematic review of prevalence and incidence studies of dementia with Lewy bodies. Age Ageing. 2005;34:561–6.
6. Van Jones SA, O'Brien JT. The prevalence and incidence of dementia with Lewy bodies: a systematic review of population and clinical studies. Psycol Med. 2014;44:673–83.
7. Yamada T, Hattori H, Miura A, et al. Prevalence of Alzheimer's disease, vascular dementia and dementia with Lewy bodies in a Japanese population. Psychiatry Clin Neurosci. 2001;55:21–5.
8. Yamada T, Kadekaru H, Matsumoto S, et al. Prevalence of dementia in the older Japanese-Brazilian population. Psychiatry Clin Neurosci. 2002;56:71–5.
9. Herrera Jr E, Caramelli P, Silveira AS, et al. Epidemiologic survey of dementia in a community-dwelling Brazilian population. Alzheimer Dis Assoc Disord. 2002;56:71–5.
10. Stevens T, Livingston G, Kitchen G, et al. Islington study on dementia subtypes in the community. Br J Psychiatry. 2002;180:270–6.
11. de Silvia HA, Gunatilake SB, Smith AD, et al. Prevalence of dementia in a semi-urban population in Sri Lanka: report from a regional survey. Int J Geriatr Psychiatry. 2003;18:711–5.
12. Rahkonen T, Eloniemi-Sulkava U, Rissanen S, et al. Dementia with Lewy bodies according to the consensus criteria in a general population aged 75 years or older. I Neurol Neurosurg Psychiatry. 2003;74:720–4.
13. Miech RA, Breitner JCS, Zandi PP, et al. Incidence of AD may decline in the early 90s for men, later for women. The Cache County study. Neurology. 2002;58:209–18.
14. McKeith IG, Galasko D, Wilcock GK, et al. Lewy body dementia-diagnosis and treatment. Br J Psychiatry. 1995;67:09–717.
15. McKeith IG, Glasko D, Kosaka K, et al. Consensus guidelines for the clinical and pathological diagnosis of dementia with Lewy bodies (DLB): report of the consortium on DLB international workshop. Neurology. 1996;47:1113–24.
16. Ikeda M, Hokoishi K, Maki N, et al. Increased prevalence of dementia in Japan: a community-based epidemiological study. Neurology. 2001;57:839–44.
17. Tognoni G, Ceravolo R, Nucciarone B, et al. From mild cognitive impairment to dementia: a prevalence study in a district of Tuscany, Italy. Acta Neurol Scand. 2005;112:65–71.
18. Galasko D, Salmon D, Gamst A, et al. Prevalence of dementia in Chamorros on Guam: relationship to age, gender, education, and APOE. Neurology. 2007;68:1772–81.
19. Molero AE, Pino-Ramirez G, Maestre GE. High prevalence of dementia in Caribbean population. Neuroepidemiology. 2007;29:107–12.

20. Fernandez Martinez M, CastroFlores J, Perez de las Heras S, et al. Prevalence of neuropsychiatric symptoms in elderly patients with dementia in Mungialde County. Dement Geriatr Cogn Disord. 2008;25:103–8.
21. Gascon-Bayarri J, Rene R, Del Barrion JL, et al. Prevalence of dementia subtypes in EI Prat de Llobregat, Catalonia, Spain: the PRATICON study. Neuroepidemiology. 2007;28:224–34.
22. Jhoo JH, Kim KW, Huh Y, et al. Prevalence of dementia and its subtypes in an elderly urban Korean population: results from the Korean Longitudinal Study on Health and Aging (KLoSHA). Dement Geriatr Cogn Disord. 2008;26:270–6.
23. Gurvit H, Emre M, Tinaz S, et al. The prevalence of dementia in an urban Turkish population. Am J Alzheimers Dis Other Demen. 2008;23:67–76.
24. Arslantas D, Oezbabalik D, Metintas S, et al. Prevalence of dementia and associated risk factors in Middle Anatolia, Turkey. J Clin Neurosci. 2009;16:1455–9.
25. Kim KW, Park JH, Kim M-H, et al. A nationwide survey on the prevalence of dementia and mild cognitive impairment in South Korea. J Alzheimer Dis. 2011;23:279–89.
26. Yusuf AJ, Baiyewu O, Sheikh TL, et al. Prevalence of dementia and dementia subtypes among community-dwelling elderly people in northern Nigeria. Int Psychogeriatrics. 2011;23:379–86.
27. Dimitrov I, Tzourio C, Milanov I, et al. Prevalence of dementia and mild cognitive impairment in a Bulgarian urban population. Am J Alzheimers Dis Other Demen. 2012;27:131–5.
28. Matsui Y, Tanizaki Y, Arima H, et al. Incidence and survival of dementia in a general population of Japanese elderly: the Hisayama study. J Neurol Neurosurg Psychiatry. 2009;80:366–70.
29. Perez F, Helmer C, Dartigues JF, et al. A 15-year population-based cohort study of the incidence of Parkinson's disease and dementia with Lewy bodies in an elderly French cohort. J Neurol Neurosurg Psychiatry. 2010;81:742–6.
30. McKeith IG, Dickson DW, Lowe J, et al. Diagnosis and management of dementia with Lewy bodies: third report of the DLB Consortium. Neurology. 2005;65:1863–72.
31. Wada-Isoe K, UemuraY SY, et al. Prevalence of dementia in the rural island town of Ama-cho, Japan. Neuroepidemiology. 2009;32:101–6.
32. Tola-Arribas MA, Yugueros MI, Garea MJ, et al. Prevalence of dementia and subtypes in Valladolid, northwestern Spain: the DEMINVALL study. PLoS One. 2013;8(10):e77688.
33. Savica R, Grossardt BR, Bower JH, et al. Incidence of dementia with Lewy bodies and Parkinson disease dementia. JAMA Neurol. 2013;70:1396–402.
34. Fujimi K, Sasaki K, Noda K, et al. Clinicopathological outline of dementia with Lewy bodies applying the revised criteria: the Hisayama study. Brain Pathol. 2008;18:317–25.
35. Litvan I, Bhatia KP, Burn DJ, et al. SIC Task Force appraisal of clinical diagnostic criteria for Parkinsonian disorders. Mov Disord. 2003;18:467–86.
36. Ferman T, Smith GE, Boeve BF, et al. DLB fluctuations: specific features that reliably differentiate from AD and normal aging. Neurology. 2004;62:181–7.

Part II
Biological Aspects

Chapter 3
Cholinergic Pathology in Dementia with Lewy Bodies

John-Paul Taylor, Daniel Collerton, Fiona LeBeau, and Elaine Perry

Abstract Cholinergic dysfunction is a major feature of dementia with Lewy bodies (DLB) and makes a significant contribution to the cognitive impairment and other challenging symptoms seen in this condition. Despite this, or indeed, because of this, manipulation of the cholinergic system can offer significant therapeutic opportunities for treating DLB, and this is reflected in the fact that cholinesterase inhibitors remain one of our best treatments in this condition. In this chapter, we will explore the pathology of cholinergic dysfunction in DLB, review findings from both post-mortem and imaging studies and place this within a clinical framework.

Keywords Cholinergic • Dementia with Lewy bodies • Acetylcholine

3.1 Introduction

To date, cholinesterase inhibitors have been our most successful therapeutic intervention in dementia with Lewy bodies (DLB) supporting the concept that cholinergic dysfunction is central to understanding DLB.

In this chapter, we will examine the salience of the cholinergic system to DLB by considering a number of perspectives including pathological evidence of dysfunction of this system, in vivo imaging data and, throughout, provide a clinical perspective which provides a useful subtext. Given the overlap between DLB and Parkinson's disease with dementia (PDD), we also make reference to this as well as make relevant comparisons with the pathology and symptoms of Parkinson's disease (PD) and Alzheimer's disease (AD) as part of our exegesis.

It is important to acknowledge that other neurotransmitter systems (e.g. dopaminergic, noradrenergic and serotonergic) are likely to be relevant in the aetiology of DLB and are emerging as potential targets for therapeutic manipulation. For example, there are case reports advocating the use of atomoxetine (norepinephrine) for fatigue and emerging double blind clinical trial data

---

J.-P. Taylor (✉) • D. Collerton • F. LeBeau • E. Perry
Institute of Neuroscience, Newcastle University, Newcastle upon Tyne NE4 5PL, UK
e-mail: john-paul.taylor@ncl.ac.uk

K. Kosaka (ed.), *Dementia with Lewy Bodies*, DOI 10.1007/978-4-431-55948-1_3

supporting the use of pimavanserin (serotonin 2A antagonist) in psychosis in PD [1, 2]. Aside from dopamine, however, their role is only partially understood. Thus, for the purposes of the present chapter, we will focus mainly on the cholinergic system and justify this given the clear therapeutic implications of targeting this system.

3.2 Pathology

Studies in post-mortem tissue of the presynaptic cholinergic enzyme detected biochemically in the cerebral cortex, and of neuronal density in the basal forebrain, identified cholinergic deficits in PD and DLB over 25 years ago [3, 4]. Studies since then have extended to consider other cholinergic nuclei and receptors.

3.2.1 Nucleus Basalis and Cerebral Cortex

Ninety percent of neurons in the nucleus basalis of Meynert (nbM) are cholinergic and send widespread cortipedal projections to the entire cortical mantle, and thus this nucleus is a key driver of cholinergic drive in the brain. It is also notable that from a Lewy body disease perspective that Friedrich Lewy first observed inclusion bodies, not in midbrain dopaminergic neurons, but in the nbM [5].

In DLB and PDD, cell loss in the nbM and cortical cholinergic deficits are at least as extensive as in AD and correlate with cognitive decline. In a recent stereological analysis of the nbM, Hall et al. (2014) [6] assessed α-synuclein pathology in demented and non-demented patients with PD, together with choline acetyltransferase activity in the hippocampus and frontal cortex. Despite variable cell loss in the region of Ch4, a major nbM subgroup supplying cholinergic input to the cortex and amygdala, cortical but not hippocampal cholinergic activity was consistently reduced in PD without dementia. This relative structural preservation of Ch4 nbM despite cortical cholinergic loss suggests that prior to neurodegenerative change, there are marked functional impairments in cholinergic activity, and this has been attributed to α-synuclein pathology reducing neurotransmitter production. Once dementia becomes manifest in PD, however, there is an increase in the severity of α-synuclein pathology in the basal forebrain and hippocampus and a further reduction in hippocampal cholinergic activity, suggesting that hippocampal cholinergic dysfunction may be a major contributor to dementia in PDD.

Lui et al. (2015) [7] in a recent review suggested that there is a caudo-rostral pattern of neuronal loss within the nbM in AD on the basis of accumulated data across a number of studies. In contrast, the pattern of neuronal loss in the nbM is not as clear in Lewy body (LB) disease, although the distinctively different neuropsychiatric and cognitive deficits seen in DLB and PDD are likely to reflect a differential pattern of nbM neuronal loss in LB disease to that seen in AD. Certainly up to

80 % depletion in Ch4 occurs in PD, and this is comparable to, or more extensive than, that seen in AD [3, 8, 9]. This is accentuated in PD patients with dementia and appears greater in the intermediate nbM region.

Interestingly, a recent study by Alexandris et al. (2015) [10] demonstrated galanin upregulation within the basal forebrain cholinergic system in PD and PDD patients. Galanin has been mooted to be an inducible neuroprotective factor, and thus increased activity of this neuropeptide may reflect a protective tissue response which is attempting to improve the survivability of residual cholinergic neurons, a phenomenon which has been observed in AD [11].

The aetiology of neuronal dysfunction in Lewy body diseases is also different to that of AD; AD is characterised by amyloid plaques and abundant neurofibrillary tangles, and whilst these pathologies can occur in DLB, LB disease is more typically characterised by α-synuclein pathology [12] which localises to presynaptic elements and reduces the efficiency of synaptic communication. Quite how these presynaptic changes impact upon cholinergic function in Lewy body diseases remains to be clarified, however. From a cortical perspective, pathological Lewy body load and reductions in choline acetyltransferase activity can be observed in PD patients with cognitive impairment, with the number of Lewy bodies negatively correlating with choline acetyltransferase activity, suggesting a potential link between the two [13].

In addition to this presynaptic pathology, postsynaptic cholinergic receptors are also affected in LB disorders. Based on radioreceptor binding in autopsy tissue, Piggott et al. (2003) [14] reported that muscarinic M1, M2 and M4 binding in the striatum correlated positively with increased Alzheimer-type pathology, with M2 cortical binding correlating with LB pathology. Loss of nicotine binding (a broad-spectrum ligand with binding to a range of nicotinic receptor subtypes) was reported in early studies of cortical and subcortical areas in DLB and PD [15, 16]. With the evolution of subtype-specific nicotinic ligands, a complex topographic pattern of nicotinic receptor alterations in relation to cognitive dysfunction and neuropsychiatric symptoms is now apparent (below).

3.2.2 Nucleus Basalis and Limbic Structures

Efferent cholinergic projections from the nbM are concentrated in limbic areas such as the hippocampus and amygdala. Dementia in PD is associated with reductions in hippocampal cholinergic activity and Ch4 cholinergic neurons [6]. Sahin et al. (2006) [17] found that the distribution pattern of pathology and cholinergic deficits in the amygdaloid complex in AD and DLB differ; cholinergic deficits, as measured by choline acetyltransferase activity, were more prominent in the amygdaloid subnuclei of basolateral and corticomedial groups in DLB, probably because of the combined involvement of both nbM and brainstem cholinergic nuclei in DLB.

3.2.3 Striatum

Broadly, pathological changes in the striatum are evident in Lewy body diseases; in particular, striatal amyloid beta has been implicated in the development of dementia in PD and DLB, independent of comorbid AD pathologies [18].

In regard to the cholinergic system, there is direct evidence that striatal nicotinic receptors are affected in DLB and PD, with nicotine binding reduced in both conditions [19]. This reduction appears to be accentuated by a history of neuroleptic medication. Muscarinic striatal receptors (M1) correlate negatively with cortical LB pathology and are reduced in DLB but not in AD [14]. Low M1 and dopamine 2 (D2) receptors in DLB imply altered regulation of the striatal projection neurons which express these receptors. Pimlott et al. (2004) [20] also identified loss of striatal nicotinic alpha4beta2 activity in DLB, which paralleled reductions in nigrostriatal dopaminergic markers. Reduced striatal binding of nicotinic alpha4beta2, comparable to that in PD, has been postulated as a potential index of early degeneration in nigrostriatal inputs in DLB. Ray et al. (2004) [21] reported parallel reductions in striatal alpha6/alpha3 nicotinic receptor and dopamine uptake sites in DLB, and Bohr et al. (2005) [22] observed reduced alpha6 nicotinic binding in the putamen and caudate in PD and DLB. Gotti et al. (2006) [23] used nicotinic subtype-specific immunochemistry to demonstrate extensive striatal deficits in alpha6 and beta3, compared to alpha4 and beta2, in PD and DLB.

In summation, therefore, there appears to be marked disturbances in striatal cholinergic function both in terms of intrinsic striatal cholinergic interneuron function and nicotinic/muscarinic receptor change. This is likely not only to have an impact on voluntary movement but also on cognitive function in Lewy body diseases [24], although this is not fully understood.

3.2.4 Thalamus

The thalamus has been posited to have a central role in the symptoms of DLB, including cognitive fluctuations and visual hallucinations, symptoms which also show a positive response to cholinergic therapies [25, 26].

The thalamus receives dual cholinergic innervation from both the nbM and pedunculopontine nucleus, and this innervation has been implicated in the mediation of cortical activation and attention. Thalamic presynaptic cholinergic deficits occur in Lewy body diseases, particularly after significant cortical and subcortical neurodegeneration when the dementia manifested after prolonged parkinsonism [27].

Topographically, it appears that, in PDD, mediodorsal thalamic choline acetyltransferase activity is reduced compared with PD and centromedian activity is lower in DLB with, as opposed to without, concomitant parkinsonism.

With respect to nicotinic receptors, Ray et al. (2004) [21] noted extensive reductions in the alpha6/alpha3 subunits in DLB in the centromedian, ventral lateral and ventroposterior medial thalamic nuclei. Thalamic nicotinic alpha6 was further compared in DLB with, and without, extrapyramidal symptoms [22]. Whilst reductions in the centromedian and parafascicular nuclei were apparent in both groups, decreased binding in the ventral lateral nucleus only occurred in those with symptoms. Reviewing evidence of thalamic cholinergic denervation in LB disorders and AD, Kotagal et al. (2012) [28] concluded that this occurs in PD, PDD and DLB but not in AD and contributes to the motor and cognitive abnormalities of LB disorders.

3.2.5 Brainstem

Seidel et al. (2014) [29], analysing α-synuclein-immunoreactive inclusion pathologies in brainstem nuclei and fibre tracts in PD and DLB, found Lewy bodies and Lewy neurites to be prevalent in the pedunculopontine nucleus in both conditions.

Schmeichel et al. (2008) [30] observed loss of cholinergic pedunculopontine tegmental nuclei/laterodorsal tegmental nuclei neurons in DLB that was not related to REM sleep behaviour disorder, and this was reinforced by the observations of Dugger et al. (2012) [31]; in the latter study, choline acetyltransferase immunohistochemistry was used to label these neurones. Neuronal losses in this region occurred in DLB, but not AD, and again, these losses were independent of REM sleep behaviour disorder. Therefore, whilst cholinergic losses within the pedunculopontine nucleus are severe in the Lewy body dementias, they do not appear to be aetiologically implicated in REM sleep behaviour disorder; rather losses in this region might associate more with gait dysfunction [32] or neuropsychiatric symptoms [33] (see below).

3.2.6 White Matter

White matter intensities in cholinergic pathways have previously been related to cognitive dysfunction in AD and PDD. In a structural imaging study using a visual rating scale, Park and colleagues (2015) [34] demonstrated that white matter hyperintensities were a feature of AD, DLB and PDD and related to the severity of cognitive impairment, although the degree of pathology was similar between the conditions. Whether this reflects specific cholinergic loss or reflects more general disease severity is not clear.

3.3 Neuroimaging

Monitoring the cholinergic system in the living human brain has followed autopsy tissue studies and has confirmed that there is extensive and clinically significant pathology in DLB and PDD. The first PET imaging study used a presynaptic marker of the vesicular transporter to detect extensive cortical loss in PDD [35]. Since then, PET imaging advances in LB disorders have been based on monitoring the catabolic cholinergic enzyme, acetylcholinesterase (AChE). This molecule was not, paradoxically, the subject of previous tissue studies, presumably reflecting its postsynaptic as well as presynaptic location and also co-localisation with non-cholinergic as well as cholinergic neurons.

3.3.1 Acetylcholinesterase Imaging

Acetylcholinesterase (AChE) imaging indicates that basal forebrain cholinergic system degeneration appears early in PD and progresses with the appearance of dementia. Hilker et al. (2005) [36] detected lower activity in frontal, parietal and temporal cortex in PDD compared to PD without dementia. Shimada et al. (2009) [37] reported cholinergic dysfunction in PD and DLB in the cerebral cortex, especially in the medial occipital cortex with deficits evident in early PD, was more widespread and profound in both PDD and DLB.

Both AChE and fluorodeoxyglucose PET imaging demonstrate severe reductions in the neocortex in DLB and PDD, with increasing signal diminution from frontal to occipital regions [38].

Marcone et al. (2012) [39], using AChE PET, observed comparable AChE reductions in AD and MCI (mild cognitive impairment) converters, with a more variable degree of cholinergic dysfunction in early DLB. Such imaging analyses are in agreement with the autopsy studies described above, in that thalamic cholinergic denervation occurs in DLB and PDD (but not AD) and that degeneration of thalamic cholinergic afferent projections is likely to contribute to LB disease-specific motor and cognitive abnormalities [28].

3.3.2 Nicotinic Receptor Imaging

According to O'Brien et al. (2008) [40], alterations in nicotinic alpha4beta2 receptor SPECT binding in DLB are distinct from perfusion deficits, with increases in nicotinic receptor binding in occipital lobe. Colloby et al. (2010) [41] followed this observation with the finding that the same nicotinic marker is a predictor of cognitive progression DLB as well as AD. Isaias et al. (2014) [42] concluded from SPECT nicotinic imaging in PD that upregulated cholinergic activity in striatal, motor and limbic cortical regions is evident at an early stage of disease, prior to cognitive decline.

3.3.3 Muscarinic Receptor Imaging

Using a ligand that primarily detects the M1 subtype, Colloby et al. (2006) [43] observed elevated muscarinic binding in the right occipital lobe in DLB and in both occipital lobes in PDD. Reduced binding was evident in PDD in frontal regions and temporal lobes bilaterally but not DLB. These patterns were independent of regional blood flow changes, suggesting that structural loss or perfusion deficits do not explain the deficits in binding. In a follow-up study, Colloby et al. (2016) [44] applied a spatial covariance approach to their imaging data to examine relative M1/M4 binding in PDD patients and demonstrated a pattern of relative decreased binding in basal forebrain, temporal, striatum, insula and anterior cingulate which was independent of perfusion changes. They posited that these reflected disturbances in cholinergic innervation of specific limbic-paralimbic and salience brain networks.

3.3.4 Volumetric, Perfusion and Metabolic Imaging

Using MRI, Kim et al. (2011) [45] reported that the volume of the substantia innominata (SI, which incorporates the cholinergic nbM) is equally reduced in PDD and DLB and more so than in AD. However, two recent studies [46, 47], whilst demonstrating grey matter loss in the SI/basal forebrain in DLB, found that this was not significantly greater than that seen in AD. In relation to disease progression, PD through to PD-MCI and PDD are associated with grey matter loss in the SI [45], although given the relatively small size of the SI and structural heterogeneity (as it contains many different nuclei), structural imaging studies can only provide inferential insights.

Other studies of atrophy and hypometabolism in DLB do not relate directly to cholinergic function, although cortical hypoperfusion/hypometabolism in mild DLB is taken to be an indicator of cholinergic dysfunction [48, 49].

3.4 Functional Implications

Cholinergic pathologies, detected with imaging during life or in post-mortem tissue, have been implicated in a broad range of clinical symptoms – cognitive, behavioural and motor – in DLB, as well as in PD or PDD.

3.4.1 Attention and Cognition

Nucleus basalis lesions in animals block electrocortical activation and impair learning and memory, providing a clear mechanistic basis for the role of cholinergic system in cognition. In particular, an emerging consensus supports the notion that automatic orienting of attention is mediated by 'bottom-up', stimulus-driven signals from cholinergic nuclei, particularly the nbM. Increases in acetylcholine in cortical targets also appear to boost signal-to-noise ratios for salient stimuli, so amplifying their detection and ensuring their attentional significance [50, 51]. Pathophysiologically, the fact that cholinergic deficits are profound in DLB and PDD compared to PD and that the prototypical cognitive profile in these dementias aligns with clinical observations of major deficits in attention in DLB [52], together with the observation that cholinergic therapies such as cholinesterase inhibitors can ameliorate these deficits, strongly supports the notion that the cholinergic system is central to cognitive and attentional impairment in the Lewy body dementias.

However, are there further data and cognitive correlates to support this conjecture? Findings from structural imaging studies are variable. Hanyu et al. (2002) [53] observed atrophy of the SI, and whilst they obtained significant correlation between SI thickness and cognition (MMSE) in AD, they did not see this in PDD. In contrast, Kim et al. (2011) [45] noted in relation to PD-related cognitive impairment (PD-MCI, PDD or DLB) but not AD a significant positive correlation between the SI volume and MMSE. Choi et al. (2012) [54] also noted that SI volume correlates with cognitive performance in PD. SI grey matter atrophy in DLB patients in another study by Colloby et al. (2016) was associated with global cognitive impairment and the severity of cognitive fluctuations. However, a similar study by Grothe et al. (2014) [46] found basal forebrain atrophy in AD but not DLB was associated with lower MMSE scores although poorer visuoperceptual function was associated with SI volume in DLB. Some of this heterogeneity in associations between basal forebrain atrophy and cognition may reflect challenges with imaging such small structures and also variability in cholinergic loss between individuals with LB disease even with the same degree of cognitive impairment.

From a functional imaging perspective, Bohnen et al. (2006) [55] reported significant correlations between the degree of in vivo cortical AChE activity and tests of attentional and executive functions in PD and PDD, but no correlation between cortical AChE activity and duration of motor disease or severity of parkinsonian motor symptoms. Lorenz et al. (2014) [56] observed that nicotinic alpha4beta2 SPECT imaging in parietal and thalamic regions correlated with impairments in memory-related and perceptual cognitive tasks in PD.

Overall, it is likely that cognitive deficits do not reflect loss of cholinergic drive to one area; rather functional imaging and electroencephalography (EEG) studies suggest that the degree and pattern of cognitive loss depends upon the interrelationship of cholinergic-related pathology across multiple regions rather than within discrete brain areas [44, 57–60].

3.4.2 Neuropsychiatric Symptoms: Hallucinations, Delusions and Behavioural Disturbances

Neuropsychiatric symptoms are core features of Lewy body disorders [61] although they commonly coexist and have complex and hard to disentangle interrelationships [62].

Early retrospective clinical-pathological analyses in post-mortem tissue identified differential cortical cholinergic enzyme and receptor activities in DLB with and without visual hallucinations [63]. Court et al. (2001) [64] noted, for example, that visual hallucinations are associated with lower levels of cortical nicotinic alpha7 subtype in DLB. Increased cingulate M2 and M4 receptors in DLB are also associated with visual hallucinations in DLB [65]. Delusions appear to be associated with different cholinergic dysfunctions; Ballard et al. (2000) [63] observed that delusions are associated with elevated cortical M1 muscarinic receptors, whilst visual hallucinations were associated with lower choline acetyltransferase. Teaktong et al. (2005) [65] associated delusions in DLB with increased cingulate M2 binding.

Correlating behavioural symptoms with the deficit of global cholinergic activity, as measured in vivo by short-latency afferent inhibition (a neurophysiological technique combining peripheral stimulation with transcranial magnetic stimulation which is sensitive to cholinergic function), Marra et al. (2012) [66] found that loss of short-latency inhibition (an indirect marker of cholinergic loss) was associated with hallucinations in DLB patients. From an imaging perspective, O'Brien et al. (2008) [67] reported that nicotinic alpha4beta2 SPECT was associated in occipital cortex with visual hallucinations.

The pedunculopontine nucleus may be particularly relevant in PD for hallucinosis. Whilst there is a primary role of pedunculopontine cholinergic drive in locomotion [32], neuropathologically, cholinergic cell loss in this nucleus has been shown in hallucinating PD although not DLB patients (Hepp et al. [68]). This is supported by imaging data using voxel-based morphometry which has demonstrated correlations between visual hallucinations in PD patients and volumetric reductions in the pedunculopontine nucleus [33].

The relationships between these multiple cholinergic changes and those seen in other neurotransmitter networks, particularly dopaminergic, remain obscure (e.g. [69]). Most current theories see a core role for the cholinergic innervation of distributed perceptual and cognitive networks in accounting for neuropsychiatric symptoms, especially complex visual hallucinations [70, 71]. For example, theories for the genesis of hallucinations see a complex interplay between attentional and perceptual impairment and subsequent compensation across the ventral visual stream, thalamus and frontal cortex, all areas with significant cholinergic loss in Lewy body disorders. Modelling of these networks is in an early stage, but accumulating evidence suggests that symptoms are associated with widely distributed pathology across a number of cortical areas and pathways (e.g. [58, 59]). This complexity may illuminate why these problems commonly co-occur and the lack of specific responses seen in treatment trials (e.g. [72]). Relating particular patterns of modulation across these networks with specific symptoms remains a challenge.

3.4.3 Fluctuations in Consciousness

Disturbances of consciousness are common in DLB. Fluctuations in attention and awareness have been associated with variations in epibatidine binding to the high-affinity nicotinic receptor in autopsy temporal cortex in DLB, being higher in those more prone to fluctuations [73]. In DLB, Ray et al. (2004) [21] detected lower nicotinic alpha6/alpha3 receptors, and Pimlott et al. (2006) [74] higher alpha4beta2 in the thalamus, in subgroups of patients affected by disturbed consciousness. Concentrated in the thalamus compared with other human brain areas, nicotinic modulation of thalamo-cortical circuitry may be a key factor in control of conscious awareness in DLB. This overlaps with associations between clinically observed cognitive fluctuations and electrocortical disturbances in the low alpha (so-called pre-alpha) and theta range in DLB and PDD patients, which are known to be contingent upon cortico-thalamic activations [75].

The mechanism underlying these fluctuations, which can occur across a number of timescales [76, 77], is not well understood, though comparisons with delirium, which is also characterised by variable alertness, suggest that cholinergic hypofunction is a common factor [78]. The role of feedforward and feedback loops between the cortex, thalamus, subcortical areas and the cerebellum in maintaining stability within attentional networks is likely to be central to understanding cognitive fluctuations within Lewy body disorders, and it is likely that cholinergic (dys)function is a key player in these processes [26, 79].

3.4.4 Motor Symptoms: Gait Disturbances

The concept that cholinergic pathology impacts on motor function in LB disorders is relatively recent. Based on AChE PET studies, Bohnen et al. (2009) [80] originally suggested that in contrast to nigrostriatal dopaminergic denervation, cholinergic hypofunction in the cortex and thalamus is associated with a propensity to falls in PD. Thalamic cholinergic activity in part represents cholinergic output of the pedunculopontine nucleus, which, as noted previously, is a key centre for gait control. Subcortical cholinergic denervation, due to degeneration of brainstem pedunculopontine nucleus neurons, may thus relate to the presence of dopamine nonresponsive gait and balance impairments including falls, in PD.

Analysing cholinergic correlates of gait speed in PD, Bohnen and colleagues (2013) [80] further tested the hypothesis that gait dysfunction results from multisystem degeneration with acetylcholinesterase PET imaging indicating slower gait speed occurred in a low cholinergic PD subgroup, compared to the normal-range cholinergic PD subgroup. Comorbid cortical cholinergic denervation was proposed to be a more robust marker of slowing of gait than nigrostriatal denervation alone. Sarter et al. (2014) [81] reviewed PET studies in PD 'fallers' and argued that falls result from interactions between loss of basal forebrain cholinergic projections to the cortex and striatal dopamine loss. Bohnen et al. (2009) [82] obtained in vivo imaging evidence that cholinergic pathology in the PPN is associated with frequent falling in PD. From the perspective of activities of daily living, there is evidence to suggest that risky driving is linked to thalamic cholinergic denervation in PD [83].

Importantly, cortical cholinergic deafferentation impairs attentional processes including monitoring of gait, posture and complex movements. There is building evidence, particularly in LB diseases, to support the notion that there is a cholinergic-mediated relationship between attention and gait function [68, 84]. This is of practical relevance; gait, falls and mobility impairments in PD are generally resistant to dopaminergic therapy, and thus cholinergic therapy could offer a viable alternative intervention for these symptoms.

Beyond such motor features, anosmia in PD and PDD has been shown to be associated with limbic cortical cholinergic denervation and Ch4 nbM pathology has been implicated [85]. In addition to this, 5-[(11)C]-methoxy-donepezil with PET imaging has recently begun to elucidate peripheral cholinergic deficits in PD demonstrating that both the small bowel and pancreas undergo significant parasympathetic denervation [86]. How this impacts on non-motor symptoms such as gastroparesis and other autonomic functions and whether this peripheral cholinergic imaging approach may offer early diagnostic opportunities remain to be explored. However, it may represent an exciting new approach for understanding Lewy body disorders. Furthermore, cholinergic pathologies may also extend to other 'non-brain' areas such as oculomotor function – which may lead to new opportunities for future clinical-pathological investigations and alternative therapeutic targets for cholinergic modulation.

3.4.5 Treatment Response

Post-mortem studies of the presynaptic cholinergic enzyme in DLB identified extremely low activity in the absence of classical AD pathology, in responders to the cholinesterase inhibitor, tacrine [87]. Graff-Radford et al. [88] in a retrospective analysis of hippocampal volume PET studies noted that patients with DLB who do not have the imaging features of coexistent AD pathology are more likely to improve cognitively with acetylcholinesterase inhibitor treatment.

Response to cholinergic treatments can also be seen on imaging. For example, Fong et al. (2011) [89] used cholinesterase inhibitor drug challenges in DLB to detect perfusion increases in temporal and parietooccipital cortex and relate these to improvements in cognitive performance on a verbal fluency task. Interestingly, Colloby et al. (2016) [44] recently demonstrated that cognitive improvement on the

MMSE to a cholinesterase inhibitor in PDD is associated with a specific covariance pattern of M1/M4 receptors which map onto key brain networks including the frontoparietal attention network and the default mode network, thus providing a new potential biomarker of cholinergic response.

3.5 Conclusion

Cholinergic pathology in DLB (and other Lewy body disorders) extends across cortical and subcortical regions, parallels cognitive decline and differentiates those affected by select noncognitive and motor symptoms. Occurring at least as extensively as in AD, and generally in the absence of classic neurofibrillary pathology of AD, a prediction over 20 years ago that 'cholinergic therapy may be particularly relevant to patients with Lewy body type dementia' [86] is still pertinent.

The distributed cholinergic pathology of Lewy body disorders, their multiple and interrelated symptomatology and the strong evidence that functional disturbances span many brain systems suggest that it is unlikely that there will be a one-to-one mapping of specific symptoms to specific cholinergic abnormalities. Instead, network models may hold the key to understanding the relationship between (cholinergic) pathology and dysfunction in these disorders.

References

1. Cummings J, Isaacson S, Mills R, et al. Pimavanserin for patients with Parkinson's disease psychosis: a randomised, placebo-controlled phase 3 trial. Lancet. 2014;383(9916):533–40. doi:10.1016/s0140-6736(13)62106-6.
2. Aarsland D, Ballard C, Rongve A, et al. Clinical trials of dementia with Lewy bodies and Parkinson's disease dementia. Curr Neurol Neurosci Rep. 2012;12(5):492–501. doi:10.1007/s11910-012-0290-7.
3. Candy JM, Perry RH, Perry EK, et al. Pathological changes in the nucleus of Meynert in Alzheimer's and Parkinson's diseases. J Neurol Sci. 1983;59(2):277–89.
4. Perry RH, Tomlinson BE, Candy JM, et al. Cortical cholinergic deficit in mentally impaired Parkinsonian patients. Lancet. 1983;2(8353):789–90.
5. Bohnen NI, Albin RL. The cholinergic system and Parkinson disease. Behav Brain Res. 2011;221(2):564–73. doi:10.1016/j.bbr.2009.12.048.
6. Hall H, Reyes S, Landeck N, et al. Hippocampal Lewy pathology and cholinergic dysfunction are associated with dementia in Parkinson's disease. Brain. 2014;137(Pt 9):2493–508. doi:10.1093/brain/awu193.
7. Liu AK, Chang RC, Pearce RK, et al. Nucleus basalis of Meynert revisited: anatomy, history and differential involvement in Alzheimer's and Parkinson's disease. Acta Neuropathol. 2015;129(4):527–40. doi:10.1007/s00401-015-1392-5.
8. Chui HC, Mortimer JA, Slager U, et al. Pathologic correlates of dementia in Parkinson's disease. Arch Neurol. 1986;43(10):991–5.

9. Perry EK, Curtis M, Dick DJ, et al. Cholinergic correlates of cognitive impairment in Parkinson's disease: comparisons with Alzheimer's disease. J Neurol Neurosurg Psychiatry. 1985;48(5):413–21.
10. Alexandris A, Liu AK, Chang RC, et al. Differential expression of galanin in the cholinergic basal forebrain of patients with Lewy body disorders. Acta Neuropathol Commun. 2015;3:77. doi:10.1186/s40478-015-0249-4.
11. Chan-Palay V. Galanin hyperinnervates surviving neurons of the human basal nucleus of Meynert in dementias of Alzheimer's and Parkinson's disease: a hypothesis for the role of galanin in accentuating cholinergic dysfunction in dementia. J Comp Neurol. 1988;273 (4):543–57. doi:10.1002/cne.902730409.
12. Cullen KM, Halliday GM. Neurofibrillary degeneration and cell loss in the nucleus basalis in comparison to cortical Alzheimer pathology. Neurobiol Aging. 1998;19(4):297–306.
13. Mattila PM, Roytta M, Lonnberg P, et al. Choline acetytransferase activity and striatal dopamine receptors in Parkinson's disease in relation to cognitive impairment. Acta Neuropathol (Berl). 2001;102(2):160–6.
14. Piggott MA, Owens J, O'Brien J, et al. Muscarinic receptors in basal ganglia in dementia with Lewy bodies, Parkinson's disease and Alzheimer's disease. J Chem Neuroanat. 2003;25 (3):161–73.
15. Perry EK, Morris CM, Court JA, et al. Alteration in nicotine binding sites in Parkinson's disease, Lewy body dementia and Alzheimer's disease: possible index of early neuropathology. Neuroscience. 1995;64(2):385–95.
16. Court J, Spurden D, Lloyd S, et al. Neuronal nicotinic receptors in dementia with Lewy bodies and schizophrenia: alpha-bungarotoxin and nicotine binding in the thalamus. J Neurochem. 1999;73(4):1590–7.
17. Sahin HA, Emre M, Ziabreva I, et al. The distribution pattern of pathology and cholinergic deficits in amygdaloid complex in Alzheimer's disease and dementia with Lewy bodies. Acta Neuropathol. 2006;111(2):115–25. doi:10.1007/s00401-005-0003-2.
18. Kalaitzakis ME, Walls AJ, Pearce RK, et al. Striatal Abeta peptide deposition mirrors dementia and differentiates DLB and PDD from other Parkinsonian syndromes. Neurobiol Dis. 2011;41(2):377–84. doi:10.1016/j.nbd.2010.10.005.
19. Court JA, Piggott MA, Lloyd S, et al. Nicotine binding in human striatum: elevation in schizophrenia and reductions in dementia with Lewy bodies, Parkinson's disease and Alzheimer's disease and in relation to neuroleptic medication. Neuroscience. 2000;98 (1):79–87.
20. Pimlott SL, Piggott M, Owens J, et al. Nicotinic acetylcholine receptor distribution in Alzheimer's disease, dementia with Lewy bodies, Parkinson's disease, and vascular dementia: in vitro binding study using 5-[(125)i]-a-85380. Neuropsychopharmacology. 2004;29 (1):108–16.
21. Ray M, Bohr I, McIntosh JM, et al. Involvement of alpha6/alpha3 neuronal nicotinic acetylcholine receptors in neuropsychiatric features of Dementia with Lewy bodies: [(125)I]-alpha-conotoxin MII binding in the thalamus and striatum. Neurosci Lett. 2004;372(3):220–5. doi:10.1016/j.neulet.2004.09.042.
22. Bohr IJ, Ray MA, McIntosh JM, et al. Cholinergic nicotinic receptor involvement in movement disorders associated with Lewy body diseases. An autoradiography study using [(125)I] alpha-conotoxinMII in the striatum and thalamus. Exp Neurol. 2005;191(2):292–300. doi:10.1016/j.expneurol.2004.10.004.
23. Gotti C, Moretti M, Bohr I, et al. Selective nicotinic acetylcholine receptor subunit deficits identified in Alzheimer's disease, Parkinson's disease and dementia with Lewy bodies by immunoprecipitation. Neurobiol Dis. 2006;23(2):481–9. doi:10.1016/j.nbd.2006.04.005.
24. Lee JE, Cho KH, Song SK, et al. Exploratory analysis of neuropsychological and neuroanatomical correlates of progressive mild cognitive impairment in Parkinson's disease. J Neurol Neurosurg Psychiatry. 2014;85(1):7–16. doi:10.1136/jnnp-2013-305062.

25. Delli Pizzi S, Maruotti V, Taylor JP, et al. Relevance of subcortical visual pathways disruption to visual symptoms in dementia with Lewy bodies. Cortex. 2014;59:12–21. doi:10.1016/j.cortex.2014.07.003.
26. Delli Pizzi S, Franciotti R, Taylor JP, et al. Thalamic involvement in fluctuating cognition in Dementia with Lewy Bodies: magnetic resonance evidences. Cerebral Cortex (New York: 1991). 2015;25(10):3682–9. doi:10.1093/cercor/bhu220.
27. Ziabreva I, Ballard CG, Aarsland D, et al. Lewy body disease: thalamic cholinergic activity related to dementia and parkinsonism. Neurobiol Aging. 2006;27(3):433–8.
28. Kotagal V, Muller ML, Kaufer DI, et al. Thalamic cholinergic innervation is spared in Alzheimer disease compared to Parkinsonian disorders. Neurosci Lett. 2012;514(2):169–72. doi:10.1016/j.neulet.2012.02.083.
29. Seidel K, Mahlke J, Siswanto S, et al. The brainstem pathologies of Parkinson's disease and dementia with Lewy bodies. Brain Pathol. 2015;25(2):121–35. doi:10.1111/bpa.12168.
30. Schmeichel AM, Buchhalter LC, Low PA, et al. Mesopontine cholinergic neuron involvement in Lewy body dementia and multiple system atrophy. Neurology. 2008;70(5):368–73. doi:10.1212/01.wnl.0000298691.71637.96.
31. Dugger BN, Murray ME, Boeve BF, et al. Neuropathological analysis of brainstem cholinergic and catecholaminergic nuclei in relation to rapid eye movement (REM) sleep behaviour disorder. Neuropathol Appl Neurobiol. 2012;38(2):142–52. doi:10.1111/j.1365-2990.2011.01203.x.
32. Pahapill PA, Lozano AM. The pedunculopontine nucleus and Parkinson's disease. Brain. 2000;123(Pt 9):1767–83.
33. Janzen J, van 't Ent D, Lemstra AW, et al. The pedunculopontine nucleus is related to visual hallucinations in Parkinson's disease: preliminary results of a voxel-based morphometry study. J Neurol. 2012;259(1):147–54. doi:10.1007/s00415-011-6149-z.
34. Park HE, Park IS, Oh YS, et al. Subcortical whiter matter hyperintensities within the cholinergic pathways of patients with dementia and parkinsonism. J Neurol Sci. 2015;353(1–2):44–8. doi:10.1016/j.jns.2015.03.046.
35. Kuhl DE, Minoshima S, Fessler JA, et al. In vivo mapping of cholinergic terminals in normal aging, Alzheimer's disease, and Parkinson's disease. Ann Neurol. 1996;40(3):399–410.
36. Hilker R, Thomas AV, Klein JC, et al. Dementia in Parkinson disease: functional imaging of cholinergic and dopaminergic pathways. Neurology. 2005;65(11):1716–22. doi:10.1212/01.wnl.0000191154.78131.f6.
37. Shimada H, Hirano S, Shinotoh H, et al. Mapping of brain acetylcholinesterase alterations in Lewy body disease by PET. Neurology. 2009;73(4):273–8. doi:10.1212/WNL.0b013e3181ab2b58.
38. Klein JC, Eggers C, Kalbe E, et al. Neurotransmitter changes in dementia with Lewy bodies and Parkinson disease dementia in vivo. Neurology. 2010;74(11):885–92. doi:10.1212/WNL.0b013e3181d55f61.
39. Marcone A, Garibotto V, Moresco RM, et al. [11C]-MP4A PET cholinergic measurements in amnestic mild cognitive impairment, probable Alzheimer's disease, and dementia with Lewy bodies: a Bayesian method and voxel-based analysis. J Alzheimers Dis. 2012;31(2):387–99. doi:10.3233/JAD-2012-111748.
40. O'Brien JT, Colloby SJ, Pakrasi S, et al. Nicotinic alpha4beta2 receptor binding in dementia with Lewy bodies using 123I-5IA-85380 SPECT demonstrates a link between occipital changes and visual hallucinations. Neuroimage. 2008;40(3):1056–63. doi:10.1016/j.neuroimage.2008.01.010.
41. Colloby SJ, Perry EK, Pakrasi S, et al. Nicotinic 123I-5IA-85380 single photon emission computed tomography as a predictor of cognitive progression in Alzheimer's disease and dementia with Lewy bodies. Am J Geriatr Psychiatry. 2010;18(1):86–90. doi:10.1097/JGP.0b013e3181b972aa.

42. Isaias IU, Spiegel J, Brumberg J, et al. Nicotinic acetylcholine receptor density in cognitively intact subjects at an early stage of Parkinson's disease. Front Aging Neurosci. 2014;6:213. doi:10.3389/fnagi.2014.00213.
43. Colloby SJ, Pakrasi S, Firbank MJ, et al. In vivo SPECT imaging of muscarinic acetylcholine receptors using (R, R) 123I-QNB in dementia with Lewy bodies and Parkinson's disease dementia. NeuroImage. 2006;33(2):423–9.
44. Colloby S, McKeith I, Burn D, et al. Cholinergic and perfusion brain networks in Parkinson's disease dementia. Neurology. 2016; pii: 10.1212/WNL.0000000000002839. [Epub ahead of print]
45. Kim HJ, Lee JE, Shin SJ, et al. Analysis of the substantia innominata volume in patients with Parkinson's disease with dementia, dementia with Lewy bodies, and Alzheimer's disease. J Mov Disord. 2011;4(2):68–72. doi:10.14802/jmd.11014.
46. Grothe MJ, Schuster C, Bauer F, et al. Atrophy of the cholinergic basal forebrain in dementia with Lewy bodies and Alzheimer's disease dementia. J Neurol. 2014;261(10):1939–48. doi:10.1007/s00415-014-7439-z.
47. Colloby SJ, Elder GJ, Rabee R, et al. Structural grey matter changes in the substantia innominata in Alzheimer's disease and dementia with Lewy bodies: a DARTEL-VBM study. Int J Geriatr Psychiatry. 2016. doi:10.1002/gps.4500.
48. Satoh M, Ishikawa H, Meguro K, et al. Improved visual hallucination by donepezil and occipital glucose metabolism in dementia with Lewy bodies: the Osaki-Tajiri project. Eur Neurol. 2010;64(6):337–44. doi:10.1159/000322121.
49. Fong T, Inouye S, Dai W, et al. Association cortex hypoperfusion in mild dementia with Lewy bodies: a potential indicator of cholinergic dysfunction? Brain Imag Behavior. 2010;5(1):25–35. doi:10.1007/s11682-010-9108-x.
50. Gratwicke J, Kahan J, Zrinzo L, et al. The nucleus basalis of Meynert: a new target for deep brain stimulation in dementia? Neurosci Biobehav Rev. 2013;37(10 Pt 2):2676–88. doi:10.1016/j.neubiorev.2013.09.003.
51. Gratwicke J, Jahanshahi M, Foltynie T. Parkinson's disease dementia: a neural networks perspective. Brain. 2015;138(Pt 6):1454–76. doi:10.1093/brain/awv104.
52. Collerton D, Burn D, McKeith I, et al. Systematic review and meta-analysis show that dementia with Lewy bodies is a visual-perceptual and attentional-executive dementia. Dement Geriatr Cogn Disord. 2003;16(4):229–37.
53. Hanyu H, Asano T, Sakurai H, et al. MR analysis of the substantia innominata in normal aging, Alzheimer disease, and other types of dementia. AJNR Am J Neuroradiol. 2002;23(1):27–32.
54. Choi SH, Jung TM, Lee JE, et al. Volumetric analysis of the substantia innominata in patients with Parkinson's disease according to cognitive status. Neurobiol Aging. 2012;33(7):1265–72. doi:10.1016/j.neurobiolaging.2010.11.015.
55. Bohnen NI, Kaufer DI, Hendrickson R, et al. Cognitive correlates of cortical cholinergic denervation in Parkinson's disease and parkinsonian dementia. J Neurol. 2006;253(2):242–7.
56. Lorenz R, Samnick S, Dillmann U, et al. Nicotinic alpha4beta2 acetylcholine receptors and cognitive function in Parkinson's disease. Acta Neurol Scand. 2014;130(3):164–71. doi:10.1111/ane.12259.
57. Kenny ER, Blamire AM, Firbank MJ, et al. Functional connectivity in cortical regions in dementia with Lewy bodies and Alzheimer's disease. Brain. 2012;135(Pt 2):569–81. doi:10.1093/brain/awr327.
58. Peraza LR, Kaiser M, Firbank M, et al. fMRI resting state networks and their association with cognitive fluctuations in dementia with Lewy bodies. NeuroImage Clinical. 2014;4:558–65. doi:10.1016/j.nicl.2014.03.013.
59. Peraza LR, Taylor JP, Kaiser M. Divergent brain functional network alterations in dementia with Lewy bodies and Alzheimer's disease. Neurobiol Aging. 2015;36(9):2458–67. doi:10.1016/j.neurobiolaging.2015.05.015.

60. Dauwan M, van Dellen E, van Boxtel L, et al. EEG-directed connectivity from posterior brain regions is decreased in dementia with Lewy bodies: a comparison with Alzheimer's disease and controls. Neurobiol Aging. 2016;41:122–9. doi:10.1016/j.neurobiolaging.2016.02.017.
61. McKeith IG, Dickson DW, Lowe J, et al. Diagnosis and management of dementia with Lewy bodies. Third report of the DLB consortium. Neurology. 2005;65:1863–72.
62. Ballard C, Aarsland D, Francis P, et al. Neuropsychiatric symptoms in patients with dementias associated with cortical Lewy bodies: pathophysiology, clinical features, and pharmacological management. Drugs Aging. 2013;30(8):603–11. doi:10.1007/s40266-013-0092-x.
63. Ballard C, Piggott M, Johnson M, et al. Delusions associated with elevated muscarinic binding in dementia with Lewy bodies. Ann Neurol. 2000;48(6):868–76.
64. Court JA, Ballard CG, Piggott MA, et al. Visual hallucinations are associated with lower alpha bungarotoxin binding in dementia with Lewy bodies. Pharmacol Biochem Behav. 2001;70 (4):571–9.
65. Teaktong T, Piggott MA, McKeith IG, et al. Muscarinic M2 and M4 receptors in anterior cingulate cortex: relation to neuropsychiatric symptoms in dementia with Lewy bodies. Behav Brain Res. 2005;161(2):299–305.
66. Marra C, Quaranta D, Profice P, et al. Central cholinergic dysfunction measured "in vivo" correlates with different behavioral disorders in Alzheimer's disease and dementia with Lewy body. Brain Stimul. 2012;5(4):533–8. doi:10.1016/j.brs.2011.08.009.
67. O'Brien JT, Colloby SJ, Pakrasi S, et al. Nicotinic [alpha]4[beta]2 receptor binding in dementia with Lewy bodies using 123I-5IA-85380 SPECT demonstrates a link between occipital changes and visual hallucinations. NeuroImage. 2008;40(3):1056–63.
68. Hepp DH, Ruiter AM, Galis Y, et al. Pedunculopontine cholinergic cell loss in hallucinating Parkinson disease patients but not in dementia with Lewy bodies patients. J Neuropathol Exp Neurol. 2013;72(12):1162–70.
69. Yarnall A, Rochester L, Burn DJ. The interplay of cholinergic function, attention, and falls in Parkinson's disease. Mov Disord. 2011;26(14):2496–503. doi:10.1002/mds.23932.
70. Onofrj M, Taylor JP, Monaco D, et al. Visual hallucinations in PD and Lewy body dementias: old and new hypotheses. Behav Neurol. 2013;27(4):479–93. doi:10.3233/BEN-129022.
71. Collerton D, Perry E, McKeith I. Why people see things that are not there: a novel perception and attention deficit model for recurrent complex visual hallucinations. Behav Brain Sci. 2005;28(6):737–57.
72. Stinton C, McKeith I, Taylor JP, et al. Pharmacological management of Lewy body dementia: A systematic review and meta-analysis. Am J Psychiatry. 2015:appiajp201514121582. doi:10.1176/appi.ajp.2015.14121582.
73. Ballard CG, Court JA, Piggott M, et al. Disturbances of consciousness in dementia with Lewy bodies associated with alteration in nicotinic receptor binding in the temporal cortex. Conscious Cogn. 2002;11(3):461–74.
74. Pimlott SL, Piggott M, Ballard C, et al. Thalamic nicotinic receptors implicated in disturbed consciousness in dementia with Lewy bodies. Neurobiol Dis. 2006;1:50–6.
75. Bonanni L, Thomas A, Tiraboschi P, et al. EEG comparisons in early Alzheimer's disease, dementia with Lewy bodies and Parkinson's disease with dementia patients with a 2-year follow-up. Brain. 2008;131(3):690–705. doi:10.1093/brain/awm322.
76. Walker MP, Ayre GA, Cummings JL, et al. The clinician assessment of fluctuation and the one day fluctuation assessment scale. Two methods to assess fluctuating confusion in dementia. Br J Psychiatry. 2000;177:252–6.
77. Walker MP, Ayre GA, Cummings JL, et al. Quantifying fluctuation in dementia with Lewy bodies, Alzheimer's disease, and vascular dementia. Neurology. 2000;54(8):1616–25.
78. Gore RL, Vardy ER, O'Brien JT. Delirium and dementia with Lewy bodies: distinct diagnoses or part of the same spectrum? J Neurol Neurosurg Psychiatry. 2015;86(1):50–9. doi:10.1136/jnnp-2013-306389.

79. Taylor JP, Colloby SJ, McKeith IG, et al. Covariant perfusion patterns provide clues to the origin of cognitive fluctuations and attentional dysfunction in dementia with Lewy bodies. Int Psychogeriatrics/IPA. 2013;25(12):1917–28. doi:10.1017/S1041610213001488.
80. Bohnen NI, Frey KA, Studenski S, et al. Gait speed in Parkinson disease correlates with cholinergic degeneration. Neurology. 2013;81(18):1611–6. doi:10.1212/WNL.0b013e3182a9f558.
81. Sarter M, Albin RL, Kucinski A, et al. Where attention falls: increased risk of falls from the converging impact of cortical cholinergic and midbrain dopamine loss on striatal function. Exp Neurol. 2014;257:120–9. doi:10.1016/j.expneurol.2014.04.032.
82. Bohnen NI, Muller ML, Koeppe RA, et al. History of falls in Parkinson disease is associated with reduced cholinergic activity. Neurology. 2009;73(20):1670–6. doi:10.1212/WNL.0b013e3181c1ded6.
83. Weathers SP, Kotagal V, Bohnen NI, et al. Risky driving and pedunculopontine nucleus-thalamic cholinergic denervation in Parkinson disease. Parkinsonism Relat Disord. 2014;20 (1):13–6. doi:10.1016/j.parkreldis.2013.08.021.
84. Rochester L, Yarnall AJ, Baker MR, et al. Cholinergic dysfunction contributes to gait disturbance in early Parkinson's disease. Brain. 2012;135(Pt 9):2779–88. doi:10.1093/brain/aws207.
85. Bohnen NI, Muller ML, Kotagal V, et al. Olfactory dysfunction, central cholinergic integrity and cognitive impairment in Parkinson's disease. Brain. 2010;133(Pt 6):1747–54. doi:10.1093/brain/awq079.
86. Gjerloff T, Fedorova T, Knudsen K, et al. Imaging acetylcholinesterase density in peripheral organs in Parkinson's disease with 11C-donepezil PET. Brain. 2015;138(Pt 3):653–63. doi:10.1093/brain/awu369.
87. Perry EK, Haroutunian V, Davis KL, et al. Neocortical cholinergic activities differentiate Lewy body dementia from classical Alzheimer's disease. Neuroreport. 1994;5(7):747–9.
88. Graff-Radford J, Boeve BF, Pedraza O, et al. Imaging and acetylcholinesterase inhibitor response in dementia with Lewy bodies. Brain. 2012;135(Pt 8):2470–7. doi:10.1093/brain/aws173.
89. Fong TG, Inouye SK, Dai W, et al. Association cortex hypoperfusion in mild dementia with Lewy bodies: a potential indicator of cholinergic dysfunction? Brain Imaging Behav. 2011;5 (1):25–35. doi:10.1007/s11682-010-9108-x.

Chapter 4
Molecular Biology of Dementia with Lewy Bodies

Masato Hasegawa

Abstract The discovery of mutation of the α-synuclein gene, *SNCA*, in familial forms of Parkinson's disease (PD) and subsequent identification of α-synuclein in the filamentous component of Lewy bodies indicated that fibrillization or conformational change of α-synuclein plays a central role in the pathogenesis of PD and dementia with Lewy bodies (DLB). Indeed, distribution and spreading of α-synuclein pathologies strongly correlate with disease manifestation and progression. Recent in vitro and in vivo experimental models clearly demonstrate that amyloid-like α-synuclein fibrils show prion-like properties and are able to convert normal α-synuclein to an abnormal form. For example, synthetic fibrils made of recombinant α-synuclein and sarkosyl-insoluble α-synuclein fibrils prepared from DLB brains both induce abnormal α-synuclein pathology in wild-type mice after direct inoculation into the brain. This prion-like propagation of α-synuclein through neuronal networks is the key mechanism of formation of α-synuclein pathology, and such spreading in the central and peripheral nervous systems may explain the disease progression. Thus, a detailed understanding of the molecular mechanisms of cell-to-cell propagation and its regulation is likely to be helpful for the development of disease-modifying therapy for DLB and PD.

Keywords Synuclein • Phosphorylation • Prion-like • Fibril • Propagation

4.1 Identification of α-Synuclein in Lewy Bodies

I first saw an autopsy brain sample from a patient with dementia with Lewy bodies (DLB) in about 1993, when I was working on biochemical analysis of tau in Alzheimer's disease (AD) at Prof. Yasuo Ihara's lab at the Brain Research Institute, University of Tokyo. One of the students was doing an immunochemical analysis of insoluble proteins prepared from several autopsy brain samples of patients with AD. Most cases were immunopositive for both anti-phospho tau and ubiquitin

M. Hasegawa (✉)
Department of Dementia and Higher Brain Function, Tokyo Metropolitan Institute of Medical Science, 2-1-6 Kamikitazawa, Setagaya-ku, Tokyo 156-8506, Japan
e-mail: hasegawa-ms@igakuken.or.jp

K. Kosaka (ed.), *Dementia with Lewy Bodies*, DOI 10.1007/978-4-431-55948-1_4

antibodies, but one case was tau negative but ubiquitin positive. I wondered if this case might have a non-AD pathology, and indeed, it later turned out that the patient had DLB.

Immunocytochemical approaches to identifying the protein elements of the Lewy bodies (LBs) were initiated in the 1980s, and neurofilaments (NFs) were suggested to be involved by Goldman et al. [1]. In 1988, Kuzuhara et al. reinvestigated the issue with various antibodies and demonstrated that antibodies to 200-kDa component of NF and tau did not stain LBs, whereas monoclonal and polyclonal antibodies to ubiquitin stained cortical LBs as intensely as Alzheimer's neurofibrillary tangles and plaque neurites [2]. They confirmed by means of immunoelectron microscopy that the antibodies labeled the filaments of LBs and concluded that ubiquitin is a good marker of LBs [2]. Later, Iwatsubo et al. purified LBs by means of fluorescence-activated particle sorting with ubiquitin antibodies. They raised ~15 monoclonal antibodies to LBs and reported that the monoclonal antibody that stained the largest number of LBs reacted with polyubiquitin chains [3], while some other mAbs (LB48, LB202, and LB204) recognized medium-molecular-mass neurofilaments [4].

In 1997, the A53T missense mutation in the *SNCA* gene was discovered in the Italian kindred and in three unrelated families of Greek origin with autosomal dominant inheritance for the PD phenotype [5], and shortly after, the *SNCA* gene product, α-synuclein, was identified as the major component of the filaments of Lewy bodies by immunohistochemistry and immunoelectron microscopy using specific antibodies to α- and β-synuclein [6, 7]. As I discuss later, Goedert et al. had cloned human α- and β-synuclein cDNA and had raised antibodies against both α- and β-synuclein [8]. I was in Michel Goedert's lab as a visiting scientist during 1996–1998, and I well remember the heated discussions about whether α-synuclein is the major component of Lewy bodies. Later, Maria Spillantini reported in Nature an immunohistochemical study of Lewy bodies with anti-α-synuclein antibodies, marking a new chapter in the history of Lewy bodies [6] (Fig. 4.1). Iwatsubo et al. also reported that one of the antibodies raised against purified Lewy bodies strongly reacted with α-synuclein and confirmed that α-synuclein is the component of Lewy bodies [9].

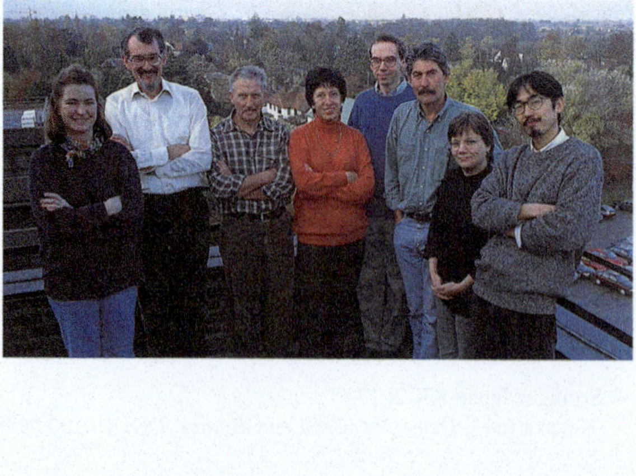

Fig. 4.1 Scientists who have worked alongside Michel Goedert in Cambridge – (from *left*) Valerie Buee-Sherrer, Tony Crowther, Ross Jakes, Maria Spillantini, Michel Goedert, Mike Smith, Molly Craxton and Masato Hasegawa in 1997

α-Synuclein is a relatively small, abundant protein of 140 amino acids, which was first identified in 1988 as a neuron-specific protein in synaptic vesicles in the electric organ of *Torpedo* [10]. The cDNA of the orthologue from rat brain was cloned, and the gene product was given the name "synuclein," which means a protein located in synapses and nuclei [10]. It is quite a coincidence that human α-synuclein cDNA was cloned independently in two laboratories (Goedert's and Ihara's labs) working on PHF and tau in neurodegenerative diseases and that I spent time working in both. Ihara et al. identified two unknown peptides, designated X and Y, in SDS-insoluble fractions prepared from AD brains by means of lysl-endopeptidase digestion followed by amino acid sequencing [11]. Ueda in Tsunao Saito's lab (UCSD) cloned the cDNA in collaboration with Ihara and reported in PNAS that it was a precursor of non-amyloid component (NACP), since one of the antisera against the peptides stained senile plaques [12]. At almost the same time, Jakes and Goedert found that monoclonal antibody 11.57 directed toward PHF-tau and fetal tau also cross-reacted with doublet bands at 19 kDa in soluble fraction of human brain [8]. They purified the proteins, determined 55-amino acid sequences, and cloned cDNAs for two homologous proteins of 140 and 134 amino acids. The former protein was a homologue of synuclein from *Torpedo* and rat, reported by Maroteaux, and the same protein as NACP reported by Ueda. The latter was a homologue of PNP14 identified by Nakajo in bovine brain [13]. Therefore, they named these two proteins α- and β-synuclein [8]. Both groups took the opportunity afforded by the cross reactivity of the antibodies to clone cDNA of synuclein.

Shortly after the identification of α-synuclein in Lewy bodies, it was reported that glial cytoplasmic inclusions (GCIs) in multiple system atrophy are also strongly immunopositive for α-synuclein antibodies [14, 15] and that α-synuclein is also the major component of the filaments of GCIs [15]. This made another major impact on the classification of neurodegenerative diseases, since three different clinical entities, i.e., olivopontocerebellar atrophy (OPCA), striatonigral degeneration (SND), and Shy-Drager syndrome (SDS), were found to comprise a disease entity characterized by oligodendrocytic α-synuclein pathology. Later, neurodegenerative diseases with α-synuclein pathologies were referred to as α-synucleinopathies. These studies demonstrated a direct link between intracellular accumulation of abnormal protein and the causative genes identified by human molecular genetics. This is also the case in frontotemporal dementia and parkinsonism linked to chromosome 17 (FTDP-17), where mutations in the *MAPT* (tau) gene in patients were discovered in 1998 [16].

4.2 Structure and Function of α-Synuclein

Synuclein is a relatively small protein characterized by the presence of five imperfect repeats of a KT(A)KE(Q)G(Q)V motif in the amino-terminal half, hydrophobic amino acids in the midportion, and an acidic C-terminal region (Fig. 4.2). The repeat region has been reported to be important for the association of synucleins with lipid membranes [17]. Three homologous proteins with the repeat sequence

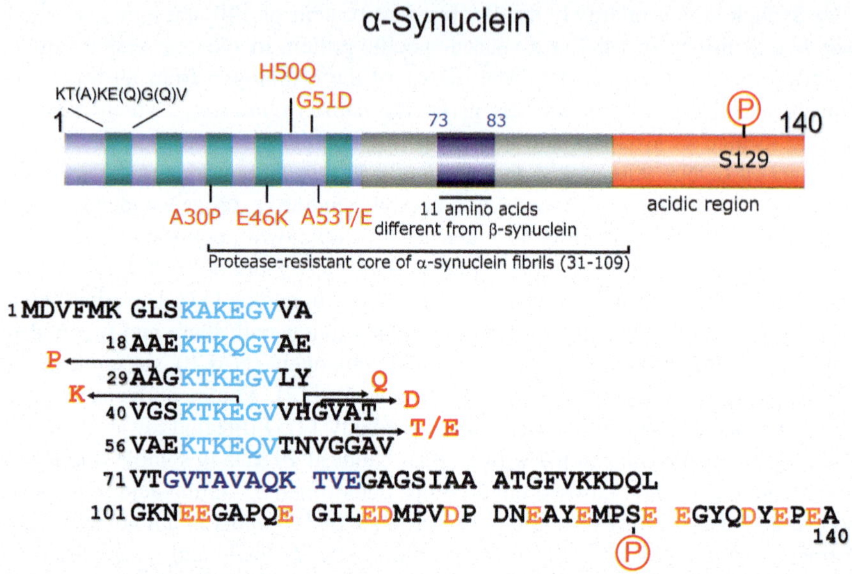

Fig. 4.2 Schematic illustration of the structure and amino acid sequence of human α-synuclein. Domain structures including five KT(A)KE(Q)G(Q)V motifs, 11 amino acids different from β-synuclein and an acidic region are illustrated. Six missense mutations identified in familial forms of PD or DLB, an abnormal phosphorylation site (Ser129) identified in pathological α-synuclein from diseased brains and the protease-resistant core of α-synuclein fibrils are shown

have been cloned and named α-, β-, and γ-synucleins; they are encoded by three independent genes [18]. β-Synuclein has 78 % homology and γ-synuclein has 58 % homology to α-synuclein in terms of DNA sequences. α-Synuclein and β-synuclein are colocalized in synaptic terminals in many regions of the brain, whereas γ-synuclein is expressed in particular kinds of neurons, such as dorsal root ganglion or non-neuronal tissues, and is overexpressed in breast cancer cells.

Electron microscopy combined with immunocytochemistry showed that α-synuclein is localized in presynaptic terminals, especially near synaptic vesicles [10]. The physiological roles of the protein remain to be clarified, but several functions have been suggested. It may be involved in (1) memory, learning, and plasticity of synapses, since expression levels of the homologue synelfin are increased only during a limited period of song learning in zebra finch [19], and (2) transport processes in vesicles, since it is localized in membranes and inhibits phospholipase D2, a regulator of the cytoskeleton and endocytosis [20]. A chaperon-like role of synuclein has also been proposed [21]. Based on analyses of knockout mice lacking both α- and β-synuclein, α-synuclein may contribute to the long-term regulation and/or maintenance of presynaptic function, as well as protection of nerve terminals against injury, and may exhibit this activity in conjunction with CSPα and SNARE proteins on the presynaptic membrane interface [22]. Since only a minor use-dependent alteration of dopamine release was observed in α-synuclein KO mice, α-synuclein is not essential for survival or for neurotransmitter release. These studies led to the idea that, consistent with its localization, α-synuclein may regulate synaptic plasticity (reviewed in [18]). No synuclein homologue has been identified in worm or fly.

4.3 Biochemical Analyses of α-Synuclein in Neurodegenerative Diseases

To investigate the molecular mechanisms of Lewy body pathogenesis, it is essential to know what are the differences between normal α-synuclein and the abnormal form in Lewy bodies. Biochemical analyses of α-synuclein from DLB and control brains demonstrated that normal α-synuclein is mostly recovered in Tris and Triton-X-soluble fractions, whereas the abnormal form is detected in sarkosyl-insoluble fraction (which is soluble in 8 M urea, 6 M guanidine hydrochloride, and SDS). Mass spectrometric analysis of α-synuclein revealed that Ser129 is abnormally phosphorylated in the sarkosyl-insoluble form [23]. Phosphorylation site-specific antibodies indicated that more than 90 % of insoluble α-synuclein is phosphorylated at Ser129, while only about 5 % is phosphorylated in normal synuclein [23]. Casein kinases 1, 2 (CK1, CK2) and G protein-coupled receptor kinases 2, 5 (GRK2, GRK5) are candidate kinases for the in vitro phosphorylation, and major kinase activities in rat brain extracts were reported to be due to CK2 [24]. The level of phosphorylation seems to be higher in the striatum than in the hippocampus in mouse brain, and it was decreased up to 57 % by cold-water-induced stress [25]. The physiological role of Ser129 phosphorylation in the brain remains unclear, but it may be a degradation signal for the ubiquitin proteasome system or it may affect some interaction of other proteins.

Other posttranslational modifications such as nitration [26] have also been reported, but their biological significance is unknown. Ubiquitination is another important modification in the abnormal phosphorylated form of α-synuclein, as confirmed by both immunochemical and mass spectrometric analyses. Because the extent of ubiquitination is less than that of phosphorylation, ubiquitination may be a later event. Ubiquitination sites of α-synuclein in Lewy bodies in PD and DLB and also glial cytoplasmic inclusions in MSA have been determined by MS analysis to be Lys12, 21, and 23, with Lys 48 multi-ubiquitination [27]. These sites are different from those found in soluble α-synuclein, suggesting that aggregated proteins may be recognized as abnormal by the ubiquitin proteasome system of the cells [27, 28].

A much more prominent feature of abnormal α-synuclein in Lewy bodies is its conformation. Ultrastructurally, it has been shown that α-synuclein in Lewy bodies and Lewy neurites consists of filamentous or fibrous forms with a width of 10 nm, which are completely different from the normal unstructured form. Furthermore, the fibrils are thioflavin S-positive, a characteristic feature of amyloid fibrils, as well as Aβ and tau fibrils [29]. As discussed later, recombinant α-synuclein forms fibrils biochemically and morphologically similar to those in diseased brains in the absence of posttranslational modification. Furthermore, X-ray diffraction analysis demonstrated that α-synuclein is assembled into fibrils with cross-β structure [30].

There is continuing debate as to whether or not the phosphorylation is a primary and causative event for the accumulation of intracellular abnormal proteins, especially for tau protein in tauopathies. However, at least in the case of α-synuclein, the results of in vitro and in vivo studies strongly suggest that phosphorylation is not a primary event leading to accumulation. Instead, the conformational change of α-synuclein is thought to be the primary event in diseased brains.

4.4 Molecular Mechanisms of Amyloid-Like Fibril Formation

α-Synuclein is natively unfolded, i.e., it is basically unstructured, with no significant secondary structures [31]. So, in considering the molecular mechanisms of PD and DLB pathogenesis and potential therapies, the key questions seem to be: "how does the unstructured protein form amyloid-like fibrils?", "how do pathogenic mutations in the α-synuclein affect the conformation and induce fibril formation?", "what are the mechanisms of toxicity of the fibrils?", and "how can we inhibit fibril formation?".

Purified recombinant α-synuclein can be easily converted to filamentous form by incubation at 37 °C with shaking at a high concentration. Conformational change from random coil to β-sheet structure can be observed by CD spectral analysis and thioflavin S fluorescence measurement. In contrast, no such conformational changes are observed with β-synuclein, whose amino acid sequence is 61 % homologous to that of α-synuclein, suggesting that the difference is critical for fibril formation. Actually, α-synuclein lacking a hydrophobic stretch of 12 amino acid residues (71VTGVTAVAQKTV82) does not form fibrils, and this sequence is essential for α-synuclein fibril formation [32]. As mentioned above, the fibrils have cross-β structure typical of amyloid fibrils [30]. MALDI-TOF mass analysis of proteinase K-resistant fragments of α-synuclein fibrils revealed that the core of α-synuclein fibrils is composed of residues 31–109 of α-synuclein [33].

To date, six missense mutations in the α-synuclein gene (A30P, E46K, H50Q, G51D, A53T, and A53E), as well as occurrence of gene duplication and triplication, have been identified in familial forms of PD and DLB [5, 34–41]. The A53T and E46K mutants form fibrils faster than wild-type α-synuclein (WT), but fibrillization of A30P is slow [42]. Instead, A30P mutant was suggested to form oligomeric protofibrils, and oligomer formation may the cause of PD [43]. However, we found that A30P mutant forms a fragile-type fibril, which resulted in accelerated nucleation-dependent fibrillization of α-synuclein compared with WT fibrils

[44]. Later, autopsy of a patient with the A30P mutation revealed abundant α-synuclein pathology in the brain, strongly suggesting that the mutation induced PD via accumulation of pathological α-synuclein fibrils, not formation of soluble oligomers [45]. These results support the idea that αsyn fibril formation causes PD and DLB.

Although α-synuclein is natively unfolded, as mentioned above, NMR analysis of the monomer revealed interactions between NAC (residues 61–95) and the C-terminal region (residues 110–130), between residues 120–130 and 105–115, and between the N-terminal region and near residue 120 [46], indicating that the protein molecule is not totally unfolded. The natively unfolded state of α-synuclein may be stabilized by long-range interactions (e.g., shielding of the hydrophobic NAC domain by the acidic C-terminal region) that inhibit aggregation or fibrillization [46]. This could be the reason why C-terminally truncated forms have higher propensities to aggregate [47]. The A30P and A53T mutations were reported to influence the stability of the native state and to favor fibril formation [48]. The conformational changes of α-synuclein in going from the monomer state to amyloid-like fibrils can be detected more easily by using site-specific α-synuclein antibodies [49]. Antibodies against the N-terminal region or NAC region of α-synuclein do not react very well with the monomer, but strongly stain the fibrils in dot blot analysis, while antibodies against the C-terminal region stain both monomer and fibrils well [49].

4.5 Seed-Dependent Aggregation of α-Synuclein

Fibrillization or conformational change of α-synuclein is thought to be the central event in the pathogenesis of PD and DLB. Assembly of protein into amyloid fibrils is usually a nucleation-dependent process that consists of nucleation followed by elongation, and α-synuclein fibrillization was also confirmed to be nucleation dependent (Fig. 4.3) [50]. Addition of seeds (a small amount of preformed fibrils) to the monomer promotes fibrillization by skipping the nucleation process. Although the precise mechanism remains to be characterized, the conversion of monomer to fibrils seems to be basically a prion-like conversion. Namely, the conformation is changed to the abnormal form by interaction of the monomer with fibril seeds. Amyloid-like fibril seeds act as a template for conversion, and multiplication of this conversion induces propagation of well-ordered homogeneous amyloid-like fibrils.

This seed-dependent conversion and fibril formation of α-synuclein have been established in culture cells by introducing fibril seeds with transfection reagents. Aggregation or fibrillization does not occur when α-synuclein is overexpressed in cultured cells by means of plasmid transfection, even if pathogenic mutants are induced, or when cells are exposed to various stresses. In contrast, abundant

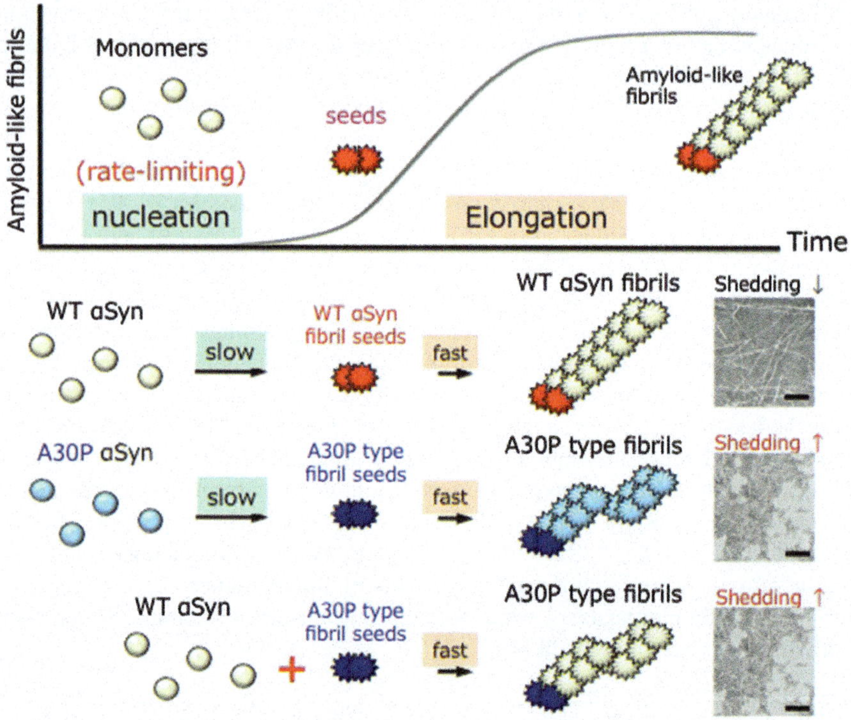

Fig. 4.3 Schematic illustration of amyloid-like fibril formation. Seed-dependent, prion-like conversion of normal proteins into abnormal forms is believed to be the basic mechanism of amyloid or amyloid-like fibril formation. Assembly of protein into fibrils is usually a nucleation-dependent process consisting of a lag phase (nucleation) and a growth phase (elongation). Wild-type (WT) α-synuclein forms amyloid-like fibrils. A30P mutant α-synuclein also forms fibrils, but their shedding propensity is higher than that of WT. When A30P seeds are added to WT α-synuclein, WT fibrils with the character and conformation of A30P fibrils are formed

α-synuclein inclusions were formed inside cells transfected with α-synuclein plasmid when preformed fibril seeds were introduced into the cells with a transfection reagent (Fig. 4.4) [51]. EM observation of the inclusions revealed that they were composed of 10-nm α-synuclein fibrils similar to those found in DLB brains. Biochemical and immunocytochemical analyses demonstrated that the aggregated α-synuclein is abnormally phosphorylated at Ser129 and partially ubiquitinated and is recovered in sarkosyl-soluble and sarkosyl-insoluble fractions; it is indistinguishable from the aggregates in DLB brains [51]. Interestingly, cells with inclusions have been shown to degenerate gradually during 3–4 days in culture. Monitoring of proteasome activities in cells using GFP-CL1 (a degron that is an effective proteasome-degradation signal) and additional biochemical analyses indicated

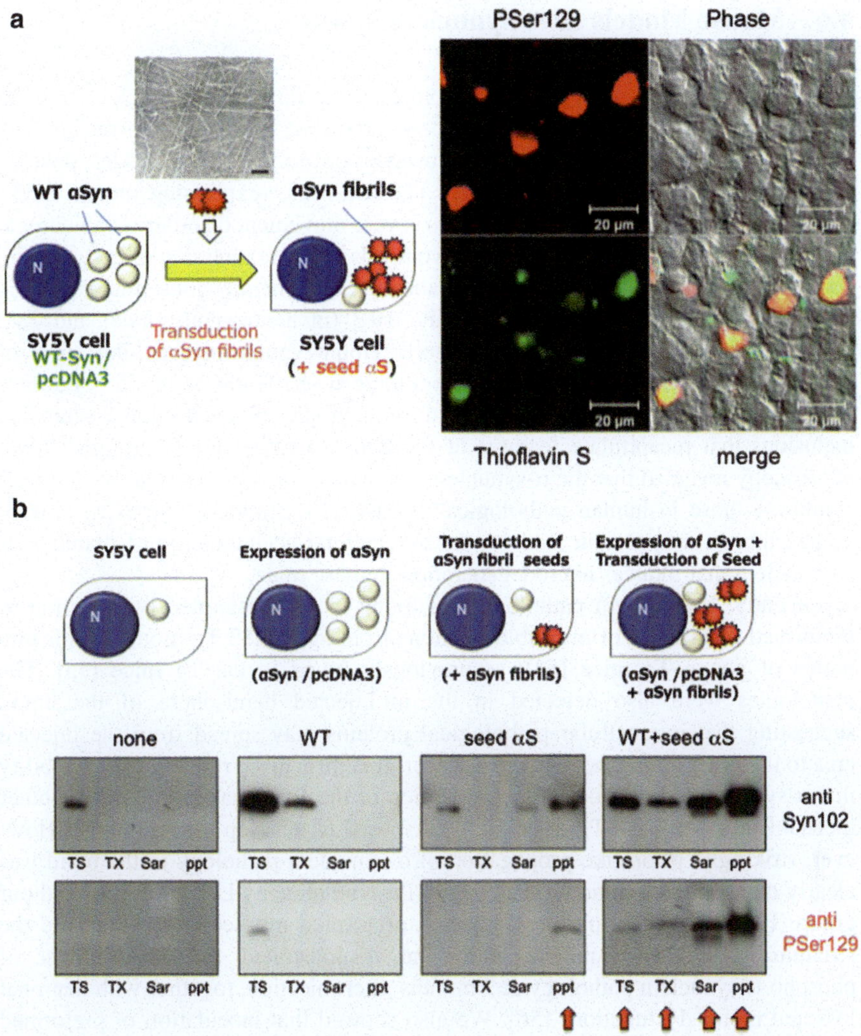

Fig. 4.4 Conversion of normal α-synuclein to abnormal form in cultured cells by transduction of preformed fibril seeds. (**a**) Seeded aggregation of α-synuclein in SH-SY5Y cells overexpressing α-synuclein, upon transfection with α-synuclein fibrils. Abundant phosphorylated, thioflavin-S-positive α-synuclein aggregates are formed. (**b**) Schematic illustration of molecular events associated with transduction of the seeds and immunoblot analyses of soluble and insoluble α-synuclein with PSer129 antibody

that proteasome dysfunction induced by abnormal α-synuclein may be one of the major causes of cell necrosis [51]. Similar seed-dependent aggregation has been observed with other intracellular pathological proteins, such as tau and TDP-43 [51, 52].

4.6 Mouse Models of α-Synucleinopathy

Many lines of transgenic mice overexpressing wild-type α-synuclein, mutant α-synuclein, or truncated forms have been produced in attempts to recapitulate the neuropathologies of PD and DLB. However, only a few mouse models develop phosphorylated α-synuclein pathology. The M83 line (expressing mutant A53T human α-synuclein) of Tg mice develops severe movement disorder with neuronal α-synuclein pathologies [53]. The relative levels of overexpression of α-synuclein, compared to endogenous protein, are about 3.3 (in hemizygous mice) and 4.6 (in homozygous mice) in the cortex and 19.3 (in hemizygous mice) and 28.2 (in homozygous mice) in the spinal cord. Homozygous mice exhibit signs of spontaneous neurological dysfunction beginning at ~8 months of age [53]. Furthermore, the mice develop age-dependent intracytoplasmic neuronal α-synuclein inclusions that recapitulate features of the human counterparts. Immunoelectron microscopy revealed that the α-synuclein inclusions contain 10–16 nm wide fibrils similar to those in human pathological inclusions [53]. Thus, overexpression of mutant human α-synuclein leads to the intracellular accumulation of filamentous α-synuclein that induces neurodegeneration in these mice.

Recently, α-synuclein pathology was found to be accelerated by injection of preformed fibril seeds or insoluble fractions from aged M83 Tg-mouse brains into brains of young Tg mice [54], as previously found in tau Tg mice [55]. The pathologies were also detected in the un-injected hemisphere of the brain, suggesting that intracellular pathological proteins may spread from the injected area to the other hemisphere [54]. However, it is difficult to rule out the possibility that α-synuclein fibrils accelerate production of the abnormal form by some other mechanism(s), because Tg mice are predisposed to develop the pathology. However, strikingly, prion-like propagation of α-synuclein pathology in the brain was clearly demonstrated in non-Tg, C57B6 wild-type mice by Luk et al. [56] and our group (Fig. 4.5) [57]. Luk et al. injected preformed mouse α-synuclein into the striatum of wild-type mouse brain and demonstrated the development of phospho-α-synuclein pathology at 3 months after injection, together with neuronal loss and motor dysfunctions [56]. We also showed that inoculation of preformed human and mouse α-synuclein fibrils into substantia nigra of wild-type mouse brain induced phosphorylated and ubiquitinated α-synuclein pathology in various brain regions and that mouse α-synuclein fibrils induced the pathology more efficiently than human α-synuclein fibrils, suggesting there may be a species barrier, as has been found in the case of infection of prion proteins [57]. Importantly, our study clearly demonstrated that mouse endogenous α-synuclein is converted to an abnormal form that is indistinguishable from the form in DLB brain by inoculation of human α-synuclein fibrils, though the injected human α-synuclein fibrils are degraded within a week after injection [57]. We also showed that sarkosyl-insoluble pellets from DLB brains, in which abnormal α-synuclein fibrils are enriched, induced similar pathologies of phospho-α-synuclein [57], strongly suggesting that pathological α-synuclein protein spreads from cell to cell by prion-like propagation

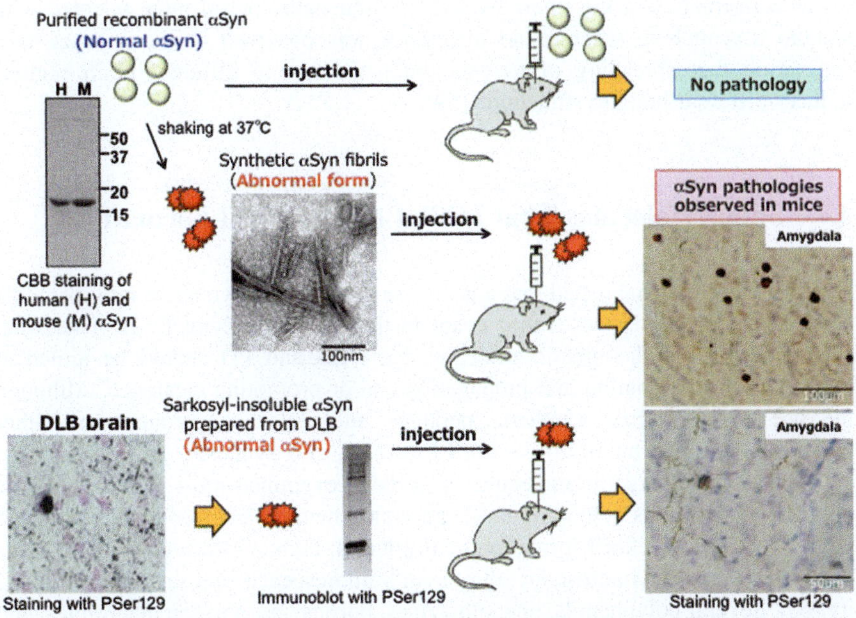

Fig. 4.5 Schematic illustration of prion-like conversion of α-synuclein in wild-type mice by inoculation of synthetic α-synuclein fibrils or sarkosyl-insoluble α-synuclein prepared from DLB brain. Widespread α-synuclein pathologies were detected with PSer129 antibody, and the pathology seems to spread through the neural networks in a time-dependent manner

in DLB brains. No such pathology was detected in mice injected with soluble α-synuclein monomer or in α-synuclein KO (deficient) mice injected with α-synuclein fibrils. Recently, Watts reported that brain homogenates from MSA brains also accelerated and induced α-synuclein pathology and motor dysfunction in the heterozygous M83 Tg mice; since α-synuclein fibrils fulfilled all the criteria for classification as prions, the name "α-synuclein prions" was proposed [58].

To find out where and how abnormal α-synuclein propagates in brain, we injected α-synuclein fibrils into three different brain regions (substantia nigra, striatum, and entorhinal cortex) and investigated the spread of pathology at 1 month after injection. In mice injected into the substantia nigra, abnormal phosphorylated α-synuclein pathology was restricted mainly to the substantia nigra, amygdala, and stria terminalis of the hemisphere on the injection side, while the pathology in mice injected in the striatum was widely distributed bilaterally throughout the brain, including the striatum, amygdala, substantia nigra, and cortex [59]. Injection of the fibrils into the entorhinal cortex induced severe pathology in the entorhinal cortex, dentate gyrus, hippocampal CA3 region, and septal nucleus [59]. These results clearly demonstrate that propagation of pathological α-synuclein occurred along neural circuits and involved transsynaptic transport. Furthermore, mice injected into the substantia nigra and striatum showed lower performance in the rotarod test compared with control mice injected with soluble α-synuclein, whereas no difference was observed in the Y-maze test, suggesting that spreading of α-synuclein pathology in different brain regions induces different brain dysfunctions [59].

4.7 Small Molecules That Inhibit α-Syn Fibril Formation

Overall, it is well established that conversion of soluble α-synuclein into insoluble amyloid-like fibrils is the central event in the pathogenesis of DLB. Therefore, disease-modifying therapeutic strategies for DLB and PD should be aimed at inhibiting fibril formation and propagation and/or promoting clearance. Although the use of antibodies, synthetic peptides, molecular chaperones, and other chemicals to inhibit amyloid-like fibril formation of α-synuclein in vitro has been considered, small organic molecules have been examined most extensively. We tested 75 compounds belonging to 12 different chemical classes for the ability to inhibit amyloid-like fibril formation of full-length human α-synuclein, which was assessed by electron microscopy, thioflavin S fluorescence, and sarkosyl insolubility [60]. Several polyphenols, phenothiazines, porphyrins, polyene macrolides, and Congo red and its derivatives BSB and FSB inhibited α-synuclein fibril formation with IC50 values in the low micromolar range [60]. Interestingly, the formation of soluble oligomeric α-synuclein was detected in the presence of inhibitory compounds [60]. Since the oligomers show intermediate features between monomer and fibrils in conformational analysis using site-specific α-synuclein antibodies, it is reasonable to speculate that the small molecules inhibit fibril formation by stabilizing the oligomers and/or blocking interaction of monomer with fibrils [49]. These soluble oligomeric species did not show any toxicity to SH-SY5Y cells, unlike α-synuclein fibrils and protofibrils. These findings suggest that these compounds may have therapeutic potential for α-synucleinopathies [49]. Further studies using cellular and mouse models will be needed, especially to investigate whether the compounds can inhibit prion-like propagation of pathological α-synuclein in vivo.

4.8 Conclusions and Perspectives

Lewy bodies and Lewy neurites are abnormal intracellular structures composed of amyloid-like fibrils of α-synuclein and associated cellular proteins and organelles and are defining characteristics of PD and DLB. Recent studies, including our work, have clearly demonstrated that both synthetic α-synuclein fibrils made of recombinant protein and sarkosyl-insoluble α-synuclein fibrils from DLB and MSA brains have prion-like ability to convert normal α-synuclein to abnormal amyloid-like fibrils in vitro and in vivo. Although the precise molecular mechanisms of this prion-like conversion and its cell-to-cell propagation remain to be clarified, it is not an exaggeration to say that the phenomenon of prion-like propagation of α-synuclein in brain is validated by the experimental models much more clearly than in the case of prion disease itself. Inhibition of α-synuclein fibril formation and propagation seems to be a solidly based strategy for developing disease-modifying therapy for DLB and other α-synucleinopathies.

Acknowledgments I gratefully acknowledge the work of past and present members of my laboratory. I also would like to thank Michel Goedert for helpful comments.

References

1. Goldman JE, Yen SH, Chiu FC, et al. Lewy bodies of Parkinson's disease contain neurofilament antigens. Science. 1983;221:1082–4.
2. Kuzuhara S, Mori H, Izumiyama N, et al. Lewy bodies are ubiquitinated. A light and electron microscopic immunocytochemical study. Acta Neuropathol. 1988;75:345–53.
3. Iwatsubo T, Yamaguchi H, Fujimuro M, et al. Purification and characterization of Lewy bodies from the brains of patients with diffuse Lewy body disease. Am J Pathol. 1996;148:1517–29.
4. Galvin JE, Lee VM, Baba M, et al. Monoclonal antibodies to purified cortical Lewy bodies recognize the mid-size neurofilament subunit. Ann Neurol. 1997;42:595–603.
5. Polymeropoulos MH, Lavedan C, Leroy E, et al. Mutation in the alpha-synuclein gene identified in families with Parkinson's disease. Science. 1997;276:2045–7.
6. Spillantini MG, Schmidt ML, Lee VM, et al. Alpha-synuclein in Lewy bodies. Nature. 1997;388:839–40.
7. Spillantini MG, Crowther RA, Jakes R, et al. alpha-Synuclein in filamentous inclusions of Lewy bodies from Parkinson's disease and dementia with Lewy bodies. Proc Natl Acad Sci U S A. 1998;95:6469–73.
8. Jakes R, Spillantini MG, Goedert M. Identification of two distinct synucleins from human brain. FEBS Lett. 1994;345:27–32.
9. Baba M, Nakajo S, Tu PH, et al. Aggregation of alpha-synuclein in Lewy bodies of sporadic Parkinson's disease and dementia with Lewy bodies. Am J Pathol. 1998;152:879–84.
10. Maroteaux L, Campanelli JT, Scheller RH. Synuclein: a neuron-specific protein localized to the nucleus and presynaptic nerve terminal. J Neurosci. 1988;8:2804–15.
11. Ihara Y, Kondo J. Polypeptide composition of paired helical filaments. Ann Med. 1989;21:121–5.
12. Ueda K, Fukushima H, Masliah E, et al. Molecular cloning of cDNA encoding an unrecognized component of amyloid in Alzheimer disease. Proc Natl Acad Sci U S A. 1993;90:11282–6.
13. Nakajo S, Omata K, Aiuchi T, et al. Purification and characterization of a novel brain-specific 14-kDa protein. J Neurochem. 1990;55:2031–8.
14. Wakabayashi K, Yoshimoto M, Tsuji S, et al. Alpha-synuclein immunoreactivity in glial cytoplasmic inclusions in multiple system atrophy. Neurosci Lett. 1998;249:180–2.
15. Spillantini MG, Crowther RA, Jakes R, et al. Filamentous alpha-synuclein inclusions link multiple system atrophy with Parkinson's disease and dementia with Lewy bodies. Neurosci Lett. 1998;251:205–8.
16. Goedert M, Jakes R, Crowther RA, et al. Intraneuronal filamentous tau protein and alpha-synuclein deposits in neurodegenerative diseases. Biochem Soc Trans. 1998;26:463–71.
17. Davidson WS, Jonas A, Clayton DF, et al. Stabilization of alpha-synuclein secondary structure upon binding to synthetic membranes. J Biol Chem. 1998;273:9443–9.
18. Goedert M, Spillantini MG, Davies SW. Filamentous nerve cell inclusions in neurodegenerative diseases. Curr Opin Neurobiol. 1998;8:619–32.

19. George JM, Jin H, Woods WS, et al. Characterization of a novel protein regulated during the critical period for song learning in the zebra finch. Neuron. 1995;15:361–72.
20. Jenco JM, Rawlingson A, Daniels B, et al. Regulation of phospholipase D2: selective inhibition of mammalian phospholipase D isoenzymes by alpha- and beta-synucleins. Biochemistry. 1998;37:4901–9.
21. Ostrerova N, Petrucelli L, Farrer M, et al. alpha-Synuclein shares physical and functional homology with 14-3-3 proteins. J Neurosci. 1999;19:5782–91.
22. Chandra S, Fornai F, Kwon HB, et al. Double-knockout mice for alpha- and beta-synucleins: effect on synaptic functions. Proc Natl Acad Sci U S A. 2004;101:14966–71.
23. Fujiwara H, Hasegawa M, Dohmae N, et al. alpha-Synuclein is phosphorylated in synucleinopathy lesions. Nat Cell Biol. 2002;4:160–4.
24. Ishii A, Nonaka T, Taniguchi S, et al. Casein kinase 2 is the major enzyme in brain that phosphorylates Ser129 of human alpha-synuclein: Implication for alpha-synucleinopathies. FEBS Lett. 2007;581:4711–7.
25. Hirai Y, Fujita SC, Iwatsubo T, et al. Phosphorylated alpha-synuclein in normal mouse brain. FEBS Lett. 2004;572:227–32.
26. Giasson BI, Duda JE, Murray IV, et al. Oxidative damage linked to neurodegeneration by selective alpha-synuclein nitration in synucleinopathy lesions. Science. 2000;290:985–9.
27. Anderson JP, Walker DE, Goldstein JM, et al. Phosphorylation of Ser-129 is the dominant pathological modification of alpha-synuclein in familial and sporadic Lewy body disease. J Biol Chem. 2006;281:29739–52.
28. Nonaka T, Iwatsubo T, Hasegawa M. Ubiquitination of alpha-synuclein. Biochemistry. 2005;44:361–8.
29. Hashimoto M, Hsu LJ, Sisk A, et al. Human recombinant NACP/alpha-synuclein is aggregated and fibrillated in vitro: relevance for Lewy body disease. Brain Res. 1998;799:301–6.
30. Serpell LC, Berriman J, Jakes R, Crowther RA, et al. Fiber diffraction of synthetic alpha-synuclein filaments shows amyloid-like cross-beta conformation. Proc Natl Acad Sci U S A. 2000;97:4897–902.
31. Weinreb PH, Zhen W, Poon AW, et al. NACP, a protein implicated in Alzheimer's disease and learning, is natively unfolded. Biochemistry. 1996;35:13709–15.
32. Giasson BI, Murray IV, Trojanowski JQ, et al. A hydrophobic stretch of 12 amino acid residues in the middle of alpha-synuclein is essential for filament assembly. J Biol Chem. 2001;276:2380–6.
33. Miake H, Mizusawa H, Iwatsubo T, et al. Biochemical characterization of the core structure of alpha-synuclein filaments. J Biol Chem. 2002;277:19213–9.
34. Appel-Cresswell S, Vilarino-Guell C, Encarnacion M, et al. Alpha-synuclein p.H50Q, a novel pathogenic mutation for Parkinson's disease. Mov Disord. 2013;28:811–3.
35. Chartier-Harlin MC, Kachergus J, Roumier C, et al. Alpha-synuclein locus duplication as a cause of familial Parkinson's disease. Lancet. 2004;364:1167–9.
36. Ibanez P, Bonnet AM, Debarges B, et al. Causal relation between alpha-synuclein gene duplication and familial Parkinson's disease. Lancet. 2004;364:1169–71.
37. Kruger R, Kuhn W, Muller T, et al. Ala30Pro mutation in the gene encoding alpha-synuclein in Parkinson's disease. Nat Genet. 1998;18:106–8.
38. Lesage S, Anheim M, Letournel F, et al. G51D alpha-synuclein mutation causes a novel Parkinsonian-pyramidal syndrome. Ann Neurol. 2013;73:459–71.
39. Pasanen P, Myllykangas L, Siitonen M, et al. Novel alpha-synuclein mutation A53E associated with atypical multiple system atrophy and Parkinson's disease-type pathology. Neurobiol Aging. 2014;35:2180 e1–5.
40. Singleton AB, Farrer M, Johnson J, et al. alpha-Synuclein locus triplication causes Parkinson's disease. Science. 2003;302:841.
41. Zarranz JJ, Alegre J, Gomez-Esteban JC, et al. The new mutation, E46K, of alpha-synuclein causes Parkinson and Lewy body dementia. Ann Neurol. 2004;55:164–73.

42. Conway KA, Harper JD, Lansbury PT. Accelerated in vitro fibril formation by a mutant alpha-synuclein linked to early-onset Parkinson disease. Nat Med. 1998;4:1318–20.
43. Conway KA, Lee SJ, Rochet JC, et al. Acceleration of oligomerization, not fibrillization, is a shared property of both alpha-synuclein mutations linked to early-onset Parkinson's disease: implications for pathogenesis and therapy. Proc Natl Acad Sci U S A. 2000;97:571–6.
44. Yonetani M, Nonaka T, Masuda M, et al. Conversion of wild-type alpha-synuclein into mutant-type fibrils and its propagation in the presence of A30P mutant. J Biol Chem. 2009;284:7940–50.
45. Seidel K, Schols L, Nuber S, et al. First appraisal of brain pathology owing to A30P mutant alpha-synuclein. Ann Neurol. 2010;67:684–9.
46. Bertoncini CW, Jung YS, Fernandez CO, et al. Release of long-range tertiary interactions potentiates aggregation of natively unstructured alpha-synuclein. Proc Natl Acad Sci U S A. 2005;102:1430–5.
47. Crowther RA, Jakes R, Spillantini MG, et al. Synthetic filaments assembled from C-terminally truncated alpha-synuclein. FEBS Lett. 1998;436:309–12.
48. Bertoncini CW, Fernandez CO, Griesinger C, et al. Familial mutants of alpha-synuclein with increased neurotoxicity have a destabilized conformation. J Biol Chem. 2005;280:30649–52.
49. Masuda M, Hasegawa M, Nonaka T, et al. Inhibition of alpha-synuclein fibril assembly by small molecules: analysis using epitope-specific antibodies. FEBS Lett. 2009;583:787–91.
50. Wood SJ, Wypych J, Steavenson S, et al. alpha-synuclein fibrillogenesis is nucleation-dependent. Implications for the pathogenesis of Parkinson's disease. J Biol Chem. 1999;274:19509–12.
51. Nonaka T, Watanabe ST, Iwatsubo T, et al. Seeded aggregation and toxicity of {alpha}-synuclein and tau: cellular models of neurodegenerative diseases. J Biol Chem. 2010;285:34885–98.
52. Nonaka T, Masuda-Suzukake M, Arai T, et al. Prion-like properties of pathological TDP-43 aggregates from diseased brains. Cell Rep. 2013;4:124–34.
53. Giasson BI, Duda JE, Quinn SM, et al. Neuronal alpha-synucleinopathy with severe movement disorder in mice expressing A53T human alpha-synuclein. Neuron. 2002;34:521–33.
54. Luk KC, Kehm VM, Zhang B, et al. Intracerebral inoculation of pathological alpha-synuclein initiates a rapidly progressive neurodegenerative alpha-synucleinopathy in mice. J Exp Med. 2012;209:975–86.
55. Clavaguera F, Bolmont T, Crowther RA, et al. Transmission and spreading of tauopathy in transgenic mouse brain. Nat Cell Biol. 2009;11:909–13.
56. Luk KC, Kehm V, Carroll J, et al. Pathological alpha-synuclein transmission initiates Parkinson-like neurodegeneration in nontransgenic mice. Science. 2012;338:949–53.
57. Masuda-Suzukake M, Nonaka T, Hosokawa M, et al. Prion-like spreading of pathological alpha-synuclein in brain. Brain. 2013;136:1128–38.
58. Watts JC, Giles K, Oehler A, et al. Transmission of multiple system atrophy prions to transgenic mice. Proc Natl Acad Sci U S A. 2013;110:19555–60.
59. Masuda-Suzukake M, Nonaka T, Hosokawa M, et al. Pathological alpha-synuclein propagates through neural networks. Acta Neuropathol Commun. 2014;2:88.
60. Masuda M, Suzuki N, Taniguchi S, et al. Small molecule inhibitors of alpha-synuclein filament assembly. Biochemistry. 2006;45:6085–94.

Part III
Clinical Aspects

Chapter 5
Clinical Diagnostic Criteria for Dementia with Lewy Bodies

Ian G. McKeith

Abstract Clinical diagnostic concepts and methods for the dementias associated with Lewy body disease have evolved over the last three decades to incorporate previously used terminologies including diffuse LB disease (DLBD) [Kosaka et al., Clin Neuropathol 3(5):185–192, 1984; Dickson et al., Acta Neuropathol 75:8–15, 1987; Lennox et al., Lancet 8633(1):323–324, 1989], LB dementia (LBD) [Gibb et al., Brain 110:1131–1153, 1987], dementia associated with cortical Lewy bodies (DCLB) [Byrne et al., Dementia 2:283–284, 1991], the LB variant of Alzheimer's disease (LBVAD) [Hansen et al., Neurology 40:1–8, 1990; Förstl et al., Br J Psychiatry 162:385–392, 1993] and senile dementia of LB type (SDLT) [Perry et al. J Neurol Sci 95:119–139, 1990]. Dementia with Lewy bodies (DLB) was eventually agreed as a term to include all of these within one set of operationalised consensus criteria [McKeith et al., Neurology 47(5):1113–1124, 1996; McKeith et al. Neurology 65(12):1863–1872, 2005]. These in turn formed the basis for the inclusion of neurocognitive disorder with Lewy bodies (NCDLB) in the latest revision of the DSM5 [APA. Diagnostic and statistical manual of mental disorders: DSM-5. American Psychiatric Association, Washington, DC, 2013]. This formal recognition of DLB as a diagnostic category equivalent to others such as Alzheimer's disease, vascular disease and frontotemporal disorder will greatly assist recognition and diagnosis of the disorder with benefit for patients and families. It will also enable clinical and research practice and impact upon reimbursement and regulatory authorities. Criteria for early and prodromal diagnosis remain in development.

Keywords Clinical • Diagnosis • Lewy • Dementia

I.G. McKeith (✉)
Newcastle University Institute for Ageing, Biomedical Research Building, Campus for Ageing and Vitality, Newcastle upon Tyne NE4 5PL, UK
e-mail: i.g.mckeith@ncl.ac.uk

K. Kosaka (ed.), *Dementia with Lewy Bodies*, DOI 10.1007/978-4-431-55948-1_5

5.1 Development of Clinical Diagnostic Criteria for DLB

5.1.1 First Reports and Preliminary Attempts at Clinical Description: Japanese and US Studies

The early history of DLB has already been detailed in chapter one. This brief review gives an account of the various clinical diagnostic schemes that have been devised and in particular how they have been refined and harmonised into a globally accepted system. Table 5.1 lists the major systems that have been proposed.

Although the first case reports specifically describing patients with dementia and LBs appeared as early as 1961 when Okazaki reported on two elderly men presenting with cognitive decline and who subsequently developed severe rigidity [12], it was another two decades before Kosaka et al. [1] reported the first significant series of 34 cases, noting a 3:1 male predominance, with memory disturbance as the presenting feature in 67 %, psychotic states in 17 % and dizziness due to orthostatic hypotension in 17 %. Progressive dementia with muscular rigidity occurred eventually in 80 %, although only 25 % of cases were diagnosed with parkinsonism. The first substantial listing of these Japanese cases in the Western literature was in 1987 by Gibb et al. [4] who added four new UK cases. The following year, Burkhardt et al. [13] listed 34 additional cases from the USA and carried out a simple meta-analysis. The most common presentation was a "neurobehavioural syndrome"; memory impairment and other cognitive deficits were typical; all but one eventually becoming demented. Psychotic features such as depression, hallucinations and paranoia were seen in ten patients (29 %), two being psychotic for many years before developing other symptoms. Parkinsonian features, the most common of which was rigidity, were usually overshadowed by dementia; in only five cases (15 %) were no extrapyramidal features present. Duration of illness was very variable (1–20 years) with an end state of severe dementia, rigidity, akinetic mutism, quadriparesis in flexion and emaciation. The most common reported cause of death was aspiration pneumonia. Based upon these observations, Burkhardt et al. were the first to attempt a general description of the

Table 5.1 Diagnostic terminology for DLB, listed in chronological order

Diffuse Lewy body disease (DLBD)	Kosaka et al. [1], Dickson et al. [2], Lennox et al. [3]
Lewy body dementia (LBD)	Gibb et al. [4]
Lewy body variant of Alzheimer's disease (LBVAD)	Hansen et al. [6], Förstl et al. [7]
Senile dementia of LB type (SDLT)	Perry et al. [8]
Dementia associated with cortical Lewy bodies (DCLB)	Byrne et al. [5]
Dementia with Lewy bodies (DLB)	McKeith et al. [9, 10]
Neurocognitive disorder with Lewy bodies (NCDLB)	APA [11]

clinical syndrome associated with diffuse Lewy body disease, distinguishing it as separate from PD with dementia. They concluded that "DLBD (diffuse Lewy body disease) should be suspected in any elderly patient who presents with a rapidly progressive dementia, followed in short order by rigidity and other parkinsonian features. Myoclonus may be present"[13].

Crystal et al. [14] in a paper entitled "Antemortem diagnosis of diffuse Lewy body disease" criticised this approach on the grounds that "extrapyramidal features occur in many patients with severe AD and since dementia occurs in many subjects with PD, the clinical criteria for the diagnosis of DLBD remain unclear". The authors proposed alternative criteria of "progressive dementia with gait disorder, psychiatric symptoms and a burst pattern on EEG at the time of moderate dementia". No particular characteristics of the pattern of cognitive impairment were noted.

Although these early clinical definitions were important in drawing attention to the existence of DLBD and describing some of its salient characteristics, neither could be regarded as satisfactory for clinical diagnostic purposes, since they were not operationalised in a way which would allow acceptable inter-rater reliability [15]. Despite the emphasis on motor disability, these early attempts did make a clear distinction between the DLBD group and patients with PD who later developed dementia, a proposition which has been maintained in the DLB consensus criteria and which de facto has encouraged the development of diagnostic criteria for PD dementia along a separate but parallel path.

5.1.2 Development of Operationalised Criteria Based Upon Individual Cohorts

At around the same time that US investigators were reporting the cases above, the Nottingham, UK, group reported the clinical characteristics of 15 new cases in considerable detail, the largest single-site series published at that time [16] and which led to the first formal proposal of operationalised criteria for dementia associated with cortical Lewy bodies (DCLB) [5]. Seven were men, the mean age at onset was 72 years and the mean duration of illness 5.5 years. Forty per cent presented with symptoms and signs of idiopathic PD, with cognitive impairment occurring 1–4 years later. A further 20 % had parkinsonism and mild cognitive impairment at presentation, and the remaining 40 % showed motor features later in their illnesses, gait disturbance and postural abnormalities being most common. These latter cases presented with neuropsychiatric features only, in various combinations of cognitive impairment, paranoid delusions and visual or auditory hallucinations. Fourteen of the 15 were demented before death, the exception presenting with classical PD and later becoming depressed, irritable and mildly forgetful with frequent falls. Fluctuating cognition with episodic confusion for which no adequate underlying cause could be found was observed in 80 % of the Nottingham cases. Byrne also drew attention to the frequent occurrence of depression (20 %) and psychosis (33 %). In retrospect many of these cases would now be classified as having PD dementia rather than DLB.

Also around the same time, the Newcastle upon Tyne group identified 14 UK cases with the neuropathological features of "senile dementia of Lewy body type" (SDLT) [8] accounting for 15 % of a series of dementia autopsies. These SDLT cases had been regarded during lifetime as clinically atypical, "causing much diagnostic perplexity". Acute onset, fluctuating course, more rapid deterioration, early and prominent hallucinatory and behavioural disturbances and associated mild parkinsonian features were present. Two further Newcastle series were reported soon after [17, 18], and depressive symptoms, unexplained falls, observed disturbances of consciousness and excessive sensitivity to side effects of neuroleptic medication were added to the list of clinical characteristics with potential to distinguish DLB pathology cases from AD.

Based upon these observations, new clinical diagnostic criteria proposed with an emphasis upon cognitive dysfunction and neuropsychiatric features which could occur in the absence of extrapyramidal motor signs, and an attempt was made to describe the typical course of illness. "The first stage is often recognised only in retrospect and may extend back 1–3 years pre-presentation with occasional minor episodes of forgetfulness, sometimes described as lapses of concentration or "switching off". A brief period of delirium is sometimes noted for the first time, often associated with genuine physical illness and/or surgical procedures. Disturbed sleep, nightmares and daytime drowsiness often persist after recovery.

Progression to the second stage frequently prompts psychiatric or medical referral. A more sustained cognitive impairment is established, albeit with marked fluctuations in severity. Recurrent confusional episodes are accompanied by vivid hallucinatory experiences, visual misidentification syndromes and topographical disorientation. Extensive medical screening is usually negative. Attentional deficits are apparent as apathy, and daytime somnolence and sleep behaviour disorder may be severe. Gait disorder and bradykinesia are often overlooked, particularly in elderly subjects. Frequent falls occur due either to postural instability or syncope.

The third and final stage often begins with a sudden increase in behavioural disturbance, leading to requests for sedation or hospital admission by perplexed and exhausted carers. The natural course from this point is variable and obscured by the high incidence of adverse reactions to neuroleptic medication. For patients not receiving, or tolerating neuroleptics, a progressive decline into severe dementia with dysphasia and dyspraxia occurs over months or years, with death usually due to cardiac or pulmonary disease. During this terminal phase, patients show continuing behavioural disturbance including vocal and motor responses to hallucinatory phenomena. Lucid intervals with some retention of recent memory function and insight may still be apparent. Neurological disability is often profound with fixed flexion deformities of the neck and trunk and severe gait impairment" [17].

5.1.3 The Lewy Body Variant of Alzheimer's Disease

The majority of case reports and series up till this time generally made reference to the atypical clinical presentations of patients with cortical LB pathology, who generally did not easily fit any of the existing diagnostic rubrics. Exceptions to this were the reports by Hansen et al. [6] working in San Diego and Förstl et al. [7] in London, both of which described patients who met clinical criteria for possible or probable Alzheimer's disease (AD). The Förstl series comprised four men and four women who did not differ from autopsy-confirmed AD controls in survival time, severity of cognitive impairment or presence of hallucinations or fluctuation. Five of the eight were recorded as having confusional states and five also developed pronounced parkinsonism at a later stage. They concluded that the mere presence of LB in a case of dementia did not seem to warrant the differentiation of a separate illness, particularly as rigidity appeared to be the only characteristic clinical feature. They regarded their patients as having "Lewy body variant of Alzheimer's disease (LBVAD)", a term which had been coined by Hansen and colleagues a few years earlier. The San Diego group had been studying clinically diagnosed AD patients meeting NINCDS-ADRDA criteria but found that 13 of 36 such cases followed to autopsy had cortical and subcortical LBs in addition to pathologically confirmed AD.

The only differences between the LBVAD and pure AD cases were that the former had a different neuropsychological profile with more severe attentional deficits, reduced verbal fluency and severely impaired visuospatial performance on block design and drawing tests. Mild extrapyramidal features with masked facies, bradykinesia and gait difficulty were also recorded. Although Hansen et al. concluded that "in some case it may be possible to diagnose LBV premortem on the basis of the clinical and neuropsychological profile", they did not extend to generating formalised diagnostic criteria [6].

5.2 Development of International Consensus Criteria

By the early 1990s, it was becoming apparent that DLB was a relatively common cause of dementia in old age and that the several research groups investigating it were adopting different terminologies which were most likely predicated on their different patient sampling biases and the relatively small size of individual case series. All of the essential clinical diagnostic elements had been described by this stage, but it was unclear how to use the information to construct a set of clinically useful diagnostic guidelines or how to conceptualise relationships between the new atypical group with AD, LBVAD or PDD. The way forward was achieved through the DLB Consortium which established itself as a collaboration of interested researchers with international and multidisciplinary membership. An account of events leading up to and including the establishment of this group has previously

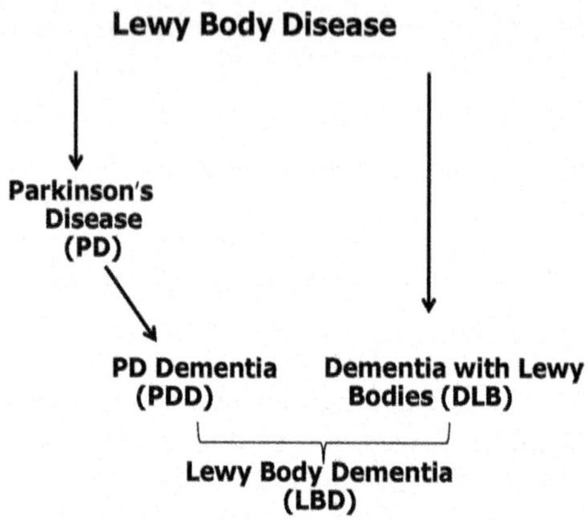

Fig. 5.1 A simple schematic shows the relationship between the terms LBD, DLB and PDD. This simple and memorable scheme should be adhered to in order to ensure consistency in diagnostic practice. This is equally important to patients and their families as it is to clinicians and researchers

been published [19]. The DLB Consortium also worked closely with the International Movement Disorder Society working groups which developed criteria for the clinical diagnosis of PD dementia [20, 21] and through a boundary exercise were able to ensure a harmonised diagnostic glossary (see Fig. 5.1) across these parts of the Lewy body disease spectrum [22].

5.2.1 *First Report of the DLB Consortium*

The consortium on DLB met for the first time in October 1995 in Newcastle upon Tyne, to agree common clinical and pathological methods and nomenclature based upon the evidence and opinion available [9]. DLB was recommended as an appropriate, generic term for those previously used by different groups and "because it acknowledges the presence of LB without specifying their relative importance in symptom formation with respect to other degenerative or vascular pathology that is simultaneously present". This seems to have been a sensible decision given subsequent advances in our understanding of α-synuclein pathology and neuritic/synaptic disruption in these patients. Lewy bodies per se are almost certainly not the cause of neuronal dysfunction and may indeed represent a neuroprotective response. Although much of the first consensus paper was devoted to describing pathological sampling and staining and scoring methods [9], it also described in some detail the particular characteristics of the cognitive impairments of DLB as differing from the dementia syndrome of AD, in which memory deficits predominate. In DLB, attentional deficits and prominent visuospatial dysfunction are the main features [23, 24], and amnestic deficits are often less evident, especially in the early stages. Probable DLB could be diagnosed according to this system (Table 5.2) if any two of the three key symptoms were present, namely, fluctuation, visual hallucinations or spontaneous motor features of parkinsonism, and possible DLB could be diagnosed if only one was present.

Table 5.2 Consensus criteria for the clinical diagnosis of probable and possible DLB – report of the first consortium meeting [9]

1. *The central feature* required for a diagnosis of DLB is progressive cognitive decline of sufficient magnitude to interfere with normal social and occupational function. Prominent or persistent memory impairment may not necessarily occur in the early stages but is usually evident with progression. Deficits on tests of attention and of frontal–subcortical skills and visuospatial ability may be especially prominent
2. *Two of the following core features* are essential for a diagnosis of probable DLB, and one is essential for possible DLB:
(a) Fluctuating cognition with pronounced variations in attention and alertness
(b) Recurrent visual hallucinations that are typically well formed and detailed
(c) Spontaneous motor features of parkinsonism
3. *Features supportive of the diagnosis are:*
(a) Repeated falls
(b) Syncope
(c) Transient loss of consciousness
(d) Neuroleptic sensitivity
(e) Systematised delusions
(f) Hallucinations in other modalities
4. *A diagnosis of DLB is less likely in the presence of:*
(a) Stroke disease evident as focal neurologic signs or on brain imaging
(b) Evidence on physical examination and investigation of any physical illness or other brain disorder sufficient to account for the clinical picture

Several retrospective and two prospective studies have examined the predictive accuracy of these original consensus clinical criteria for probable DLB [25, 26]. These reported that the specificity of a probable DLB clinical diagnosis is high at autopsy, typically around 90 %, but that sensitivity of case detection is lower at an average around 40 % but with considerable variability between sites. This means that the criteria in their 1996 format were most useful for confirmation of diagnosis (a low false-positive rate) but that many cases were missed (high false-negative rate). The initial interpretation of these findings was that either the clinical criteria were lacking either in their content or in adequate operationalisation which allowed clinicians to use them adequately. The core feature, fluctuation, was particularly singled out as hard to recognise or quantify. An alternative and not mutually exclusive view was that all DLB patients simply did not have the same clinical presentation, those with a significant degree of Alzheimer pathology being speculated as having a more Alzheimer-like clinical onset and course.

The other key issue tackled by the first consortium report was the relationship between DLB and PD dementia. A "one-year rule" was proposed by which it was suggested that "if dementia occurs within 12 months of the onset of extrapyramidal motor symptoms, the patient should be assigned a primary diagnosis of possible DLB and this will be strengthened by the presence of additional core or additional features. If the clinical history of parkinsonism is longer than 12 months, PD with dementia (clinically DLB or other) will usually be a more appropriate diagnostic label" [9]. Although the one-year rule has continued to be hotly debated over the last 20 years, it has proved useful in the clinical setting and will probably continue to do so until empirical data become available to improve upon it.

5.2.2 Second Report of the DLB Consortium

The Second International DLB Workshop briefly met in July 1998 in Amsterdam. The objectives were to review developments since publication of the consensus guidelines and to determine whether these yet required to be modified. It was recommended that the clinical consensus criteria should continue to be used in their current format with the addition of two new supportive features, namely, rapid eye movement (REM) sleep behaviour disorder (RBD) and depression [27].

5.2.3 Third Report of the DLB Consortium

In order to address the perceived insensitivity of the DLB diagnostic criteria outlined above, the DLB Consortium met again in 2003 in Newcastle to resolve improving the identification of cases ante-mortem. No major amendments to the three core features of DLB were proposed, but better methods for their clinical assessment were recommended. A new category of features "suggestive" of DLB was described, comprising REM sleep behaviour disorder (RBD) [28], severe neuroleptic sensitivity [18] and abnormal dopamine transporter neuroimaging [29]. If one or more of these suggestive features is present, in addition to one or more core features, a diagnosis of probable DLB can be made – see Table 5.3. Possible DLB can be diagnosed if one or more suggestive features are present in a patient with dementia even in the absence of any core features. The revised criteria are also more explicit about the importance to be attached to clinical and radiological evidence of cerebrovascular disease.

These improved criteria have been suggested to detect 25 % more DLB cases than the previous version [30], although a retrospective application of the new criteria to an autopsy-verified sample reported that cases with Braak stage 5 and 6 Alzheimer pathology were still unlikely to be detected ante-mortem. Such cases tend to lack core or suggestive DLB features, clinically resemble AD [31] and lend credence to the original LBVAD concept. It has also been shown that the DLB clinical syndrome is modified by the severity of Alzheimer neuritic pathology, while β-amyloid load has no effect [32]. This is consistent with the proposal made by the third consortium group that the likelihood of a patient having the typical DLB clinical syndrome is "directly related to the severity of Lewy-related pathology and inversely related to the severity of concurrent AD-type pathology". Given that AD-type pathology is frequently present in DLB, there will therefore be a significant number of patients who will always prove very difficult to identify solely

Table 5.3 Revised consensus criteria for the clinical diagnosis of probable and possible DLB – report of the third consortium meeting [10]

1. *Central feature* (essential for a diagnosis of possible or probable DLB)
Dementia defined as progressive cognitive decline of sufficient magnitude to interfere with normal social or occupational function. Prominent or persistent memory impairment may not necessarily occur in the early stages but is usually evident with progression. Deficits on tests of attention, executive function and visuospatial ability may be especially prominent
2. *Core features* (two core features are sufficient for a diagnosis of probable DLB, one for possible DLB):
Fluctuating cognition with pronounced variations in attention and alertness
Recurrent visual hallucinations that are typically well formed and detailed
Spontaneous features of parkinsonism
3. *Suggestive features* (if one or more of these are present in the presence of one or more core features, a diagnosis of probable DLB can be made. In the absence of any core features, one or more suggestive features are sufficient for possible DLB. Probable DLB should not be diagnosed on the basis of suggestive features alone):
REM sleep behaviour disorder
Severe neuroleptic sensitivity
Low dopamine transporter uptake in basal ganglia demonstrated by SPECT or PET imaging
4. *Supportive features* (commonly present but not proven to have diagnostic specificity):
Repeated falls and syncope
Transient, unexplained loss of consciousness
Severe autonomic dysfunction, e.g. orthostatic hypotension, urinary incontinence
Hallucinations in other modalities
Systematised delusions
Depression
Relative preservation of medial temporal lobe structures on CT/MRI scan
Generalised low uptake on SPECT/PET perfusion scan with reduced occipital activity
Abnormal (low uptake) MIBG myocardial scintigraphy
Prominent slow wave activity on EEG with temporal lobe transient sharp waves
5. *A diagnosis of DLB is less likely*
In the presence of cerebrovascular disease evident as focal neurological signs or on brain imaging
In the presence of any other physical illness or brain disorder sufficient to account in part or in total for the clinical picture
If parkinsonism only appears for the first time at a stage of severe dementia
6. *Temporal sequence of symptoms*
DLB should be diagnosed when dementia occurs before or concurrently with parkinsonism (if it is present). The term Parkinson's disease dementia (PDD) should be used to describe dementia that occurs in the context of well-established Parkinson's disease. In a practice setting, the term that is most appropriate to the clinical situation should be used, and generic terms such as LB disease are often helpful. In research studies in which distinction needs to be made between DLB and PDD, the existing one-year rule between the onset of dementia and parkinsonism DLB continues to be recommended. Adoption of other time periods will simply confound data pooling or comparison between studies. In other research settings that may include clinicopathologic studies and clinical trials, both clinical phenotypes may be considered collectively under categories such as LB disease or α-synucleinopathy

on clinical grounds alone. This group, who are best described pathologically as AD+LB or as LBVAD [6], can probably only be reliably identified by additional investigations and biomarkers, and the lack of success of clinicians and clinically based criteria alone should not be regarded as failure.

5.2.4 *Further Reports of the DLB Consortium*

The DLB Consortium met for the fourth time in Yokohama in 2006 under the leadership of Professor Kosaka [33], and the opportunity was particularly taken to review advances in tissue and imaging biomarkers. The recommendation was to leave the relatively recently modified consensus criteria unchanged in order to facilitate their uptake into practice and to avoid unnecessary change. The consortium held a further Consortium event in December 2015 and is likely to publish an updated report in 2016. The likely topics of clinical diagnostic interest will include review and update of the clinical and pathological diagnostic criteria and a reconsideration of progress made in genetics, imaging and tissue biomarker profiling.

5.3 New Diagnostic Concepts

5.3.1 *DSM V*

Although the DLB consensus criteria were constructed for both research and general clinical use, it is only recently that they have been formally incorporated into the formally recognised diagnostic classification systems. DSM 5 [11] now contains categories for major and mild "neurocognitive disorder with Lewy bodies" that are based upon the 2006 consensus criteria, both in the diagnostic features listed and the possible/probable distinction. DSM 5 also contains a separate category of major and mild "neurocognitive disorder due to Parkinson's disease", which uses the previously stated one-year rule to distinguish it from DLB. It is hoped that ICD 11 will similarly incorporate DLB into its dementia subtype classification and together these changes should assist case detection rates, clinical service development, reimbursement and research funding.

5.3.2 *Pre-dementia and Prodromal Diagnosis of DLB*

Possibly the most significant clinical development in the whole dementia field over the last decade has been a shift away from diagnosing at a mild/moderate symptomatic stage to prodromal or even presymptomatic diagnosis. The main justification for this shift to earlier diagnosis is that preventative treatment will only be effective if given before extensive neurochemical and anatomic pathological changes have occurred in the brain. It follows that trials of potential preventative agents will only be possible once reliable methods of prodromal diagnosis have been established.

Efforts to start developing diagnostic methods and criteria for Lewy body disease are already underway [34]. Since we do not yet know why some cases progress to PD, and others to DLB, very early identification of LB disease would identify individuals at risk of an uncertain future clinical course and progression. Criteria for the identification of early cases at high risk of progression to a dementia syndrome of the DLB type might be made at a stage when an individual has at least one clinical feature suggestive of prodromal DLB, e.g., cognitive or neuropsychiatric features, and at least one biomarker supportive of Lewy body disease. Given the large number of potential prodromal symptoms and existence of several biomarker candidates, it is anticipated that formal criteria for prodromal DLB are still some way off. The MCI–DLB category is however already being used informally in some memory clinic settings, with evidence that non-amnestic MCI subjects are more likely to progress to DLB rather than AD, particularly if they have additional DLB core or suggestive features [32]. DSMV also contains criteria for "mild neurocognitive disorder with Lewy bodies" (see above), although these have not yet been validated.

References

1. Kosaka K, Yoshimura M, Ikeda K, et al. Diffuse type of Lewy body disease: progressive dementia with abundant cortical Lewy bodies and senile changes of varying degree – a new disease? Clin Neuropathol. 1984;3(5):185–92.
2. Dickson DW, Davies P, Mayeux R, et al. Diffuse Lewy body disease. Neuropathological and biochemical studies of six patients. Acta Neuropathol. 1987;75:8–15.
3. Lennox G, Lowe J, Byrne EJ, et al. Diffuse Lewy body disease. Lancet. 1989;8633(1):323–4.
4. Gibb WRG, Esiri MM, Lees AJ. Clinical and pathological features of diffuse cortical Lewy body disease (Lewy body dementia). Brain. 1987;110:1131–53.
5. Byrne EJ, Lennox G, Godwin-Austen RB, et al. Dementia associated with cortical Lewy bodies. Proposed diagnostic criteria. Dementia. 1991;2:283–4.
6. Hansen L, Salmon D, Galasko D, et al. The Lewy body variant of Alzheimer's disease: a clinical and pathologic entity. Neurology. 1990;40:1–8.
7. Förstl H, Burns A, Luthert P, et al. The Lewy-body variant of Alzheimer's disease. Clinical and pathological findings. Br J Psychiatry. 1993;162:385–92.
8. Perry RH, Irving D, Blessed G, et al. Senile dementia of Lewy body type. A clinically and neuropathologically distinct form of Lewy body dementia in the elderly. J Neurol Sci. 1990;95:119–39.
9. McKeith IG, Galasko D, Kosaka K, et al. Consensus guidelines for the clinical and pathologic diagnosis of dementia with Lewy bodies (DLB): report of the consortium on DLB international workshop. Neurology. 1996;47(5):1113–24.

10. McKeith I, Dickson D, Emre M, et al. Dementia with Lewy bodies: diagnosis and management: third report of the DLB consortium. Neurology. 2005;65(12):1863–72.
11. APA. Diagnostic and statistical manual of mental disorders: DSM-5. Washington, DC: American Psychiatric Association; 2013.
12. Okazaki H, Lipkin LE, Aronson SM. Diffuse intracytoplasmic ganglionic inclusions (Lewy type) associated with progressive dementia and quadriparesis in flexion. J Neuropathol Exp Neurol. 1961;20:237–44.
13. Burkhardt CR, Filley CM, Kleinschmidt-DeMasters BK, et al. Diffuse Lewy body disease and progressive dementia. Neurology. 1988;38:1520–8.
14. Crystal HA, Dickson DW, Lizardi JE, et al. Antemortem diagnosis of diffuse Lewy body disease. Neurology. 1990;40:1523–8.
15. Hansen LA, Galasko D. Lewy body disease. Curr Opin Neurol Neurosurg. 1992;5:889–94.
16. Byrne EJ, Lennox G, Lowe J, et al. Diffuse Lewy body disease: clinical features in 15 cases. J Neurol Neurosurg Psychiatry. 1989;52:709–17.
17. McKeith IG, Perry RH, Fairbairn AF, et al. Operational criteria for senile dementia of Lewy body type (SDLT). Psychol Med. 1992;22:911–22.
18. McKeith I, Fairbairn A, Perry R, et al. Neuroleptic sensitivity in patients with senile dementia of Lewy body type. Br Med J. 1992;305:673–8.
19. McKeith IG. Consensus guidelines for the clinical and pathologic diagnosis of dementia with Lewy bodies (DLB): report of the consortium on DLB international workshop. J Alzheimers Dis. 2006;9:417–23.
20. Emre M, Aarsland D, Brown R, et al. Clinical diagnostic criteria for dementia associated with Parkinson disease. Mov Disord. 2007;e-pub ahead of print.
21. Dubois B, Burn D, Goetz C, et al. Diagnostic procedures for Parkinson's disease dementia: recommendations from the movement disorder society task force. Mov Disord. 2007;22 (16):2314–24.
22. Lippa C, Duda JE, Grossman M, et al. DLB and PDD boundary issues: diagnosis, treatment, molecular pathology, and biomarkers. Neurology. 2007;68:812–9.
23. Salmon D, Galasko D. Neuropsychological aspects of Lewy body dementia. In: Perry R, McKeith I, Perry E, editors. Dementia with Lewy bodies. New York: Cambridge University Press; 1996. p. 99–113.
24. Salmon DP, Galasko D, Hamilton JM, et al. Cognitive profiles differ across disease course in autopsy-proven dementia with Lewy bodies and Alzheimer's disease. Neurobiol Aging. 2002;23:S130.
25. McKeith IG, Ballard CG, Perry RH, et al. Prospective validation of consensus criteria for the diagnosis of dementia with Lewy bodies. Neurology. 2000;54:1050–8.
26. Litvan I, Bhatia KP, Burn DJ, et al. SIC Task Force appraisal of clinical diagnostic criteria for Parkinsonian disorders. Mov Disord. 2003;18(5):467–86.
27. McKeith IG, Perry EK, Perry RH. Report of the second dementia with Lewy body international workshop. Neurology. 1999;53(5):902–5.
28. Boeve B, Silber M, Ferman T, et al. Association of REM sleep behavior disorder and neurodegenerative disease may reflect an underlying synucleinopathy. Mov Disord. 2001;16:622–30.
29. Walker Z, Costa DC, Walker RWH, et al. *In vivo* demonstration of dopaminergic degeneration in dementia with Lewy bodies using 123I-FP-CIT and SPET. Joint meeting of international Psychogeriatric Association and Royal College of Psychiatrists', Faculty of Old Age on Non-Alzheimer Cognitive Impairment, 4–7 April 2000; 2000:23.
30. Aarsland D, Rongve A, Nore SP, et al. Frequency and case identification of Dementia with Lewy bodies using the revised consensus criteria. Dement Geriatr Cogn Disord. 2008;26 (5):445–52.
31. Weisman D, Cho M, Taylor C, et al. In dementia with Lewy bodies, Braak stage determines phenotype, not Lewy body distribution. Neurology. [Article]. 2007;69(4):356–9.

32. Tiraboschi P, Attems J, Thomas A, et al. Clinicians' ability to diagnose dementia with Lewy bodies is not affected by beta-amyloid load. Neurology. 2015;84(5):496–9.
33. Kosaka K. Lewy body disease and dementia with Lewy bodies. Proc Jpn Acad Series B Phys Biol Sci. 2014;90(8):301–6.
34. Donaghy PC, McKeith IG. The clinical characteristics of dementia with Lewy bodies and a consideration of prodromal diagnosis. Alzheimer's Res Ther 2014; (6)4. doi:10.1186/alzrt274.

Chapter 6
Cognitive Impairments of Dementia with Lewy Bodies

Etsuro Mori

Abstract Progressive cognitive impairment is essential for the diagnosis of dementia with Lewy bodies (DLB). Deficits of attention function, executive function, and visuospatial function are characteristic of DLB, whereas memory function is relatively preserved. Cognitive fluctuations and complex visual hallucinations are core features of DLB, in which cognitive impairments are deeply involved. This chapter summarizes the way to detect the deficits in each cognitive domain and the features of the deficits in DLB, discussing the neural mechanisms of the deficits.

Keywords Cognitive impairment • Neuropsychological test • Cognitive fluctuations • Visual hallucinations

6.1 Features of Cognitive Impairment

The presence of progressive cognitive impairment is essential for the diagnosis of dementia with Lewy bodies (DLB) on the current diagnostic criteria, although psychiatric symptoms may precede it [1]. As indicated in the diagnostic criteria, deficits on the tests of the attention, executive function, and visuospatial function are prominent, whereas memory is relatively preserved [1]. In fact, the results of a large number of studies as well as systematic reviews are consistent; visual perception, attention, and executive function are defective in DLB, and episodic memory and language functions are relatively preserved both in comparison with other cognitive domains and in comparison with Alzheimer's disease (AD) [2–5].

The features can be shown even on screening tests such as the Mini-Mental State Examination (MMSE). Ala et al. [6], using the scores of only three MMSE subitems, reported a cutoff value of 5 (5 or smaller) on the index (attention – recall × 5/3 + construction × 5) and differentiated DLB from AD with a sensitivity of 82 % and a specificity of 81 %, while Hanyu et al. [7], using the same index,

E. Mori (✉)
Department of Behavioral Neurology and Cognitive Neuroscience, Tohoku University Graduate School of Medicine, 2-1, Seiryo-machi, Aoba-ku, Sendai 980-8575, Japan
e-mail: morie@med.tohoku.ac.jp

K. Kosaka (ed.), *Dementia with Lewy Bodies*, DOI 10.1007/978-4-431-55948-1_6

reported a sensitivity of 72 % and a specificity of 75 % with a different cutoff value of 3. The small value of the index is likely to be suggestive of DLB rather than AD, although the clinical utility of the index should be withheld unless the diagnostic accuracy and the reliability of the index are confirmed in large cohorts.

In any case, it is requisite in the differential diagnosis to assess the characteristics of cognitive impairment with neuropsychological tests, which helps to differentiate this disorder from AD. In addition, there is a place where neuropsychological tests contribute in evaluations of cognitive fluctuations and complex visual hallucinations, which are core diagnostic features of DLB. This chapter summarizes the way to detect the deficits in each cognitive domain and the features of the deficits in DLB, discussing the neural mechanisms of the deficits.

6.2 Attention

Attention refers to a function to limit the sensory input to the narrow range containing the potentially most important stimuli by increasing the sensitivity to those stimuli in the recognition and focus of awareness [8]. Therefore, the concept of attention is broad that includes from the level of arousal to the level of voluntary goal-directed behavior [9]. As the multiple network systems connecting the brain stem, thalamus, basal ganglia, limbic system, parietal association cortex, and prefrontal cortex, and a plurality of neurotransmitters are involved in the neural basis of attention, the lesions in various brain regions may produce various types of attentional disorders. Attentional deficits of arousal level, such as sustained attention and vigilance aspects, i.e., failure of the tonic attention, are caused by a damage to the ascending reticular activating system in the brain stem. A damage of the diffuse thalamocortical projection system causes a failure of the phasic attention, such as deficits in selective or focused attention. Attention disorder caused by damage to the frontal lobe is a disorder of the selectivity of the voluntary behavior, affecting planned actions of a complex behavior, resulting in inflexibility, perseveration, and vulnerability to interference. The cingulate is a limbic part of the attentional network and has a role in motivating the detection of stimuli and maintaining the operating force. Damage to the parietal lobe causes deficits of receptive aspects of attention related to the localization of spatial stimuli: unilateral spatial neglect of the opposite side in unilateral lesions, especially in right-sided lesions, or visual inattention and simultanagnosia, such as Bálint syndrome, in bilateral lesions.

The compromise of attention in DLB is noteworthy because it may be the basis of fluctuating cognition, a characteristic of DLB, as is in the diagnostic criteria [1]. The simple and useful clinical tests for attention include digit span, spatial span, and serial 7's. It is true that attention is defective in DLB than in AD, but few studies have demonstrated that the difference can be seen between DLB and AD in these tests. On the tests that require more attention, for example, Wechsler Adult Intelligence Scale-Revised Digit Symbol subtest [10] and selective attention or dual task [11], the performance in DLB patients was reportedly poorer than AD patients. Relatively low performance on these tests is supportive of a diagnosis of DLB.

The responsible lesions of the attention deficits in DLB would be cholinergic systems of the basal forebrain (nucleus basalis of Meynert, diagonal band of Broca, and medial septal nuclei) and of the brain stem ascending reticular activating system (pedunculopontine nucleus and laterodorsal tegmental nucleus) projecting cholinergic neurons to the cerebral cortex and thalamus [12, 13]. It is known that damage to the cholinergic neurons in the brain stem nuclei causes failure of attention and arousal [14]. In the clinical trials of rivastigmine [15] and donepezil [16], significant improvements were noted on the attentional tasks. The relationship between the Lewy bodies of the cortex and cognitive impairment has not been elucidated [17], the pathological changes associated with Lewy bodies in the prefrontal lobe and cingulate gyrus [18] might involve in deficits of the active sides of the attention such as concentration, attention switching, and distractibility. The Lewy body pathology also affects the parietal lobe [18], which might cause a failure of the receptive aspects of attention, such as the spatial localization of the stimulus.

6.3 Executive Function

Executive function is a product of the coordinated operation of various neural systems and is essential for achieving a particular goal in a flexible and appropriate manner, which requires complex cognitive operations such as reasoning, judgment, and decision-making [19]. The prefrontal cortex is known to be a key structure for the performance of executive functions, which is rather than a specific area for a particular function such as perception, motor, or long-term memory, and beyond those areas, so to speak super functional areas. The coordinated operation of perceptual, motor, memory, and other cognitive systems is essential for performing cognitive functions and socially adaptive behavior, such as anticipation, planning, monitoring, reasoning, decision-making, initiation, cognitive flexibility, set-shifting, and response inhibition. Damage to the prefrontal lobe may lead to dysexecutive syndrome, a diverse set of changes in cognitive, behavioral, or emotional domains.

There are a great number of neuropsychological tests that are developed usually based on cognitive psychology model. A substantial number of studies have documented the frequency and variability of executive disorders in patients with dementia and have demonstrated that disorders of executive functions are the most frequent cognitive deficits among them including DLB and AD. Simple frontal lobe function tests that can be utilized at the bedside are usually used in clinics, such as the verbal fluency test, sequential manual and writing tasks (Luria), Go-NoGo test, and Stroop test. Also, a test battery that combines simple tests, Frontal Assessment Battery [20], is often used.

Some studies have documented the frequency and variability of executive disorders in DLB, by using the neuropsychological tests for executive functions.

It has been reported that executive functions were more impaired in DLB than in AD; the performance on the Stroop test, Wisconsin card sorting test, and phonetic verbal fluency test were lower in DLB than in AD [11]. However, a possible difference in the executive function deficit between DLB and AD may not be detected according to the choice of the executive function tests, probably due to differences in the required cognitive abilities to carry out the tests [21]. Moreover, it is a prerequisite that the background cognitive functions required to run an executive function test are preserved. If background cognitive functions are impaired, the performance of the executive function test is greatly affected therewith. This is the case in DLB. During administering those tests in DLB, it may be difficult for patients with DLB to maintain attention and arousal; they may be easily distracted to irrelevant stimuli, hardly shift their set between issues, and be affected by confabulations and perseverations [22].

It has been pointed out that disorders of executive functions remain poorly defined. Assessment of executive disorders is highly variable, and the relevance of performance indices is poorly defined [23]. Dysexecutive behavioral disorders are usually not included in the evaluation, although they tend to be prominent and can even correspond to the entire dysexecutive syndrome. In any event, it seems challenging to differentiate DLB from AD actually by the performance of the cognitive executive function tests.

6.4 Visuoperceptual and Visuospatial Functions

The visual cortex of the brain is responsible for processing visual information. The primary visual cortex (also known as V1 and the striate cortex) receives visual sensory inputs from the retina via the lateral geniculate body. Then, the flow of visual information from the primary visual cortex to other cortical areas depends on the type of information being processed. Information necessary to detect, identify, and use color and shape is sent to ventral visual association cortices in the inferior temporal lobe (ventral stream), and information used to locate objects and detect their motion is sent to the dorsal visual association cortices in the parietal lobe (dorsal stream) [24]. The ventral stream processes information about the "what" of the visual stimulus. Damage to the ventral visual association cortex produces deficits in complex visual perception tasks, including visual agnosia, prosopagnosia, alexia, and so on. The dorsal stream processes information about the "where" of the visual stimulus. Damage to the dorsal visual association cortex results in deficits in spatial orientation, motion detection, and guidance of visual tracking eye movements.

Both the ventral and dorsal visual pathways, from the occipital lobe including the primary visual cortex and visual association cortex to the subsequent temporal lobe and to the parietal lobe, are responsible for the visuoperceptual deficits and visuospatial deficits. In patients with DLB, it is well known that glucose metabolism and blood flow are reduced in these regions on functional neuroimagings

[25–27]. Although the mechanism causing the occipital dysfunction is not yet resolved, one possible explanation is pathological changes such as spongiform change [28] or Lewy body pathology [29], and the other explanation is the loss of cholinergic innervation to the occipital and temporal lobes [30, 31].

A number of studies have demonstrated that DLB has deficits of both elementary and complex visuoperceptual functions and visuospatial and visuoconstructional functions [2, 3, 32, 33]. Visuoperceptual and visuospatial dysfunctions were disproportionately severe in DLB, and the diagnostic value of them is high. Elementary and complex visual perception, such as line-length discrimination, line-angle discrimination, line orientation, figure size discrimination, shape discrimination, overlapping figure identification, and incomplete fragmented letter reading (characters of the Visual Object and Space Perception), are defective in DLB as compared with AD, as well as visuospatial function such as visual counting and direction of movement [11, 32, 33]. Relatively severe visuoconstructive disability, which is detected even with simple tests, such as the intersecting pentagon copying [34], clock drawing test [35], and Bender-Gestalt test [36], and the block design test [10], is also useful in the differential diagnosis between DLB and AD (Fig. 6.1).

In addition, some visuoperceptual deficits are reportedly involved in the development of visual hallucinations and misidentification delusions [32, 33]. Mori et al. [32] found that visual form identification ability was significantly worse in DLB patients with visual hallucinations than in those without them; visual size discrimination ability and visual counting were worse in those with television misidentification delusions than those without them. Similar results were obtained by Mosimann et al. [33] who demonstrated that in DLB and PDD those with visual hallucinations had lower performance on the tests of form identification, recognition of line angle, and direction of movement than those without them. Taken together, these data suggest that, visuoperceptual deficits are underlying visual hallucinations and misidentification delusions with a visual component, which are distinctive features of DLB.

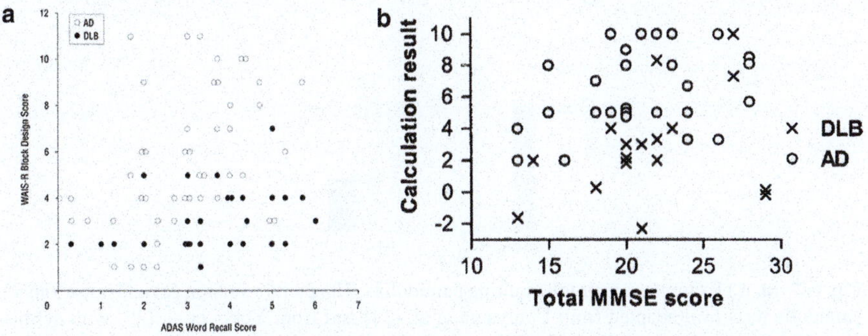

Fig. 6.1 Differentiation between DLB and AD DLB by using neuropsychological tests. (**a**) ADAS word recall score and WAIS-R blocks design score. (**b**) Total MMSE score and MMSE calculation/attention score (Reprinted from Shimomura et al. [10] and Ala et al. [6] with permission)

6.5 Visual Hallucinations and Illusions

Visual hallucinations are defined as the visual perception of an object or event in the absence of an external stimulus. Presence of repeated visual hallucinations is an important clue to the diagnosis of DLB. Examination of visual hallucination is made by interview with caregivers, often utilizing a structured questionnaire such as the Neuropsychiatric Inventory (NPI) [37], as well as asking patient. However, when asking directly to the patient, the sensitivity would be low and the severity rating would be difficult because of the patient's lack of awareness of hallucinations to be unreal or loss of memory for the experience of hallucinations. When interviewing caregivers, the different awareness and understanding of hallucinations of the caregivers would affect the assessment of the problem. Informants may often be absent. To overcome such problems, the pareidolia test has been developed as a tool directly evaluating visual hallucinations as like a performance on neuropsychological tests (Fig. 6.2) [38, 39].

Visual illusions are defined as the false visual perception of an object or event that is actually different. Although visual illusions are theoretically and conceptually different from visual hallucinations, visual illusions are very close experiences to visual hallucinations, are sometimes practically indistinguishable from visual

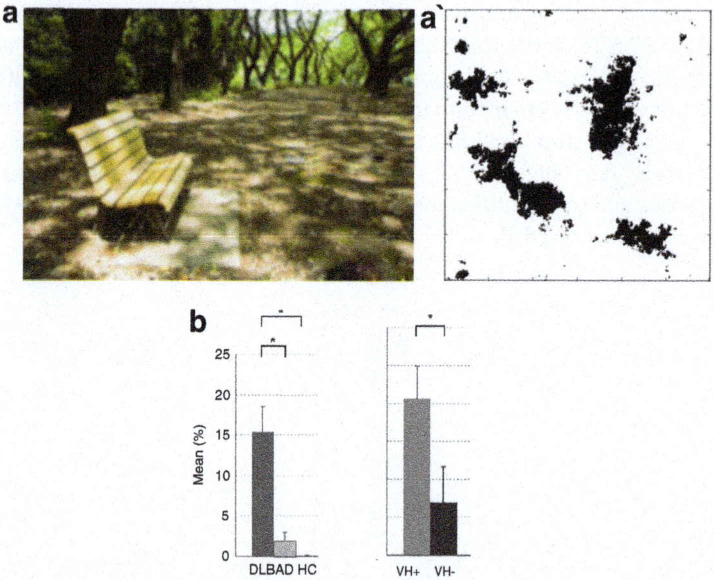

Fig. 6.2 (**a, a′**) Examples of stimuli eliciting pareidolias. The picture version (**a**) and noise version pareidolia tests (a′) (adapted from Uchiyama et al. [38] and from Yokoi et al. [39] with permission). (**b**) The numbers of pareidolias elicited by the noise version pareidolia test. Comparison between patients with DLB, patients with AD, and healthy controls (*left*) and comparison between those who had visual hallucinations and without them in patients with DLB (*right*). $*p < 0.05$ (Reprinted from Yokoi et al. [39] with permission)

hallucinations, and are also common in DLB. Among illusions, the experience of pareidolia is phenomenologically close to visual hallucinations. Pareidolias are illusions of meaningful objects such as faces and animals and are thought to arise from ambiguous forms embedded in visual scenes. For instance, patients with dementia with Lewy bodies may incorrectly see a person in a curtain or perceive blobs on the wall as faces. Uchiyama et al. [38] and Yokoi et al. [39] developed pareidolia stimuli with scenery pictures and noise figures to evoke and measure pareidolic illusions in patients with DLB and demonstrated that the number of pareidolic responses is correlated with the severity of visual hallucinations. The number of pareidolic responses on either version of the test was significantly greater in patients with DLB than in those with AD and healthy aged individuals, and the picture pareidolia test distinguished DLB from AD with a sensitivity of 100 % and a specificity of 88 %, and the noise pareidolia test with a sensitivity of 71 % and a specificity of 80 %. Cholinergic enhancement reduced the number of pareidolias on the latter test [39]. The pareidolia test can be used as a surrogate indicator of visual hallucinations in DLB and as a diagnostic tool for DLB [40].

6.6 Memory

Squire and Zola-Morgan [41] classified human memory into declarative memory and non-declarative memory; the former is memory that can be consciously recalled and described as an image or language, and the latter includes skills or procedural memory that cannot be consciously recalled as well as subconscious memory like priming and conditioning. Declarative memory is further divided into episodic memory and semantic memory. Episodic memory is the memory of specific events that individuals experienced, in which the episode is stored along with the temporal and spatial context, that is the situation when encountered. Semantic memory is equivalent to knowledge, i.e., organized memories for languages, concepts, and facts. Amnesia is a disorder of episodic memory, which includes anterograde amnesia where the ability to memorize new things is impaired and retrograde amnesia where ability to recall events that occurred before the development of the amnesia is impaired.

The human episodic memory based on the networks involving the medial temporal lobe including the hippocampus, thalamus, and basal forebrain and the lesions of any components in the networks lead to anterograde amnesia [42]. The medial limbic circuit (Papez circuit), i.e., hippocampus – fornix – mammillary body – mammillothalamic tract – anterior thalamic nucleus – anterior thalamic peduncle – cingulate gyrus (cingulate) – entorhinal cortex – hippocampus, is involved in encoding and consolidation; the ventrolateral limbic circuit, i.e., amygdala – ventral amygdalofugal tract – dorsomedial thalamic nucleus – anterior thalamic peduncle – basal forebrain/prefrontal cortex – uncinate fasciculus – amygdala, is believed to be involved in emotional memory (memory for emotional events). Other regions involving in episodic memory include the retrosplenial cortex, anterior temporal lobe, and prefrontal cortex.

It had been considered that degeneration of cholinergic neurons within the basal forebrain causes amnesia in AD [43, 44]. If that is the case, degeneration of cholinergic neurons of the basal forebrain might account for memory impairment in DLB, as DLB is characterized by a more profound degeneration of cholinergic neurons of the basal forebrain than in AD [45, 46]. However, the fact is that episodic memory is less impaired in DLB than in AD. Evidence is accumulating indicating that the medial temporal lobe including the hippocampus is responsible for memory impairment in AD [6, 10, 11, 47–50]. Atrophy of the medial temporal lobe is milder in DLB [51], which is consistent with milder impairment of episodic memory in DLB than AD.

Relatively preserved episodic memory is apparent not only on the everyday events but also on the memory tests. In general, recognition memory is disproportionately spared relative to both recall. The feature that episodic memory deficits are relatively mild suggests DLB rather than AD. Relatively milder memory impairment in DLB than in AD is evident on the memory items in the MMSE, DRS, and ADAS [6, 10, 47, 48], as well as on the various memory tests, for example, Wechsler Memory Scale-Revised (WMS-R) logical memory [11], California Verbal Learning Test (CVLT) [49], and Buschke Selective Reminding Test (BSRT) [21]. Visual memory is reportedly impaired more than verbal memory in DLB [21], which may be explained by the visuoperceptual deficits. Although impairment of episodic memory may not stand out in the early stage of the disease, it will eventually come out with the progression. In some patients with DLB, episodic memory is severely impaired, which is explained by the superimposed AD pathology on the DLB pathology [50].

Semantic memory and procedural memory are also impaired in AD. The anterior temporal lobe is crucial for semantic memory. Semantic memory is also relatively preserved in DLB [48]. Results of the category verbal fluency test and naming test that depends on semantic memory are comparably defective between DLB and AD [4, 21, 49, 50]. One report pointed out that phonetic and category verbal fluency in DLB was comparatively defective in DLB, while the former was relatively preserved than the latter in AD [48]. Procedural memory, the ability to learn skills that become automatic, involves the basal ganglia, cerebellum, and supplementary motor cortex. Procedural memory deficits are most commonly reported in patients with Parkinson disease among neurodegenerative diseases, independent of other cognitive dysfunction or dopaminergic medication [52, 53], while it has been reported that patients with mild AD can acquire motor, perceptual, and cognitive skills. [54] Therefore, procedural memory is likely to be defective in DLB and may be a distinctive feature from AD, although there were no studies addressing procedural memory in DLB.

6.7 Language

Language is a typically localized and lateralized function, which is processed in several association areas including Wernicke's area and Broca's area usually located in the dominant hemisphere. As those areas are subject to be involved in dementing illness, impairment in language is a common finding among individuals with dementia and can be a presenting symptom, particularly in AD as well as primary progressive aphasia. Identification of language impairment is important in dementia, as it aids in the accurate diagnosis of a specific type of dementia, alters the prognosis, and changes the management.

In AD, with progression of the disease, naming and verbal fluency may be impaired. In some patients with AD, language disorder may disproportionally stand out, and moreover a type of primary progressive aphasia, logopenic progressive aphasia, may emerge [55]. As for DLB, language functions are largely intact, although there may be difficulties in finding words and understanding complex sentences. A few case reports described patients with DLB presenting with logopenic progressive aphasia, in whom AD pathology was superimposed [56–58]. Such a symptom is exceptional so far, and there are no reports of patients presenting logopenic progressive aphasia or any other type of primary progressive aphasia whose pathology is not compromised by AD pathology. It is unknown whether DLB presents with primary progressive aphasia.

6.8 Fluctuations of Cognitive Function

Cognitive fluctuations with variation in attention and arousal, such as daytime sleepiness, staring spells, decreased awareness of surroundings, illogical thoughts, and incoherent behaviors, are a key feature of DLB. Although cognitive fluctuations are not specific for DLB, they are more prevalent in DLB; they occur in approximately 20 % of individuals with AD [59] and in 35–50 % of those with vascular dementia [60], while the prevalence increases to around 90 % in those with DLB [1]. Moreover, cognitive fluctuations in DLB have particular characteristics that are distinguishable from fluctuations occurring in AD. Bradshaw et al. [61] reported that fluctuating cognition in DLB had a spontaneous, periodic, transient quality, which appeared to reflect an interruption in the ongoing flow of awareness or attention that impacted on functional abilities, while fluctuations in AD frequently highlighted episodes of memory failure or a diminished capacity to cope with the cognitive demands of the immediate environment.

Cognitive fluctuations are not only of significant diagnostic importance but also of functional impact on patients in terms of significant independent effects on activities of daily living and increased care burden for caregivers [62]. However, their accurate identification and assessment present a major challenge. No operational criteria of cognitive fluctuations have been indicated in the diagnostic criteria, which is the most difficult to determine among the core symptoms of DLB [63]. There is no clear biomarker of cognitive fluctuations. Several instruments to measure cognitive fluctuations have been developed. Structured interview and questionnaire to caregivers, such as the Clinician Assessment of Fluctuation [64], One Day Fluctuation Assessment Scale [65], Mayo Fluctuations Composite Scale [66], Cognitive Fluctuation Inventory [67], and Dementia Cognitive Fluctuation Scale [68], are simple techniques and of clinical value to differentiate DLB from AD. The other technique to measure fluctuations is to utilize variance of simple reaction time and choice reaction time during attentional tasks. It measures the variation of the attention within a short period of time and can be a surrogate marker of fluctuating cognition [69], of which results correlated with those of the abovementioned structured interviews [69, 70]. These instruments are reportedly effective in differentiating DLB from AD [69, 70]. However, these have not been adequately tested as yet for reliability and validity, and the use of the reaction time tests in a clinical setting as a marker of cognitive fluctuations is limited because of the lack of available equipment and trained staffs [71].

The underlying mechanism of cognitive fluctuations is poorly understood. Which brain areas contribute to cognitive fluctuations is still unknown, and no obvious structural brain changes have been associated with cognitive fluctuations in DLB. Recent studies including functional neuroimaging studies suggested that cognitive fluctuations in DLB are associated with changes in the neural networks involving cholinergic and dopaminergic systems within the thalamus, which is the central to attentional function [72–75]. A cholinergic involvement in cognitive fluctuations in DLB is supported by results of a clinical trial of cholinesterase inhibitor, where donepezil significantly improved Cognitive Fluctuation Inventory score compared with placebo [16].

References

1. McKeith IG, Dickson DW, Lowe J, et al. Diagnosis and management of dementia with Lewy bodies: third report of the DLB consortium. Neurology. 2005;65:1863–72.
2. Simard M, van Reekum R, Cohen T. A review of the cognitive and behavioural symptoms in dementia with Lewy bodies. J Neuropsychiatry Clin Neurosci. 2000;12:425–50.
3. Tröster AI. Neuropsychological characteristics of dementia with Lewy bodies and Parkinson's disease with dementia: differentiation, early detection, and implications for "mild cognitive impairment" and biomarkers. Neuropsychol Rev. 2008;18:103–19.
4. Collerton D, Burn D, McKeith I, et al. Systematic review and meta-analysis show that dementia with Lewy bodies is a visual-perceptual and attentional-executive dementia. Dement Geriatr Cogn Disord. 2003;16:229–37.
5. Metzler-Baddeley C. A review of cognitive impairments in dementia with Lewy bodies relative to Alzheimer's disease and Parkinson's disease with dementia. Cortex. 2007;43:583–600.
6. Ala TA, Hughes LF, Kyrouac GA, et al. The Mini-Mental State exam may help in the differentiation of dementia with Lewy bodies and Alzheimer's disease. Int J Geriatr Psychiatry. 2002;17:503–9.

7. Hanyu H, Shimizu S, Hirao K, et al. Differentiation of dementia with Lewy bodies from Alzheimer's disease using Mini-Mental State examination and brain perfusion SPECT. J Neurol Sci. 2006;250:97–102.
8. Geschwind N. Disorders of attention: a frontier in neuropsychology. Philos Trans R Soc Lond. 1982;B298:173–85.
9. Mesulam M-M. Spatial attention and neglect: parietal, frontal and cingulate contributions to the mental representation and attentional targeting of salient extrapersonal events. Philos Trans R Soc Lond B. 1999;354:1325–46.
10. Shimomura T, Mori E, Yamashita H, et al. Cognitive loss in dementia with Lewy bodies and Alzheimer disease. Arch Neurol. 1998;55:1547–52.
11. Calderon J, Perry RJ, Erzinclioglu SW, et al. Perception, attention, and working memory are disproportionately impaired in dementia with Lewy bodies compared with Alzheimer's disease. J Neurol Neurosurg Psychiatry. 2001;70:157–64.
12. Tiraboschi P, Hansen LA, Alford M, et al. Early and widespread cholinergic losses differentiate dementia with Lewy bodies from Alzheimer disease. Arch Gen Psychiatry. 2002;59:946–51.
13. Perry E, Walker M, Grace J, et al. Acetylcholine in mind: a neurotransmitter correlate of consciousness? Trends Neurosci. 1999;22:273–80.
14. Cyr M, Parent MJ, Mechawar N, et al. Deficit in sustained attention following selective cholinergic lesion of the pedunculopontine tegmental nucleus in rat, as measured with both post-mortem immunocytochemistry and in vivo PET imaging with [^{18}F] fluoroethoxybenzovesamicol. Behav Brain Res. 2015;278:107–14.
15. McKeith I, Del Ser T, Spano P, et al. Efficacy of rivastigmine in dementia with Lewy bodies: a randomised, double-blind, placebo-controlled international study. Lancet. 2000;356:2031–6.
16. Mori E, Ikeda M, Kosaka K, et al. Donepezil for dementia with Lewy bodies: a randomized, placebo-controlled trial. Ann Neurol. 2012;72:41–52.
17. McKeith I, Mintzer J, Aarsland D, et al. Dementia with Lewy bodies. Lancet Neurol. 2004;3:19–28.
18. Harding AJ, Broe GA, Halliday GM. Visual hallucinations in Lewy body disease relate to Lewy bodies in the temporal lobe. Brain. 2002;125:391–403.
19. Alvarez JA, Emory E. Executive function and the frontal lobes: a meta-analytic review. Neuropsychol Rev. 2006;16:17–42.
20. Dubois B, Slachevsky A, Litvan I, et al. The FAB: a Frontal Assessment Battery at bedside. Neurology. 2000;55:1621–6.
21. Noe E, Marder K, Bell KL, et al. Comparison of dementia with Lewy bodies to Alzheimer's disease and Parkinson's disease with dementia. Mov Disord. 2004;19:60–7.
22. Doubleday EK, Snowden JS, Varma AR, et al. Qualitative performance characteristics differentiate dementia with Lewy bodies and Alzheimer's disease. J Neurol Neurosurg Psychiatry. 2002;72:602–7.
23. Godefroy O, Azouvi P, Robert P, et al. Dysexecutive syndrome: diagnostic criteria and validation study. Ann Neurol. 2010;68:855–64.
24. Goodale MA, Milner AD. Separate visual pathways for perception and action. Trends Neurosci. 1992;15:20–5.
25. Imamura T, Ishii K, Sasaki M, et al. Regional cerebral glucose metabolism in dementia with Lewy bodies and Alzheimer's disease. Neurosci Lett. 1997;235:49–52.
26. Ishii K, Imamura T, Sasaki M, et al. Regional cerebral glucose metabolism in dementia with Lewy bodies and Alzheimer's disease. Neurology. 1998;51:125–30.
27. Ishii K, Yamaji S, Kitagaki H, et al. Regional cerebral blood flow differences between dementia with Lewy bodies and AD. Neurology. 1999;53:413–6.
28. Higuchi M, Tashiro M, Arai H, et al. Glucose hypometabolism and neuropathological correlates in brains of dementia with Lewy bodies. Exp Neurol. 2000;162:247–56.
29. Kasanuki K, Iseki E, Fujishiro H, et al. Neuropathological investigation of the hypometabolic regions on positron emission tomography with [18F] fluorodeoxyglucose in patients with dementia with Lewy bodies. J Neurol Sci. 2012;314:111–9.

30. Shimada H, Hirano S, Shinotoh H, et al. Mapping of brain acetylcholinesterase alterations in Lewy body disease by PET. Neurology. 2009;73:273–8.
31. Klein JC, Eggers C, Kalbe E, et al. Neurotransmitter changes in dementia with Lewy bodies and Parkinson disease dementia in vivo. Neurology. 2010;74:885–92.
32. Mori E, Shimomura T, Fujimori M, et al. Visuoperceptual impairment in dementia with Lewy bodies. Arch Neurol. 2000;57:489–93.
33. Mosimann UP, Mather G, Wesnes KA, et al. Visual perception in Parkinson disease dementia and dementia with Lewy bodies. Neurology. 2004;63:2091–6.
34. Ala TA, Hughes LF, Kyrouac GA, et al. Pentagon copying is more impaired in dementia with Lewy bodies than in Alzheimer's disease. J Neurol Neurosurg Psychiatry. 2001;70:483–8.
35. Gnanalingham KK, Byrne EJ, Thornton A. Clock-face drawing to differentiate Lewy body and Alzheimer type dementia syndromes. Lancet. 1996;347:696–7.
36. Murayama N, Iseki E, Yamamoto R, et al. Utility of the Bender Gestalt test for differentiation of dementia with Lewy bodies from Alzheimer's disease in patients showing mild to moderate dementia. Dement Geriatr Cogn Disord. 2007;23:258–63.
37. Cummings JL, Mega M, Gray K, et al. The neuropsychiatric inventory: comprehensive assessment of psychopathology in dementia. Neurology. 1994;44:2308–14.
38. Uchiyama M, Nishio Y, Yokoi K, et al. Pareidolias: complex visual illusions in dementia with Lewy bodies. Brain. 2012;135:2458–69.
39. Yokoi K, Nishio Y, Uchiyama M, et al. Hallucinators find meaning in noises: Pareidolic illusions in dementia with Lewy bodies. Neuropsychologia. 2014;56:245–54.
40. Mamiya Y, Nishio Y, Watanabe Y, et al. The pareidolia test: a simple neuropsychological test measuring visual hallucination-like illusions. PLOS ONE, in press.
41. Squire LR, Zola-Morgan S. The neuropsychology of memory: new links between humans and experimental animals. Ann N Y Acad Sci. 1985;444:137–49.
42. Lim C, Alexander MP. Stroke and episodic memory disorders. Neuropsychologia. 2009;47:3045–58.
43. Whitehouse PJ, Price DL, Clark AW, et al. Alzheimer disease: evidence for selective loss of cholinergic neurons in the nucleus basalis. Ann Neurol. 1981;10:122–6.
44. Coyle JM, Price DL, DeLong MR. Alzheimer's disease: a disorder of cortical cholinergic innervation. Science. 1983;219:1184–90.
45. Fujishiro H, Umegaki H, Isojima D, et al. Depletion of cholinergic neurons in the nucleus of the medial septum and the vertical limb of the diagonal band in dementia with Lewy bodies. Acta Neuropathol. 2006;111:109–14.
46. Grothe MJ, Schuster C, Bauer F, et al. Atrophy of the cholinergic basal forebrain in dementia with Lewy bodies and Alzheimer's disease dementia. J Neurol. 2014;261:1939–48.
47. Aarsland D, Litvan I, Salmon D, et al. Performance on the dementia rating scale in Parkinson's disease with dementia and dementia with Lewy bodies: comparison with progressive supranuclear palsy and Alzheimer's disease. J Neurol Neurosurg Psychiatry. 2003;74:1215–20.
48. Lambon Ralph MA, Powell J, Howard D, et al. Semantic memory is impaired in both dementia with Lewy bodies and dementia of Alzheimer's type: a comparative neuropsychological study and literature review. J Neurol Neurosurg Psychiatry. 2001;70:149–56.
49. Simard M, van Reekum R, Myran D, et al. Differential memory impairment in dementia with Lewy bodies and Alzheimer's disease. Brain Cogn. 2002;49:244–9.
50. Kraybill ML, Larson EB, Tsuang DW, et al. Cognitive differences in dementia patients with autopsy-verified AD, Lewy body pathology, or both. Neurology. 2005;64:2069–73.
51. Hashimoto M, Kitagaki H, Imamura T, et al. Medial temporal and whole-brain atrophy in dementia with Lewy bodies: a volumetric MRI study. Neurology. 1998;51:357–62.
52. Yamadori A, Yoshida T, Mori E, et al. Neurological basis of skill learning. Brain Res Cogn Brain Res. 1996;5:49–54.
53. Sarazin M, Deweer B, Merkl A, et al. Procedural learning and striatofrontal dysfunction in Parkinson's disease. Mov Disord. 2002;17:265–73.
54. Hirono N, Mori E, Ikejiri Y, et al. Procedural memory in patients with mild Alzheimer's disease. Dement Geriatr Cogn Disord. 1997;8:210–6.

55. Gorno-Tempini ML, Brambati SM, Ginex V, et al. The logopenic/phonological variant of primary progressive aphasia. Neurology. 2008;71:1227–34.
56. Caselli RJ, Beach TG, Sue LI, et al. Progressive aphasia with Lewy bodies. Dement Geriatr Cogn Disord. 2002;14:55–8.
57. Harris JM, Gall C, Thompson JC, et al. Classification and pathology of primary progressive aphasia. Neurology. 2013;81:1832–9.
58. Teichmann M, Migliaccio R, Kas A, et al. Logopenic progressive aphasia beyond Alzheimer's–an evolution towards dementia with Lewy bodies. J Neurol Neurosurg Psychiatry. 2013;84:113–4.
59. Escandon A, Al-Hammadi N, Galvin JE. Effect of cognitive fluctuation on neuropsychological performance in aging and dementia. Neurology. 2010;74:210–7.
60. Roman GC, Tatemichi TK, Erkinjuntti T. Vascular dementia: diagnostic criteria for research studies: report of the NINDS-AIREN international workshop. Neurology. 1993;43:250–60.
61. Bradshaw J, Saling M, Hopwood M, et al. Fluctuating cognition in dementia with Lewy bodies and Alzheimer's disease is qualitatively distinct. J Neurol Neurosurg Psychiatry. 2004;75:382–7.
62. Ballard CG, Walker MP, O'Brien JT, et al. The characterisation and impact of 'fluctuating' cognition in dementia with Lewy bodies and Alzheimer's disease. Int J Ger Psychiatry. 2001;16:494–8.
63. McKeith IG. Dementia with Lewy bodies. Br J Psychiatry. 2002;180:144–7.
64. Walker MP, Ayre GA, Perry EK, et al. Quantification and characterization of fluctuating cognition in dementia with Lewy bodies and Alzheimer's disease. Dement Geriatr Cogn Disord. 2000;11:327–35.
65. Walker MP, Ayre GA, Cummings JL, et al. The clinician assessment of fluctuation and the one day fluctuation assessment scale. Two methods to assess fluctuating confusion in dementia. Br J Psychiatry. 2000;177:252–6.
66. Ferman TJ, Smith GE, Boeve BF, et al. DLB fluctuations: specific features that reliably differentiate DLB from AD and normal aging. Neurology. 2004;62:181–7.
67. Hashimoto M, Manabe Y, Mori E, et al. Content validity and inter-rater reliability of the cognitive fluctuation inventory. Brain Nerve. 2014;66:175–83.
68. Lee DR, McKeith I, Mosimann U, et al. The dementia cognitive fluctuation scale, a new psychometric test for clinicians to identify cognitive fluctuations in people with dementia. Am J Geriatr Psychiatry. 2014;22:926–35.
69. Walker MP, Ayre GA, Cummings JL, et al. Quantifying fluctuation in dementia with Lewy bodies, Alzheimer's disease, and vascular dementia. Neurology. 2000;54:1616–25.
70. Ballard C, Walker M, O'Brien J, et al. The characterisation and impact of 'fluctuating' cognition in dementia with Lewy bodies and Alzheimer's disease. Int J Geriatr Psychiatry. 2001;16:494–8.
71. Lee DR, Taylor JP, Thomas AJ. Assessment of cognitive fluctuation in dementia: a systematic review of the literature. Int J Geriatr Psychiatry. 2012;27:989–98.
72. Pimlott SL, Piggott M, Ballard C, et al. Thalamic nicotinic receptors implicated in disturbed consciousness in dementia with Lewy bodies. Neurobiol Dis. 2006;21:50–6.
73. Peraza LR, Kaiser M, Firbank M, et al. fMRI resting state networks and their association with cognitive fluctuations in dementia with Lewy bodies. Neuroimage Clin. 2014;4:558–65.
74. Delli Pizzi S, Franciotti R, Taylor JP, et al. Thalamic involvement in fluctuating cognition in dementia with Lewy bodies: Magnetic resonance evidences. Cereb Cortex. 2014. doi:10.1093/cercor/bhu220.
75. Piggott MA, Ballard CG, Dickinson HO, et al. Thalamic D2 receptors in dementia with Lewy bodies, Parkinson's disease, and Parkinson's disease dementia. Int J Neuropsychopharmacol. 2007;10:231–4.

Chapter 7
Behavioral and Psychological Symptoms of Dementia

Yuta Manabe and Kenji Kosaka

Abstract Behavioral and psychological symptoms of dementia (BPSD) are observed in all forms of dementia. We discuss representative forms of BPSD such as hallucination and delusion, depression, and rapid eye movement (REM) sleep behavior disorder (RBD) observed in patients with dementia with Lewy bodies (DLB). The most representative BPSD for DLB is visual hallucination. McKeith et al. reported that 80 % of DLB cases involved visual hallucination. Delusions occur more frequently in DLB, compared with Alzheimer's disease (AD). These in the patients with DLB are characterized by delusional misidentification either as a continuation of visual hallucinations or related to delusions resulting from visual misidentification of places, people, or surroundings. Depression is one of the first symptoms of DLB and is listed in the CDLB guidelines as one of the supportive features. One suggestive sign of DLB is rapid eye movement (REM) sleep behavior disorder (RBD), which is significantly more common in the patients with DLB than other forms of neurodegenerative dementia. RBD also occurs earlier than cognitive dysfunction and primary core symptoms such as parkinsonism and visual hallucination.

Keywords Visual hallucination • Delusional misidentification • Depression • Rapid eye movement • Sleep behavior disorder

Y. Manabe (✉)
Dementia Diagnostic Center, Yokohama Shintoshi Neurosurgery Hospital, 433, Eda-chou, Aoba-ku, Yokohama, Kanagawa 225-0013, Japan

Department of General Internal Medicine and Emergency Medicine, Fujita Health University School of medicine, 1-98, Dengakugakubo, Kutsukake-chou, Toyoake, Aichi 470-1192, Japan

Clinic Ian Center Minami, 40-3, Chuou, Chigasaki, Tuzuki-ku, Yokohama, Kanagawa 224-0032, Japan
e-mail: manabe.epikuros@gmail.com

K. Kosaka
Clinic Ian Center Minami, 40-3, Chuou, Chigasaki, Tuzuki-ku, Yokohama, Kanagawa 224-0032, Japan

Department of Psychiatry, Yokohama City University School of Medicine, Yokohama, Kanagawa, Japan

K. Kosaka (ed.), *Dementia with Lewy Bodies*, DOI 10.1007/978-4-431-55948-1_7

7.1 Introduction

Behavioral and psychological symptoms of dementia (BPSD) are observed in all forms of dementia, regardless of the pathology [1], and are frequently the greatest cause of caregiver breakdown. There are many forms of the condition as well as a wide variety of causative factors, including neuropathological factors, neurotransmitter imbalances, genetic factors, environmental factors, patient disposition, or psychological factors of patients or families. Below we discuss representative forms of BPSD observed in patients with dementia with Lewy bodies (DLB).

7.2 Visual Hallucinations

The most representative BPSD for DLB is visual hallucination. This is described as a core symptom in the revised clinical diagnosis guidelines [2] published by the Consortium on Dementia with Lewy Bodies (CDLB). McKeith et al. reported that 80 % of DLB cases involved visual hallucination [3], which could be one factor leading to caregiver breakdown even for patients with relatively intact cognitive function.

The CDLB guidelines describe concrete and vivid, repeated visual hallucination. These are highly varied and may range from small animals ("the wall is covered with small bugs moving around") to people ("there is a woman with red lipstick in the bathroom staring at me") to fantasy-based images ("there are dwarves walking around my bed"). Here we would like to focus on both the characteristics of visual hallucinations in DLB cases as well as their mechanism of occurrence. As described by Harding et al. [4] and Yamamoto et al. [5], visual hallucination in cases of DLB resulted from neuropathological factors such as Lewy pathology in areas of the visual cortices such as the amygdaloid nucleus and ventral visual pathway; these were also factors responsible for pareidolia. Nagahama et al. [6] also provided further neuropathological findings in their report of decreased cerebral blood flow in the dorsal and ventral visual pathway according to single photon emission computed tomography (SPECT) imaging of cases of DLB with visual hallucination.

Regardless of specific mechanism, it is significant that DLB-related visual hallucination fundamentally differ from those due to schizophrenia with no organic abnormalities. One good example is a DLB patient with visual hallucination of "men in white clothes dancing and singing in the garden." In this case, the visual hallucination was thought to be caused by motion of the white lace curtains in the patient's room; the visual hallucination ceased rapidly when the room's lights were brightened and the curtains were removed. This patient's specific visual hallucination was a result of adding a layer of meaning from inner experience to the pareidolia caused by the moving white curtains. The background described above provides a good explanation for the particular usefulness of acetylcholinesterase inhibitors for DLB-related visual hallucination [7], as well as the mitigation of symptoms possible by altering the patient's physical environment.

The category of visuoperceptual disorders also includes other symptoms, such as illusory perception, for example, perceiving stains on the wall as bugs; metamorphosis, in which perceived objects appear to distort or move; and the sensed-presence effect (leibhaftiges Bewußtsein) of feeling the presence of somebody who is not really there.

The CDLB guidelines describe nonvisual types of hallucination as additional indications for DLB, but the incidence of these is low compared to visual hallucination. Some patients present with auditory hallucination, but often it should properly be classified as delusional misidentification. For example, a woman with jealous delusion of her husband having an affair reported hearing her name mentioned in a television program in the form of "Mrs. A [patient name], whose husband is cheating on her..." It has been reported [3] that about 45 % of DLB patients experience auditory hallucination (including musical), but lack of follow-up study means that actual incidence rates remain unknown.

7.3 Delusions

Delusions occur more frequently in DLB, compared with Alzheimer's disease (AD) [3]. However, rather than being typified by delusions of theft, these are characterized by delusional misidentification either as a continuation of visual hallucinations or related to delusions resulting from visual misidentification of places, people, or surroundings [8]. Representative examples include putting snacks out for nonexistent children who have come over to play, phantom boarders, or believing that one's spouse has been replaced by an impostor (Capgras syndrome). Ellis et al. [9] have proposed an interesting hypothesis for mechanisms underlying Capgras syndrome: they hypothesize that faces are recognized normally, but lack of affect usually associated with those individual faces (feelings of affinity, like, or dislike) lead to the conclusion that while the perceived appearance is the same, the person inside must be different. Based on a meta-analysis, Collerton et al. considered DLB a form of visual-perceptual and attentional-executive dementia, which always exhibited frontal lobe function disorders such as attention disorders and executive function disorders [10]. This view also fully supports the hypothesis of Ellis et al. [9] in explaining the mechanism behind delusional misidentification of people: patients are unable to reflect on their own erroneous cognition and come to conclusions such as "this person has my wife's face, but inside they are somebody else."

Nagahama et al. [11] reported findings using SPECT that symptoms related to delusional misidentification of people were correlated with reduced cerebral blood flow in the bilateral opercular parts of the inferior frontal gyri, the left insular cortex, the hippocampus, and the nucleus accumbens. Finally, delusions in the usual sense of the word, such as delusions of theft, are also observed in DLB patients, although not as frequently as in AD.

7.4 Depression

Depression is one of the first symptoms of DLB and is listed in the CDLB guidelines as one of the supportive features. There was the interesting report on the symptoms of DLB in pre-dementia phase that Fujishiro et al. [12] retrospectively investigated the clinical courses, including olfactory dysfunction, dysautonomia, depression, and rapid eye movement sleep behavior disorder, of 90 patients with probable DLB. According to this report, Lewy body-related symptoms were present in 79 of 90 patients (87.8 %) with probable DLB before or at the time of memory loss onset, and they concluded that one of the LB-related symptoms was depression. Some researches indicate a higher frequency of depression for DLB than for AD, while some reports have described major depression episodes in 40 % of DLB patients [8, 13, 14]. Delving into the neuropathological background behind Parkinson's disease (PD), Frisina et al. [15] describe significant neuronal cell loss in the ceruleus nucleus, the substantia nigra pars compacta, and the dorsal nucleus of the vagal nerve in patients exhibiting depressive symptoms. Furthermore, in their study of correlation of affected sites between PD and depression using [18F]-fluorodeoxyglucose-positron emission tomography (PET), Mentis et al. [16] conclude that glucose metabolism is reduced in the lateral frontal and anterior limbic cortices of PD patients exhibiting depression. In addition, Remy et al. [17] report that depression in PD patients is related to the loss of dopamine and noradrenaline innervation in the limbic system in their study using [11C]RTI-32 PET. These findings suggest that the dysfunctions of the fronto-subcortical and catecholaminergic system are related to PD-related depression. In a study of the selective 5-HT1A serotonin receptor agonist such as [(3)H]8-hydroxy-2-dipropylaminotetralin in 10 patients with DLB, 17 patients with PD with dementia (PDD), and 9 control patients, there was a relationship between depression and increased serotonin 1A receptor in the Brodmann area 36. These findings are relevant for the serotonergic system, which has been considered a significant factor behind major depression. Such results implicate raphe nucleus degeneration and dysfunction as underlying mechanisms for DLB-related depression [18]. Given the neuropathological homologies between PD and DLB [19, 20], the same mechanisms are likely responsible for depression due to both conditions.

7.5 REM Sleep Behavior Disorder

One suggestive sign of DLB is rapid eye movement (REM) sleep behavior disorder (RBD), which is significantly more common in the patients with DLB than other forms of neurodegenerative dementia [21]. RBD also occurs earlier than primary core symptoms such as parkinsonism and visual hallucination. In a neuropathological study of 15 RBD patients, Boeve et al. [22, 23] found that the onset of RBD preceded cognitive dysfunction or parkinsonism by 2–29 years in 10 patients and that 12 patients were diagnosed as having DLB. In his other neuropathological study [24] of 170 patients with RBD, 160 (94 %) were diagnosed as having α-synucleinopathy (including 19 cases with multiple system atrophy). These studies indicate a close relationship between RBD and α-synucleinopathy. The study of RBD according to the concept of the likelihood, which indicates a neuropathological relationship with clinical symptoms of DLB, shows a greater incidence of DLB in patients with RBD. In contrast, there is a lower incidence of high-likelihood AD pathology in patients with RBD. Therefore, MRI imaging and macroscopic findings from autopsied brains do not show remarkable atrophy in the parietotemporal lobe and the hippocampal region [25].

RBD occurs when the inhibitory mechanism of muscle tonus that usually functions during REM sleep, when skeletal muscle activity is reduced, becomes impaired. This results in behavior mirroring that of the dream, which could be anything from laughing gently or talking, to more extreme behaviors such as screaming, thrashing violently, or even striking bed partners. Accurate diagnosis of RBD requires a polysomnography to confirm REM sleep without atonia (RWA), but in practice the limited number of hospitals offering this test makes definitive diagnosis difficult. Therefore, the preferred approach is to use the RBD screening questionnaire (RBDSQ) [26] developed by Stiasny-Kolster et al. to confirm RBD. Further, the sleep-talking test [27] developed by Honda et al. demonstrated usefulness for differentiating AD and DLB. They conclude that the sleep-talking yielded high specificity (81.2 %) and some sensitivity (61.8 %) for the differential diagnosis of DLB from AD. Furthermore, loud sleep-talking may improve the specificity (96.9 %).

References

1. Reisberg B, Franssen E, Sclan SG, et al. Stage-specific incidence of potentially remediable behavioral symptoms in aging and Alzheimer's disease: a study of 120 patients using the BEHAVE-AD. Bull Clin Neurosci. 1989;54:95–112.
2. McKeith IG, Dickson DW, Lowe J, et al. Diagnosis and management of dementia with Lewy bodies third report of the DLB consortium. Neurology. 2005;65:1863–72.
3. McKeith I, Fairbairn A, Perry R, et al. Neuroleptic sensitivity in patients with senile dementia of Lewy body type. BMJ. 1992;305:673–8.
4. Harding AJ, Broe GA, Halliday GM, et al. Visual hallucinations in Lewy body disease relate to Lewy bodies in the temporal lobe. Brain. 2002;125:391–403.

5. Yamamoto E, Iseki E, Murayama N, et al. Correlation in Lewy pathology between the claustrum and visual areas in brains of dementia with Lewy bodies. Neurosci Lett. 2007;415:219–24.
6. Nagahama Y, Okina T, Suzuki N, et al. Neural correlates of psychotic symptoms in dementia Lewy bodies. Brain. 2010;133:557–67.
7. McKeith I, Del Ser T, Spano P, et al. Efficacy of rivastigmine in dementia with Lewy bodies: a randomised, double-blind, placebo-controlled international study. Lancet. 2000;356:2031–6.
8. Ballard C, Holmes C, McKeith I, et al. Psychiatric morbidity in dementia with Lewy bodies: a prospective clinical and neuropathological comparative study with Alzheimer's disease. Am J Psychiatry. 1999;156:1039–45.
9. Ellis HD, Lewis MB. Capgras delusion: a window on face recognition. Trends Cogn Sci. 2001;5:149–56.
10. Collerton D, Burn D, McKeith I, et al. Systematic review and meta-analysis show that dementia Lewy bodies is a visual-perceptual and attentional-executive dementia. Dement Geriatr Cogn Disord. 2003;16:229–37.
11. Nagahama Y, Okina T, Suzuki N, et al. Neural correlates of psychotic symptoms in dementia with Lewy bodies. Brain. 2010;133:557–67.
12. Fujishiro H, Iseki E, Nakamura S, et al. Dementia with Lewy bodies: early diagnostic challenges. Psychogeriatry. 2013;13:123–38.
13. Simard M, van Reekum R, Cohen T, et al. A review of the cognitive and behavioral symptoms in dementia with Lewy bodies. J Neuropsychiatry Clin Neurosci. 2000;12:425–50.
14. Geser F, Wenning GK, Poewe W, et al. How to diagnose dementia with Lewy bodies: state of the art. Mov Disord. 2005;20:11–20.
15. Frisina PG, Haroutunian V, Libow IS. The neuropathological basis for depression in Parkinson's disease. Parkinsonism Relat Disord. 2009;15:144–8.
16. Mentis MJ, McIntosh AR, Perrine K, et al. Relationships among the metabolic patterns that correlate with mnemonic, visuospatial, and mood symptoms in Parkinson's disease. Am J Psychiatry. 2002;159:746–54.
17. Remy P, Doder M, Lees A, et al. Depression in Parkinson's disease: loss of dopamine and noradrenaline innervation in the limbic system. Brain. 2005;128:1314–22.
18. Sharp SI, Ballard CG, Ziabreva I, et al. Cortical serotonin 1A receptor levels are associated with depression in patients with dementia with Lewy bodies and Pakinson's disease dementia. Dement Geriatr Cogn Disord. 2008;26:330–8.
19. Kosaka K, Oyanagi S, Matsushita M, et al. Presenile dementia with Alzheimer-, Pick- and Lewy-body changes. Acta Neuropathol. 1976;36:221–33.
20. Kosaka K, Yoshimura M, Ikeda K, et al. Diffuse type of Lewy body disease: progressive dementia with abundant cortical Lewy bodies and senile changes of varying degree–a new disease? Clin Neuropathol. 1984;3:185–92.
21. Honda K, Hashimoto M, Yatabe Y, et al. The usefulness of monitoring sleep talking for the diagnosis of dementia with Lewy bodies. Int Psychogeriatr. 2013;25:851–8.
22. Boeve BF, Silber MH, Ferman TJ, et al. REM sleep behavior disorder in Parkinson's disease and dementia with Lewy bodies. J Geriatr Psychiatry Neurol. 2004;17:146–57.
23. Boeve BF, Silber MH, Parisi JE, et al. Synucleinopathy pathology and REM sleep behavior disorder plus dementia or parkinsonism. Neurology. 2003;61:40–5.
24. Boeve BF, Silber MH, Ferman TJ, et al. Clinicopathological correlations in 172 cases of rapid eye movement sleep behavior disorder with or without a coexisting neurologic disorder. Sleep Med. 2013;14:754–62.
25. Murray ME, Ferman TJ, Boeve BF, et al. MRI and pathology of REM sleep behavior disorder in dementia with Lewy bodies. Neurology. 2013;81:1681–9.
26. Stiasny-Kolster K, Mayer G, Schafer S, et al. The REM sleep behavior disorder screening questionnaire—a new diagnostic instrument. Mov Disord. 2007;22:2386–93.
27. Honda K, Hashimoto M, Yatabe Y, et al. The usefulness of monitoring sleep talking for the diagnosis of Dementia with Lewy bodies. Int Psychogeriatr. 2013;25:851–8.

Chapter 8
Parkinson Symptoms in Dementia with Lewy Bodies

Yoshikuni Mizuno

Abstract Parkinsonism in dementia with Lewy bodies (DLB) is reviewed. Frequencies of tremor, wearing off, and dyskinesia seem to be lower than those of PD. This may in part due to older age of onset in DLB compared to PD. In addition, the presence of dementia and hallucination may make use of higher doses of levodopa difficult. This may result in lower frequencies of wearing off and dyskinesia. However, not many studies were done to compare parkinsonism in DLB and PD. We do not know how much of DLB patients are suffering from gait disturbance, retropulsion, freezing, falls, camptocormia, Pisa syndrome, drop head, drooling, dysphagia, small voice, micrographia, wearing off, dyskinesia, and so on. Among the non-motor spheres, data on autonomic disturbances, pain, olfaction, fatigue impulse control disorders, and dopamine dysregulation syndromes are spares. Further studies are necessary.

Keywords Parkinson's disease • Dementia with Lewy bodies • Treatment

8.1 Introduction

Parkinsonism is one of the three major core features for the diagnosis of dementia with Lewy bodies (DLB). Fluctuating cognition and visual hallucinations are two other core features. To make a diagnosis of DLB for a given patient, dementia and parkinsonism have to start at about the same time when the parkinsonism is present [1].

Fair numbers of patients with dementia without parkinsonism exist, and in such a case, the presence of recurrent visual hallucinations suggests DLB [1]. Other suggestive features include REM sleep behavior disorders, severe neuroleptic sensitivity, and low dopamine transporter uptake in basal ganglia demonstrated by SPECT and PET imaging. The author should like to include low meta-iodo-

Y. Mizuno (✉)
Department of Neurology, Juntendo University School of Medicine, Hongo 2-1-1, Bunkyo-ku, Tokyo 113-8421, Japan
e-mail: y_mizuno@juntendo.ac.jp

K. Kosaka (ed.), *Dementia with Lewy Bodies*, DOI 10.1007/978-4-431-55948-1_8

benzylguanidine (MIBG) uptake into cardiac sympathetic nerve terminals as the fourth suggestive feature. Ten other supportive features are listed.

8.2 Prevalence of Dementia with Lewy Bodies

It is not very well known how frequent DLB is. Matsui et al. [2] followed 828 subjects without dementia for 17 years, and among them 275 developed dementia and 251 were examined by either autopsy or neuroimaging. Incidence of Alzheimer's disease (AD) was estimated to be 14.6 (124 out of 275) per 1000 per year and that of DLB 1.4 (12 out of 275) per 1000 per year. Therefore, DLB is estimated to be approximately 10 % of AD.

Ikejima et al. [3] examined 3394 elderly subjects in seven rural areas in Japan. Among them, 768 patients were demented and 67.4 % had AD and 4.6 % DLB, a similar ratio in the number of AD to DLB. Wada-Isoe et al. [4] studied the subjects 65 or older in a small rural island town. They found 148 demented patients, and the prevalence of dementia was estimated to be 16.4 % in elderly individuals at 65 years or older and 104 (70.3 %) out of 148 had AD and 8 (5.4 %) had DLB.

In outside of Japan, prevalence of dementia was reported as 5.5 % of 65 or older individuals in Spain [5], and among the 270 patients that they studied, 77.7 % had AD and 7.6 % DLB; the ratio of AD and DLB was approximately 10:1. Farina et al. [6] studied DLB alone in Italy; they found the prevalence of DLB to be 4.8 % of demented population, about the same order as in Spain. Aarsland et al. [7] studied 196 patients in early stage demented individuals and found that 65 % had AD and 20 % DLB. This is the highest value for DLB in reference to AD.

Kobayashi et al. [8] studied 60 patients with diminished uptake of MIBG into the heart without dementia or parkinsonism but with at least one psychiatric symptom such as depression, hallucination, or others. Therefore, all the patients had Lewy body disease but not necessarily DLB. Among them 27 patients had depression, but only one patient developed parkinsonism, 16 visual hallucinations, and 17 other psychiatric symptoms. At the final diagnosis, 21 out of 60 developed dementia and diagnosed as DLB. Among them 11 patients developed parkinsonism and 10 did not. Out of the 16 patients with visual hallucination, 15 developed DLB. Therefore, about 50 % of DLB patients do not have parkinsonism at a cross-sectional study.

8.3 Clinical Features of Parkinsonism in Parkinson's Disease

It is not well known how different the parkinsonism is in DLB from parkinsonism in Parkinson's disease (PD) and PD with dementia (PDD). Not many studies were done in good numbers to compare features of parkinsonism between PD and DLB.

In PDD, dementing symptoms appear on the well-established parkinsonism. Many patients with PD are believed eventually develop cognitive decline after a certain period, a few years to more than 10–20 years from the onset of parkinsonism. The clinical feature of dementia in PD is very similar to that of DLB; they show fluctuating cognition and visual fluctuation. Let me start with clinical features of parkinsonism in PD and PDD.

8.3.1 Mode of Onset

Onset is insidious. The age of onset is usually 55–70 years of age, but onset as early as 8 and as late as 80 are known. The younger age of onset is at times associated with familial cases.

8.3.2 Four Major Symptoms of Parkinson's Disease

In moderately advanced PD patients, usually four major symptoms are seen, that is, rest tremor, rigidity, bradykinesia, and postural instability (Table 8.1). These four symptoms are considered to have independent modes of pathogenesis in the brain. Usually, the diagnosis of PD is made the presence of bradykinesia and at least one of the remaining three major symptoms [9].

8.3.3 Tremor

Presenting symptom in PD is in about 50 % unilateral rest tremor in the hand or the leg, mostly in the hand. But in DLB tremor is less frequent than in PD. In the clinical course, 75–80 % of PD patients will develop tremor. The tremor in PD is in most cases rest tremor. The tremor is between 4 and 6 cycles per second. The tremor is most often seen while the patient is walking or sitting. When the patient moves his or her shaking hand or taking the posture such as stretching arms in front, the tremor will stop or decrease its severity. But occasionally stretching the arms in front will induce much larger and prominent tremor; there is a brief period (approximately less than 10 s) of tremor ceasing. The tremor will become much larger and vigorous as long as the patient takes the arm-stretched posture, and often the tremor is asymmetric. Such tremor is called as reemergent tremor, and the presence of reemergent tremor indicates the clinical diagnosis of PD [10], although the reemergent tremor is rare in PD.

Table 8.1 Motor symptoms of Parkinson's disease

Rest tremor	Freezing
Rigidity	Freezing
Bradykinesia	Festination
Reptile stare	Abnormal posture
Masked face	Camptocormia
Small voice	Pisa syndrome
Dysphagia	Head drop
Bradykinesia	Loss of automatic acts
Micrographia	Drooling
Shuffling gait	Aspiration
Postural instability	Loss of arm swing
Retro-, ante-, latero-pulsion	Loss of two motor acts
Stooped posture	

8.3.4 Rigidity

Rigidity is a form of increase in the muscle tone. When a muscle is passively stretched slowly, for instance, flexing and extending the wrist joint on one side, the examiner feels a resistance to the flexion and the extension in rigidity. This resistance is rather constant at all the flexed or extended period. This is a differentiating point from spasticity where the resistance is strong in the beginning but will soon melt away as the flexion or extension is continued. This is called a clasp-knife phenomenon in spasticity. In rigidity, sometimes the resistance is not continuous but noncontinuous interspersed with a tremor-like rhythm. This is called cogwheel rigidity and is usually seen in the upper extremity examination in PD, at times also in the lower extremity examination. Truncal rigidity can be tested by flexion of the neck in a supine position or rotating the trunk to the right and left in a sitting or a standing position.

8.3.5 Bradykinesia

Bradykinesia denotes slowness of movement. Every movement in PD becomes slow. Akinesia denotes loss of spontaneous or automatic movement. For instance, a PD patient sitting in a chair for a certain period may not move his or her hands or legs spontaneously, or there may be a marked reduction in such a spontaneous movement. Hypokinesia denotes smallness of movements. Any movement becomes smaller than normal. At times, the term bradykinesia is used to inclusively denote bradykinesia, akinesia, and hypokinesia. To exam whether or not the patient has bradykinesia, just watching the patient when he or she enters the examining room is suffice. The patient may walk slowly, may shuffle the legs, have no arm swing, have a stooped posture, have a loss of facial expression (masked face), have a reduced eye blinking, and have a reduced searching eye movement (reptile staring). Frequently, the patient has an asymmetric presentation of these symptoms; usually the side where the disease started is more involved than the other.

The voice becomes small, monotonous, and poor in intonation. At times, the pitch of the voice becomes higher than before the patient was afflicted with parkinsonism. The speech ultimately becomes mumbling and unintelligible difficult to understand. Handwriting is also affected. Initially, the size of the letter is not small but the patient continues writing; the size of the letter becomes smaller and smaller. This is called micrographia. When the patient walks, usually the arm swing is diminished or lost.

In examination of bradykinesia, we usually ask the patient to do finger tapping, rapid alternating movement, opening and closing the hands, tapping the floor with the heel with the knee up in the air as possible (foot agility), and tapping the floor with the tip of toes. In these tests, the rate of the speed in repetitive movements is reduced and the size of the movement is small. Each of these movements should be tested one extremity at one time; otherwise, subtle asymmetry of the movement may be missed.

8.3.6 Postural Instability

Postural instability can be tested by the pull test. In the test of retropulsion, ask the patient to stand up with feet apart at about the shoulder's width. Then, the examiner stands behind the patient and explains to the patient what is going to happen. Then the examiner put his or her both arms on the shoulders of the patient. Then the examiner pulls the shoulders of the patient backward with the strength that will induce a step backward in a normal person. If the patient steps backward more than two steps or would fall backward if unsupported, the patient is said to have retropulsion. At times, the patient would fall backward without stepping even one step. In a similar way, ante-pulsion and latero-pulsion can be tested for the examiner standing in front of the patient.

8.3.7 Abnormalities in Posture

The posture of PD shows a stooped posture. The patient shows a bend forward posture mainly in the upper part of the thoracic spine. Perhaps this is a compensatory posture that the patient has a tendency to fall backward. The thoracolumbar region is straight in uncomplicated PD. If this part takes a bend forward posture upon standing, it is called camptocormia. The cause of camptocormia is not well known. It may be a dystonic posture originating from the brain of PD patients. At times, a focal myositic lesion is found in the paravertebral region [11]. But this myositic change is believed to be a secondary phenomenon due to a long-standing flexed posture. Camptocormia may be seen as an untoward symptom of dopamine agonists, particularly of non-ergot dopamine agonists [12]. The head drop or antecollis is a strong anteflexion of the head so that the chin is almost touching the chest wall. This is more common in multiple system atrophy than in PD. The cause is not known. Pisa syndrome is a bend of the spine toward the right or left. Slight Pisa syndrome is frequently seen in PD. Pisa syndrome is thought to be a result of dystonia. But at times, dopamine agonists may induce Pisa syndrome [13].

8.3.8 Gait

Gait disorder in PD is a result of bradykinesia and postural instability. The typical feature of gait disorder in a moderately advanced PD patient takes a form of stooped postured, shuffling gait without arm swing looking downward with flexed neck. Some asymmetrical features may be soon. For instance, arm swing and shuffling gait is less involved on one side of the body. The patient is able to walk up and down the staircase rather easily.

8.3.9 Freezing

Freezing of gait is seen in moderately advanced PD patients. While walking, suddenly the feet are routed to the ground. The patient is unable to raise legs. Meanwhile the upper half of the body would move forward, and the bend forward posture will become extreme so that the patient must fall down to the floor. This freezing tends to occur more frequently within the house rather than outside of the house. Narrow places such as a toilet, a corner of the corridor, or a kitchen tend to precipitate freezing. Also, it can happen in front of the chair that he or she wants to sit down and the patient may fall down to the chair without moving feet.

Outside of the house, freezing of gait can occur, but it is more frequently in the form of festination. Here the patient with PD, while walking, the stride becomes smaller and smaller and the pace of walking is getting faster and faster. At the same time, the stooped posture will become prominent more and more, and ultimately the patient has to hold such an object as an electric pole to stop; otherwise, the patient may fall down to the ground. Both freezing and festination occur more frequently during off period compared to on period of levodopa intake, but it may also occur during on period. Therefore, dopamine deficiency is the most important mechanism for the freezing and the festination, but unknown additional mechanism must be working, as they may happen during on period of levodopa treatment.

8.3.10 Loss of Automatic Movements

Moderately advanced PD patients may have drooling. The saliva unconsciously comes out of the mouth, particularly when the patient is engaged in other acts such as watching TV, walking, or eating. The amount of the saliva is not increased in PD. Normal persons unconsciously swallow the saliva. This unconscious act of saliva swallowing is difficult for PD patients. Difficulties of unconscious motor acts can be seen frequently in daily life. For instance, loss of arm swing seems to be one example. Gait tends to become shuffling when the patient does not consciously pay attention to his or her feet. Aspiration is another example of loss of automatic movement.

8.3.11 Loss of Two Motor Acts

The patient with PD has a difficulty in doing two independent motor acts simultaneously in each hand. For instance, drinking a cup of coffee while reading a newspaper in the breakfast may be difficult to do. Another example is carrying a tray with dishes of soup to the dining table from the kitchen; this patient may fall down during the way. She has to pay attention to the arms so that she would not spill the soup; her attention to the feet becomes weak and she would fall down by stumbling to some object. For PD patient, it is important to do one motor act at one time.

8.3.12 Motor Fluctuations

In PD, usually the patients are doing well for the first 5 years after starting levodopa therapy without severe motor fluctuations such as wearing off or dyskinesia. After 5 years, those patients start to have motor fluctuations, and after 10 years of treatment with levodopa, more than 60 % of the patients are facing wearing off, and this percentage is becoming larger as the treatment period prolongs. Frequently on time from levodopa may last only 3 h or less and these patients may have to take levodopa six times or more to keep them in on time. Still they have on and off fluctuation. Furthermore, about 50 % of the levodopa-treated patients for more than 10 years may suffer from on-time dyskinesia. The patients may not notice a mild dyskinesia, but caregivers notice even a mild dyskinesia and feel uneasy. In a recent article from China [14], wearing off after 10 years of levodopa treatment was reported to be 68.3 % and dyskinesia 19.3 %. According to our unpublished data, the prevalence of wearing off was 81.7 % in patients with 10–15 years from the onset and dyskinesia 63.3 %.

8.4 Parkinsonism in DLB

In DLB, the rest tremor is less encountered than PD. In DLB, the rest tremor is seen in about 25 % of the patients. This difference may in part due to the difference in age of onset between PD and DLB. The age of onset in PD is usually between 55 and 70, while that of DLB is usually 65 or above. Burn et al. [15] studied clinical symptoms of parkinsonism in PD, PDD, and DLB. The mean age of onset was 67.4 in PD and PDD combined and 74.6 in DLB. Clinical dichotomy of PD into two forms is accepted by most of the movement disorder specialists. Jankovic and Kapadia [16] classified PD into two forms: tremor-dominant form and postural instability-gait disturbance (PIGD) form. The tremor-dominant form tends to progress more slowly than the rigid-akinetic form [16]. Dementia is more frequent in the rigid-akinetic form. Burn et al. [15] studied 38 PD, 43 PDD, and 26 DLB patients for subtypes of parkinsonism. Postural instability-gait difficulty (PIGD) subtype was more common in the PDD (88 % of cases) and the DLB (69 % of cases) groups compared with the PD group (38 % of cases). They also reported that cognitive decline in 2-year period was greater in the PIPG subtype [17].

Other difference is in the frequency of motor fluctuation. Here, again the age of onset seems to have an influence on the frequency of motor fluctuation. Frequencies of motor fluctuations tend to be higher in PD patients with young age of onset. In DLB, no such report is available on motor fluctuations with levodopa treatment. Perhaps, lower frequencies of motor fluctuation in DLB as compared with PD may be due to the higher age of onset, due to the shorter period of levodopa treatment in DLB, and due to dementia and hallucination, which may be limiting factors in increasing the dosage of levodopa. In PD, duration of levodopa treatment and the age of onset are important factors for motor fluctuations. Schrag and Quinn [18] reported incidence of wearing off to be 40 % and that of dyskinesia 28 % in a community-based population of PD, and the total number of PD was 124. What they found was those PD patients with wearing off were 68.8 years in average and the years of treatment with levodopa was 7.4 years, while those without wearing off had an average age of 73.3 years and the years of treatment with levodopa was 3.5 years. Thus, younger age of onset of PD and the longer duration of levodopa treatment tend to induce wearing-off phenomenon. The higher age of onset of DLB seems to be a factor for lower incidence of wearing off; however, the frequency of wearing off and dyskinesia has to be investigated in DLB.

Otherwise, parkinsonism in PD and parkinsonism in DLB are essentially similar.

8.5 Non-motor Symptoms in PD and in DLB

Many non-motor symptoms are known in PD and DLB (Table 8.2).

Table 8.2 Non-motor symptoms of parkinsonism and dementia with Lewy bodies

Autonomic disturbances	Disturbance of affect
Constipation	Anxiety
Nocturnal urinary frequency	Depression
Impotence	Apathy
Orthostatic hypotension	Sensory symptoms
Postprandial hypotension	Hyposmia
Edema	Pain
Sweating	Loss of taste sensation
Sleep disorders	Fatigue
Insomnia	ICD and DA dysregulation syndrome
REM sleep behavior disorder	Hallucination, delusion
Restless legs syndrome	Violent behavior, hypersexual behavior, psychosis
Disturbance of awakening	Dementia
Excessive daytime sleepiness	
Sudden onset of sleep	

8.5.1 *Autonomic Disorders*

The initial symptom in PD and DLB is in most cases constipation. The onset of constipation may precede the onset of parkinsonism or dementia for years or more than 10 years. In addition to constipation, diverse symptoms of autonomic disturbances frequently occur in PD and DLB including nocturnal polyuria, sexual disturbances, hypotension and orthostatic hypotension, postprandial hypotension, swinging blood pressure, profuse sweating, pretibial edema, and so on. As the pathology of PD and DLB seems to start in the peripheral autonomic nerves including the dorsal motor nuclei of the vagal nerves and climb up in the brain stem eventually involving the cerebral cortices [19], autonomic dysfunctions seem to be the first symptom of PD and DLB. Autonomic dysfunctions in DLB are covered in another chapter of this book.

8.5.2 *Sleep Disorders*

8.5.2.1 Insomnia

Difficulty in falling asleep, frequent awakenings during night, and difficulty in falling asleep toward the early morning are the causes of insomnia. Depression, anxiety, pain in some place, difficulty in rolling over, dystonia, and urinary frequency including prostate hypertrophy or cancer may become a cause of difficulty in falling asleep. Difficulty in falling asleep in uncomplicated PD patients is not very common. However, more frequently difficulty of falling asleep after wakening up in the midnight is encountered in PD. Difficulty in falling asleep should be treated properly. One may use a sleeping pill which has to be taken 30 min before the patient wants to asleep. Short-acting sleeping pills such as zolpidem (5–10 mg), zopiclone (7.5–10 mg), brotizolam (0.25 mg), or triazolam (0.125– 0.25 mg) are recommended.

The most frequent cause for awakening during night is urinary urgency. The urinary urgency occurs for both men and women. This probably due to lesion in the parasympathetic innervation to the detrusor muscles of the bladder. Secondary causes for frequent awakening during night include prostate hypertrophy or cancer, dystonia, pain, difficulty in rolling over, and spasm of the legs. For men, when frequent awakening takes place, prostate cancer should be ruled out by examination of prostate antigen in the blood; if the prostate antigen is more than 4, the patient should be introduced to an urology specialist. For frequent awakening during night, one may use a longer sleeping pill such as flunitrazepam (0.5–2 mg), nitrazepam (5–10 mg), estazolam (1–4 mg), or nimetazepam (3–5 mg) before sleep, or the very short-acting sleeping pill, triazolam (0.125– 0.25 mg), can be given when the patient wakes up in the midnight and complains of difficulty in falling asleep.

8.5.2.2 REM Sleep Behavior Disorder

When people have rapid eye movement (REM) sleep, usually he or she is silently sleeping without any movement in the limbs or in the vocalization. Muscle tones are hypotonic. He or she is dreaming without moving limbs or vocalization. The content of the dream is usually not scary. In the central nervous diseases such as PD, DLB, or MSA where the substantia nigra is involved, muscle tone will not disappear during REM sleep. The patient may be acting out the content of the dream. The dream is usually a scary one. The patient may shout or vigorously move his or her arms or legs as if he or she may be trying to fight or escape the scary content of the dream. The patient usually does not remember what he or she was doing during night. But at times, the patient may be awakening by the voice. Usually RBD appears before the motor symptoms of parkinsonism. Frequency of RBD in PD is reported as 30 % or above [20] and 60 % or above in DLB [21, 22]. The responsible lesion for RBD is not well elucidated yet; however, the sub-locus coeruleus area is thought to be responsible in PD [23]. Therefore, this structure is considered to be involved in PD and DLB before the substantia nigra is involved. RBD is thought to be a symptom, which appears earlier than motor symptoms of parkinsonism. RBD may be a prodromal symptom of other CNS disorders such as multiple system atrophy, progressive supranuclear palsy, corticobasal degeneration, or Alzheimer's disease [24]. However, frequencies of RBD in other disorders are low except for multiple system atrophy [25].

8.5.2.3 Restless Legs Syndrome

Restless legs syndrome consists of an abnormal urge to move the limbs and improvement with voluntary movement of the affected limb. The prevalence of restless legs syndrome varies from 0.1 to 10 % among different ethnic populations [26, 27]. In Japan, prevalence in general population is not so high, approximately 2.3 %, but in PD it rose up to 12 % [28]. It is not well known why in PD frequency of restless legs symptom is higher than normal population. As iron deficiency in the hypothalamic neurons has been postulated as a causative event in restless legs syndrome [29]. This iron deficiency may be an explanation for it: the amount of nigral iron is reported to be reduced [30]. In restless legs syndrome, usually dopaminergic treatment is effective [31]. Therefore, there may be some similarity in the underlying pathology in restless legs syndrome and PD. In DLB, no study has ever been done on the prevalence of restless legs syndrome with enough number of the patients and controls; however, the frequency of restless legs syndrome appears to be lower in DLB compared to other central nervous system diseases, particularly PD. Guarnieri et al. [32] compared frequencies of sleep-related problems in the central nervous system disorders, in which restless legs syndrome in DLB/PDD was practically zero, while frequencies were around 5 % in other diseases of the central nervous system including AD.

8.5.3 Excessive Daytime Sleepiness and Sudden Onset of Sleep

8.5.3.1 Excessive Daytime Sleepiness

Despite good night sleep, patients with PD and DLB may feel excessive daytime sleepiness [33]. Treatment by a dopamine agonist may induce excessive daytime sleepiness. Non-ergot dopamine agonists tend to induce excessive daytime sleepiness, but ergot dopamine agonists as well. At times, levodopa also induces excessive daytime sleepiness. Particularly, if the patient develops cognitive impairment, the patient may sleep while eating foods.

8.5.3.2 Sudden Onset of Sleep (SOS)

Here the patient falls into sleep suddenly without prodromal symptoms of sleep [34]. If this happens while the patient is driving a car, there is a risk of a traffic accident with a possible injury or fatality to persons involved. This may be an extreme example of excessive daytime sleepiness. The patient may have drowsy sensation initially, but he or she may not be able to remember this sensation because of falling asleep.

8.5.4 *Anxiety, Depression, and Apathy*

8.5.4.1 Anxiety

Anxiety is a common symptom of PD and DLB, but little attention has been paid in anxiety in DLB. Most often, patients with PD worry about the future of their life. What will happen in the future is they may become unable to walk, they may have to be taken care of their children, and drugs for parkinsonism may become unable to improve their symptoms in the future: these are the common questions of the patients with PD. In addition, they may have family problems, social problems, problems related to their works, and so on. Furthermore, some of the patients may have ill-defined anxieties not related to actual matters. Borroni et al. [35] studied the frequency of BPSD (behavioral and psychological symptoms of dementia) in DLB and found that anxiety was the most common BPSD in DLB (67.4 %) followed by depression (61.9 %). Hynninen et al. [36] studied 169 patients with dementia of various causes. Dementia was found in 19.5 % of them; they stated that patients with DLB reported anxiety more often compared to AD. In the treatment of anxiety symptoms, first of explanation of the anxiety that the patient has is very important. Here the opportunistic attitude is recommended. A minor tranquilizer can be used for moderately severe anxiety.

8.5.4.2 Depression

Depression is another important BPSD in DLB. It may have an onset before the cognitive symptoms in DLB. Depression is discussed in detail in another chapter of this book.

8.5.4.3 Apathy

Apathy is a diminished motivation and interest, expressed by a decrease in goal-related aspects of overt behavior, thought content, and flattening of thought [37]. Apathy may be seen in depressed or demented patients. But apathy can be seen in PD without accompanying depression or dementia [38].

8.5.5 *Sensory Symptoms*

8.5.5.1 Hyposmia and Anosmia

The prevalence of impaired olfactory function in PD ranges from 55 to 94 % [39–41]. Baba et al. [41] classified the patients with PD according to those with severe hyposmia and those without severe hyposmia. They took 44 patients with PD without dementia and they followed them for 3 years. They used the odor stick identification test for Japanese (OSIT-J), and patients with OSIT-J scores </= 4 were defined as having severe hyposmia and >5 as having non-severe hyposmia. The patients with severe olfactory dysfunction developed dementia with 3-year observation period. Ten patients out of 24 with severe hyposmia developed dementia and none in 20 patients without severe anosmia. They concluded that severe olfactory dysfunction is a prodromal sign of dementia. In DLB, the prevalence of hyposmia was reported as 65 %, whereas in AD it was 23 % [42]. The number of studies on hyposmia in DLB is very limited but I believe that hyposmia is very frequent in DLB.

8.5.5.2 Pain and Dysesthesia

Pain is a very common symptom in PD, more often lumbar pains. Any kind of pain can occur and its prevalence is approximately 70 % [43–45]. The pain may be due to complications such as protrusions of lumbar discs, spinal canal stenosis, compression fractures of the vertebrae, marked scoliosis, arthroses of the spine, and others. The pain may also occur as a complication of PD. Here, the pain coincides with the off time of levodopa therapy. The pain can be at any place, but more often on the side first involved in PD. The pain can be relieved by levodopa intake. In this case, treatment should be directed to the better treatment of wearing off.

Although it is rare, dysesthesia may be the first symptom in one of the limbs before the tremor sets in in PD. In this case, treatment of the tremor usually alleviates the dysesthesia, but when he or she develops wearing off, the dysesthesia comes back when the patient is in off state.

8.5.6 Fatigue

Fatigue is a common symptom in PD [46] but no study has been done on the fatigue in DLB. Fatigue is considered to be a non-motor symptom of parkinsonism. But it may be seen in association with motor symptoms. For instance, by finger tapping, initially the patient may move the index finger on the thumb in fairly good amplitude; the width of finger tapping may become smaller and smaller. This may be considered an example of fatigue. In handwriting, the size of letters may become smaller and smaller as the patient tries to do handwriting until the end. This is another example of fatigue. In a daily life, fatigue can be seen in walking, cooking, cleaning the house, and so on. The patient may feel fatigue after 5 or 10 min of the same work. But after a brief rest for 1 or 2 min, the patient may feel better and is able to continue the work. The responsible lesion of fatigue is not well elucidated and there is no good therapy.

8.5.7 Impulse Control Disorders and Dopamine Dysregulation Syndromes

Impulse control disorders seen in PD consist of gambling, shopping, binge eating, and hypersexual behaviors; dopamine dysregulation syndromes consist of drug abuse and punding. Punding is a Swedish slug meaning block head. It consists of a repetitive stereotyped behavior such as manipulating electric cords or handbag items, repetitive handwritings, or collecting small items [47]. The patient is unable to stop the movement and it appears that the patient is relieved by something else such as anxiety by doing so. Punding behaviors were seen in patients with amphetamine addicts. Similar behaviors have been seen in patients with PD. Impulse control disorders and dopamine dysregulation syndromes tend to occur in younger patients with PD treated with non-ergot dopamine agonists [48, 49]. Some of those patients have a tendency to one of such behavior disorders since younger ages. No study has been done on the impulse control disorders and dopamine dysregulation syndrome in dementia with Lewy bodies. Perhaps the frequencies of impulse control disorders and dopamine dysregulation syndromes are lower in DLB than PD because of later age of onsets in DLB

8.5.8 Hallucination and Delusions

Visual hallucination is a very important symptom in the diagnosis of DLB. It is listed in one of the major criteria [1]. Visual hallucination may be seen without levodopa and it may not be related to levodopa treatment. But levodopa treatment at times aggravates the hallucination. Hallucination in DLB is well formed and detailed. Hallucination is discussed in detail in this book.

8.5.9 Violent Behaviors, Hypersexual Behaviors, and Psychosis

The patients with PD at times go into violent behaviors, hypersexual behaviors, or psychosis. Frequently, these patients have cognitive declines (PDD). Lowering dopaminergic drugs as possible and the use of quetiapine may be necessary in these patients. Usually, those patients recover from the violent behaviors or hypersexual behaviors by appropriate therapy. The patients with DLB also may go into these behavior problems. They are discussed in detail in another chapter in this book.

8.5.10 Dementia

Patients with PD may develop dementia (PDD). Incidence of dementia in PD is going up as the disease progresses. Aarsland et al. [50] reported that at the initial examination, prevalence of dementia was 26 % with the average disease duration of 9.2 +/− 5.2 years in 224 patients with PD; however, it rose up to 51.6 % in 4 years and to 78.2 % in 8 years of observation. Lifelong frequency rises further and it is reported to be 90 % or above. Therefore, in average 17 years of observation, prevalence of dementia is approximately 80 %. The dementia of PD patients is that of dysexecutive dementia and fluctuating cognition in the awareness and the judgment. Dementia in PD is very similar to that of DLB. Dementia of DLB is discussed in detail in other chapters of this book.

8.6 Treatment of Parkinsonism in DLB

As in DLB, dementia is the prerequisite; levodopa is the choice of treatment for parkinsonism, if the parkinsonism requires drug treatment. As the currently available drugs for the treatment of parkinsonism is all symptomatic, the patient with DLB with parkinsonism should be treated only when his or her disability reaches a certain point. Levodopa should be given 100 mg each twice or three times after each meal initially. In case this dose does not alleviate the disability of the patient from parkinsonism, levodopa can be given shortly before each meal. Levodopa can be given up to 200 mg tid before meal in case no untoward effect is encountered. Attention should be paid to hallucination and dementia, whether or not levodopa treatment aggravates them.

References

1. McKeith IG, Dickson DW, Lowe J, et al. Consortium on DLB. Diagnosis and management of dementia with Lewy bodies: third report of the DLB Consortium. Neurology. 2005;65:1863–72.
2. Matsui Y, Tanizaki Y, Arima H, et al. Incidence and survival of dementia in a general population of Japanese elderly: the Hisayama study. J Neurol Neurosurg Psychiatry. 2009;80:366–70.
3. Ikejima C, Hisanaga A, Meguro K, et al. Multicentre population-based dementia prevalence survey in Japan: a preliminary report. Psychogeriatrics. 2012;12:120–3.
4. Wada-Isoe K, Uemura Y, Nakashita S, et al. Prevalence of dementia and mild cognitive impairment in the rural island town of Ama-cho, Japan. Dement Geriatr Cogn Dis Extra. 2012;2:190–9.
5. Tola-Arribas MA, Yugueros MI, Garea MJ, et al. Prevalence of dementia and subtypes in Valladolid, northwestern Spain: the DEMINVALL study. PLoS One. 2013;8:e77688.
6. Farina E, Baglio F, Caffarra P, et al. Frequency and clinical features of Lewy body dementia in Italian memory clinics. Acta Biomed. 2009;80:57–64.

7. Aarsland D, Rongve A, Nore SP, et al. Frequency and case identification of dementia with Lewy bodies using the revised consensus criteria. Dement Geriatr Cogn Disord. 2008;26:445–52.
8. Kobayashi K, Nakano H, Akiyama N, et al. Pure psychiatric presentation of the Lewy body disease is depression-an analysis of 60 cases verified with myocardial meta-iodobenzylguanidine study. Int J Geriatr Psychiatry. 2014. doi:10.1002/gps.4214.
9. Hughes AJ, Daniel SE, Kilford L, et al. Accuracy of clinical diagnosis of idiopathic Parkinson's disease: a clinico-pathological study of 100 cases. J Neurol Neurosurg Psychiatry. 1992;55:181–4.
10. Jankovic J, Schwartz KS, Ondo W. Re-emergent tremor of Parkinson's disease. J Neurol Neurosurg Psychiatry. 1999;67:646–50.
11. Schäbitz WR, Glatz K, Schuhan C, et al. Severe forward flexion of the trunk in Parkinson's disease: focal myopathy of the paraspinal muscles mimicking camptocormia. Mov Disord. 2003;18:408–14.
12. Azher SN, Jankovic J. Camptocormia: pathogenesis, classification, and response to therapy. Neurology. 2005;65:355–9.
13. Galati S, Möller JC, Städler C. Ropinirole-induced Pisa syndrome in Parkinson disease. Clin Neuropharmacol. 2014;37:58–9.
14. Chen W, Xiao Q, Shao M, et al. Prevalence of wearing-off and dyskinesia among the patients with Parkinson's disease on levodopa therapy: a multi-center registry survey in mainland China. Transl Neurodegener. 2014;3:26.
15. Burn DJ, Rowan EN, Minett T, et al. Extrapyramidal features in Parkinson's disease with and without dementia and dementia with Lewy bodies: a cross-sectional comparative study. Mov Disord. 2003;18:884–9.
16. Jankovic J, Kapadia AS. Functional decline in Parkinson disease. Arch Neurol. 2001;58:1611–5.
17. Burn DJ, Rowan EN, Allan LM, et al. Motor subtype and cognitive decline in Parkinson's disease, Parkinson's disease with dementia, and dementia with Lewy bodies. J Neurol Neurosurg Psychiatry. 2006;77:585–9.
18. Schrag A, Quinn N. Dyskinesias and motor fluctuations in Parkinson's disease. A community-based study. Brain. 2000;123:2297–305.
19. Braak H, Del Tredici K, Rüb U, et al. Staging of brain pathology related to sporadic Parkinson's disease. Neurobiol Aging. 2003;24:197–211.
20. Schenck CH, Bundlie SR, Mahowald MW. Delayed emergence of a Parkinsonian disorder in 38% of 29 older men initially diagnosed with idiopathic rapid eye movement sleep behaviour disorder. Neurology. 1996;46:388–93.
21. Ferman TJ, Boeve BF, Smith GE, et al. Inclusion of RBD improves the diagnostic classification of dementia with Lewy bodies. Neurology. 2011;77:875–82.
22. Murray ME, Ferman TJ, Boeve BF, et al. MRI and pathology of REM sleep behavior disorder in dementia with Lewy bodies. Neurology. 2013;81:1681–9.
23. Boeve BF, Silber MH, Saper CB, et al. Pathophysiology of REM sleep behaviour disorder and relevance to neurodegenerative disease. Brain. 2007;130:2770–88.
24. Olsen EJ, Boeve BF, Silber MH. Rapid eye movement sleep behavior disorder: demographic, clinical and laboratory findings in 93 cases. Brain. 2000;123:331–9.
25. Gagnon JF, Postuma RB, Mazza S, et al. Rapid-eye-movement sleep behaviour disorder and neurodegenerative diseases. Lancet Neurol. 2006;5:424–32.
26. Högl B, Kiechl S, Willeit J, et al. Restless legs syndrome: a community-based study of prevalence, severity, and risk factors. Neurology. 2005;64:1920–4.
27. Tan EK, Seah A, See SJ, et al. Restless legs syndrome in an Asian population: a study in Singapore. Mov Disord. 2001;16:577–9.
28. Nomura T, Inoue Y, Miyake M, et al. Prevalence and clinical characteristics of restless legs syndrome in Japanese patients with Parkinson's disease. Mov Disord. 2006;21:380–4.

29. Paulus W, Trenkwalder C. Less is more: pathophysiology of dopaminergic- therapy-related augmentation in restless legs syndrome. Lancet Neurol. 2006;5:878–86.
30. Schmidauer C, Sojer M, Seppi K, et al. Transcranial ultrasound shows nigral hypoechogenicity in restless legs syndrome. Ann Neurol. 2005;58:630–4.
31. Trenkwalder C, Hening WA, Montagna P, et al. Treatment of restless legs syndrome: an evidence-based review and implications for clinical practice. Mov Disord. 2008;23:2267–302.
32. Guarnieri B, Adorni F, Musicco M, et al. Prevalence of sleep disturbances in mild cognitive impairment and dementing disorders: a multicenter Italian clinical cross-sectional study on 431 patients. Dement Geriatr Cogn Disord. 2012;33:50–8.
33. Verbaan D, van Rooden SM, Visser M, et al. Nighttime sleep problems and daytime sleepiness in Parkinson's disease. Mov Disord. 2008;23:35–41.
34. Paus S, Brecht HM, Köster J, et al. Sleep attacks, daytime sleepiness, and dopamine agonists in Parkinson's disease. Mov Disord. 2003;18:659–67.
35. Borroni B, Agosti C, Padovani A. Behavioral and psychological symptoms in dementia with Lewy-bodies (DLB): frequency and relationship with disease severity and motor impairment. Arch Gerontol Geriatr. 2008;46:101–6.
36. Hynninen MJ, Breitve MH, Rongve A, et al. The frequency and correlates of anxiety in patients with first-time diagnosed mild dementia. Int Psychogeriatr. 2012;24:1771–8.
37. Pluck GC, Brown RG. Apathy in Parkinson's disease. J Neurol Neurosurg Psychiatry. 2002;73:636–42.
38. Starkstein SE, Merello M, Jorge R, et al. The syndromal validity and nosological position of apathy in Parkinson's disease. Mov Disord. 2009;24:1211–6.
39. Boesveldt S, Verbaan D, Knol DL, et al. A comparative study of odor identification and odor discrimination deficits in Parkinson's disease. Mov Disord. 2008;23:1984–90.
40. Berendse HW, Roos DS, Raijmakers P, et al. Motor and non-motor correlates of olfactory dysfunction in Parkinson's disease. J Neurol Sci. 2011;310:21–4.
41. Baba T, Kikuchi A, Hirayama K, et al. Severe olfactory dysfunction is a prodromal symptom of dementia associated with Parkinson's disease: a 3 year longitudinal study. Brain. 2012;135:161–9.
42. Olichney JM, Murphy C, Hofstetter CR, et al. Anosmia is very common in the Lewy body variant of Alzheimer's disease. J Neurol Neurosurg Psychiatry. 2005;76:1342–7.
43. Rana AQ, Saeed U, Sufian Masroor M, et al. A cross-sectional study investigating clinical predictors and physical experiences of pain in Parkinson's disease. Funct Neurol. 2013;28:297–304.
44. Kassubek J, Chaudhuri KR, Zesiewicz T, et al. Rotigotine transdermal system and evaluation of pain in patients with Parkinson's disease: a post hoc analysis of the RECOVER study. BMC Neurol. 2014;14:42.
45. Cury RG, Galhardoni R, Fonoff ET, et al. Effects of deep brain stimulation on pain and other nonmotor symptoms in Parkinson disease. Neurology. 2014;83:1403–9.
46. Friedman JH, Brown RG, Comella C, et al. Fatigue in Parkinson's disease: a review. Mov Disord. 2007;22:297–308.
47. Miwa H, Kondo T. Increased writing activity in Parkinson's disease: a punding-like behavior? Parkinsonism Relat Disord. 2005;11:323–5.
48. Weintraub D, Siderowf AD, Potenza MN, et al. Association of dopamine agonist use with impulse control disorders in Parkinson disease. Arch Neurol. 2006;63:969–73.
49. Voon V, Hassan K, Zurowski M, et al. Prevalence of repetitive and reward-seeking behaviors in Parkinson disease. Neurology. 2006;67:1254–7.
50. Aarsland D, Andersen K, Larsen JP, et al. Prevalence and characteristics of dementia in Parkinson disease: an 8-year prospective study. Arch Neurol. 2003;60:387–92.

Chapter 9
Autonomic Symptoms in Dementia with Lewy Bodies

Satoshi Orimo

Abstract In patients with dementia with Lewy bodies (DLB) as well as Parkinson's disease, Lewy bodies and Lewy neurites are observed in not only the central nervous system but also the peripheral autonomic nervous system. The peripheral autonomic nervous system innervates various organs such as the esophagus, stomach, intestines, heart, urinary bladder, and skin. Thus, various kinds of symptoms, signs, and abnormal autonomic test findings are observed in patients with DLB. Because of this, Lewy body disease is often viewed as a systemic disorder. Severe autonomic dysfunction is one of the supportive features in the revised diagnostic criteria for DLB. Three of the other supportive features including repeated falls, syncope, and transient loss of consciousness can also be partly attributed to the presence of autonomic dysfunction. Furthermore, reduced cardiac *meta*-iodobenzylguanidine (MIBG) uptake is also indicative of DLB and represents disturbances of the cardiac sympathetic nerve, implying autonomic dysfunction. Autonomic dysfunction occurs to a lesser extent in Alzheimer disease, vascular dementia, and frontotemporal dementia. Therefore, the presence of autonomic dysfunction is an important feature that differentiates DLB from other dementias.

Keywords Orthostatic hypotension • Postprandial hypotension • Urinary frequency • Constipation • Lewy bodies

9.1 Introduction

In patients with dementia with Lewy bodies (DLB), Lewy bodies and Lewy neurites immunostained by α-synuclein are observed in both the central and peripheral nervous systems [1, 2]. The same is true in Parkinson's disease (PD). The peripheral autonomic nervous system, including sympathetic and parasympathetic nerves, innervates various organs such as the esophagus, stomach, intestine, heart, urinary bladder, and skin (Fig. 9.1). As such, various symptoms and abnormal autonomic

S. Orimo (✉)
Department of Neurology, Kanto Central Hospital, 6-25-1 Kami-Yoga, Setagaya-ku, 158-8531 Tokyo, Japan
e-mail: sorimo0307@nifty.com; orimo@kanto-ctr-hsp.com

K. Kosaka (ed.), *Dementia with Lewy Bodies*, DOI 10.1007/978-4-431-55948-1_9

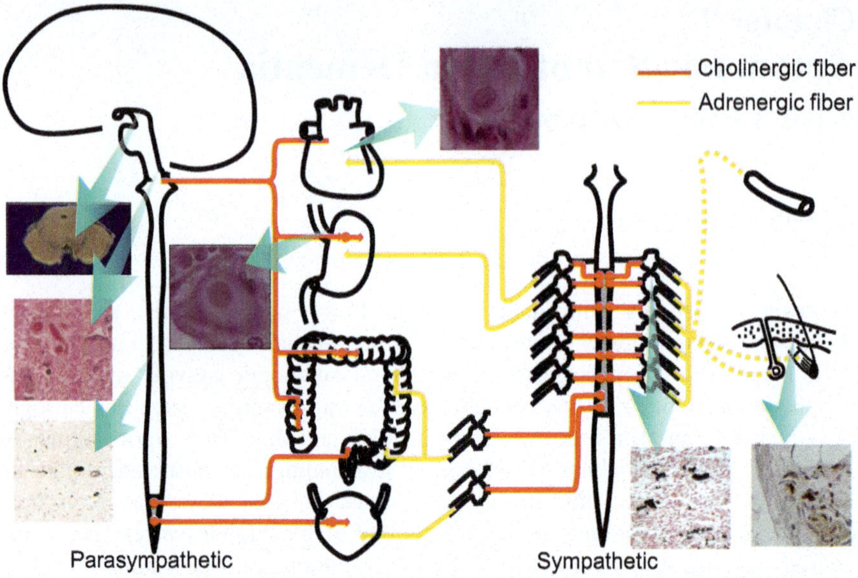

Fig. 9.1 In patients with Lewy body disease, Lewy bodies and Lewy neurites are observed in not only the central nervous system but also the peripheral autonomic nervous system. The peripheral autonomic nervous system, including sympathetic and parasympathetic nerves, innervates various organs such as the esophagus, the stomach, the intestine, the heart, the urinary bladder, and the skin

test findings are observed in patients with DLB. Lewy body disease is often considered a systemic disorder. Autonomic dysfunction is a well-known feature of α-synucleinopathies, including PD, DLB, and multiple system atrophy (MSA). Severe autonomic dysfunction is one of the supportive features in the revised diagnostic criteria for DLB [3], along with repeated falls, syncope, and transient loss of consciousness, which can also be partly attributed to autonomic dysfunction [3]. Reduced cardiac *meta*-iodobenzylguanidine (MIBG) uptake is also observed in patients with DLB [4, 5] and is indicative of a DLB diagnosis [3]. It represents disturbances of the cardiac sympathetic nerve due to degeneration [6], implying autonomic dysfunction. Autonomic dysfunction occurs to a lesser extent in Alzheimer disease (AD), vascular dementia (VaD), and frontotemporal dementia (FTD) [7]. Therefore, the presence of autonomic dysfunction is an important clinical feature that can differentiate DLB from other dementias.

9.2 Anatomical Structures Involved in Autonomic Dysfunction

Anatomical structures involved in autonomic dysfunction include: forebrain components, the hypothalamus, brainstem components, spinal cord components, and the peripheral autonomic nervous system [8, 9]. Relevant forebrain structures include the insular cortex, the anterior cingulate cortex, and the amygdala. Brainstem components include the periaqueductal gray matter of the midbrain, parabrachial nucleus, locus coeruleus, nucleus of the solitary tract, dorsal motor nucleus of the vagus, ventrolateral medulla, nucleus ambiguous, and nucleus raphe pallidus. Spinal cord structures include the intermediolateral cell column, the sacral parasympathetic nucleus, and the Onuf nucleus [8]. The peripheral autonomic nervous system includes parasympathetic and sympathetic ganglia, as well as parasympathetic and sympathetic nerves, which innervate various organs.

Different structures of the forebrain can be affected in AD and FTD [10, 11]. The hypothalamus and parts of the brainstem are involved in PD, PD with dementia (PDD), and Lewy body disease [12–14]. Spinal cord structures are involved in incidental Lewy body disease (iLBD), PD, PDD, and DLB [2, 15–18]. In the peripheral autonomic nervous system, Lewy bodies and Lewy neurites are found in various bodily regions. In iLBD, PD, and DLB, Lewy bodies and Lewy neurites can be found in the sympathetic ganglia [1, 2, 16, 19]. In iLBD and PD, Lewy bodies and Lewy neurites can be found in the stomach and distal part of the esophagus [20]. In iLBD patients, Lewy bodies and Lewy neurites are also found in Meissner's plexus and the sympathetic trunk in 82 % of patients [16] and in the epicardial nerve fascicle in 90 % of patients [21]. In one study, Lewy bodies were also found in the sinoatrial node from 33 to 50 % of patients with Lewy body disease [22]. Degeneration of the cardiac nerve fibers in the right atrium and conducting system of the heart has also been observed in Lewy body disease [23]. Minguez-Castellanos examined surgical specimens from 100 patients without apparent neurological disorder, ranging in age from 44 to 84 years, and reported that α-synuclein aggregates were found in the abdominopelvic autonomic plexuses in 9 % of the whole sample, but were more common in vesicoprostatic (26.1 %) than in digestive tract specimens (3.9 %) [24]. Navarro-Otano examined surgical heart specimens from 91 patients without parkinsonism ranging in age from 31 to 84 years and reported that α-synuclein aggregates were found in the epicardial fat tissues in 7.7 % of the whole sample [25]. Recently, Gelpi performed a postmortem histopathological study of the brain and peripheral tissues from 28 patients. All 15 patients with DLB demonstrated α-synuclein aggregates in the peripheral autonomic nervous system via lesions in the stellate, sympathetic ganglia (100 %), the vagus nerve (86.7 %), gastrointestinal tract (86.7 %), adrenal gland, and/or surrounding fat (53.3 %), heart (100 %), and genitourinary tract (13.3 %) [26]. These reports confirm that lesions of the peripheral autonomic nervous system and parts of the central autonomic system cause various symptoms and abnormal findings upon autonomic testing in patients with DLB, even in the very early stages.

9.3 Autonomic Symptoms

Horimoto and colleagues reported autonomic symptoms and signs in nearly all 29 autopsy-confirmed patients with DLB that they investigated [27]. Prior to death, urinary incontinence was observed in 97 % of the patients, constipation in 83 %, hypotension in 66 %, syncope in 28 %, and urinary retention in 28 %. Some autonomic symptoms occur prior to cognitive decline and are thought to be prodromal symptoms of DLB, including constipation (−9.2 years before onset) and orthostatic hypotension (OH) (−1.2 years before onset) [28]. OH is defined as a reduction of systolic blood pressure (BP) of at least 20 mm Hg or a reduction of diastolic BP of at least 10 mm Hg within 3 min of standing [29]. The defining symptom of OH is syncope. Syncope is the abrupt and transient loss of consciousness associated with the absence of postural tone, followed by complete and usually rapid spontaneous recovery.

9.3.1 Case Presentation

An 81-year-old man had been suffering from severe constipation. He was admitted to the hospital because of paralytic ileus at 71, 75, and 79 years of age. Upon discharge, he was given medicine for constipation. He also had frequency of urination. Around 80 years of age, he started experiencing occasional hallucinations, stumbling while walking, and his head began to bend forward. Visual hallucinations included viewing small bits of garbage as insects and rolled-up cords as snakes. The patient also felt dizziness upon standing up. He came to our hospital and was diagnosed with probable DLB because of dementia (Mini-Mental State Examination score = 23), recurrent vivid hallucinations, parkinsonism, OH, and reduced cardiac MIBG uptake. The results of a Schellong test showed severe OH (Table 9.1). He was successfully treated with donepezil for dementia and hallucination; amezinium for OH; solifenacin for frequency of urination; mosapride, magnesium oxide, and Daikenchuto (a traditional Chinese medicine) for severe constipation; and levodopa/carbidopa for parkinsonism. He showed several autonomic symptoms and signs prior to cognitive/neuropsychological symptoms.

9.3.2 Cardiovascular Autonomic Symptoms

9.3.2.1 The Control of Blood Pressure

When BP changes, BP is physiologically stabilized by three time-dependent mechanisms. Acutely, both sympathetic and parasympathetic input regulate

Table 9.1 Schellong test

10 min after the supine position	
	BP146/76 mm Hg HR78/m
Immediately after standing	
	BP 73/52 mm Hg HR86/m,dizziness
1 min)	BP 96/63 mm Hg HR86/m
2 min)	BP102/65 mm Hg HR93/m
3 min)	BP111/65 mm Hg HR88/m
4 min)	BP108/69 mm Hg HR89/m
5 min)	BP108/73 mm Hg HR89/m
Supine	
1 min)	BP148/80 mm Hg HR88/m
2 min)	BP157/83 mm Hg HR83/m
3 min)	BP154/80 mm Hg HR82/m

baroreceptors that can control BP within a few seconds or minutes. Intermediate BP control occurs within a few minutes and can last a few hours and is caused by vasoconstriction due to cardiopulmonary pressure reflexes and the release of vasopressin humoral factor. The renin-aldosterone system exerts long BP control within a few hours and can last days. The acute phase of neurologic control of BP is mainly achieved by the baroreceptor circuit. When a person stands, around 500–800 ml of blood pools in the lower extremities and visceral circulation, which causes reductions in venous return, cardiac output, and arterial BP, which results in the unloading of the baroreceptors. Reduced baroreceptor activity then leads to increased BP in two ways. One is to inhibit the vagal activity of the heart; the other is to stimulate peripheral and cardiac sympathetic activity. Finally, noradrenaline is released from the sympathetic nerve endings, resulting in increased peripheral arterial resistance, heart rate, and contractility of the heart. Neurogenic OH can occur due to disturbances anywhere in this circuit. In a study of patients with limbic or neocortical stage DLB, Lewy bodies and Lewy neurites were found in the ventrolateral medulla, which controls sympathetic output. Despite this, the number of tyrosine hydroxylase- and tryptophan hydroxylase-immunoreactive neurons was not significantly reduced compared to control subjects [14]. Thus, in DLB, OH may be primarily caused by involvement of sympathetic ganglia and postganglionic sympathetic nerves, rather than ventrolateral medulla neurons [14].

9.3.2.2 Symptoms and Signs Related to OH

Syncope can increase the risk for bone fracture or head trauma due to fall. Another symptom of OH is orthostatic intolerance, manifested by transient postural dizziness, lightheadedness, blurred vision, cognitive slowing, fatigue, weakness of the legs, and loss of attention. In elderly subjects, OH may occur in various non-neurogenic conditions such as dehydration and volume depletion and may be caused by various kinds of drugs, including alcohol, alpha blockers (terazosin), antidepressant drugs (selective serotonin receptor reuptake inhibitors, trazodone, monoamine oxidase inhibitors, tricyclic antidepressants), antihypertensive drugs (sympathetic blockers), antiparkinsonism drugs (levodopa, pramipexole, ropinirole), antipsychotic drugs (olanzapine, risperidone), beta-blocker drugs (propranolol), diuretic drugs (hydrochlorothiazide, furosemide), muscle relaxant drugs (tizanidine), narcotic analgesic drugs (morphine), phosphodiesterase inhibitors (sildenafil, tadalafil), and vasodilator drugs (hydralazine, nitroglycerin, calcium channel blockers) [30]. All these conditions may also aggravate preexisting OH [31, 32]. Cholinesterase inhibitors (donepezil, rivastigmine, and galantamine) may cause syncope due to bradyarrhythmia [33]. Furthermore, long-standing hypotension may worsen the process of dementia [34, 35]. In patients with DLB, OH is found in 42–70 % [7, 36, 37] and symptomatic OH is found in 31–50 % [7, 36–38] of patients. Syncope is found in 17 % of patients [28] and was found present before death in 28 % of autopsy-confirmed patients with DLB [27]. Patients with persistent OH have a significantly shorter survival time compared to those with no or nonpersistent OH [38]. OH is less frequent in patients with AD and FTD [7].

9.3.2.3 Postprandial Hypotension

Postprandial hypotension (PPH) is a reduction in BP during or after food intake and is sometimes observed in patients with autonomic dysfunction. Symptoms include cognitive slowing, loss of attention, dizziness, and decreased consciousness during or after food intake. PPH can be a risk for aspiration or suffocation. The pathophysiology of PPH is related to splanchnic vasodilation and the release of vasodilatory gut peptides such as neurotensin and is not accompanied by compensatory changes in cardiac output or skeletal muscle resistance vessels [39]. PPH is defined as a reduction of systolic BP of more than 20 mm Hg while being in the supine position [40]. In our studies, the incidence of PPH in DLB was 3/27 (11.1 %) compared to 1/15 (0.07 %) in AD [41]. Figure 9.2 shows a 24-h ambulatory electrocardiogram (ECG) and BP of an 85-year-old man with DLB. PPH is clearly found after breakfast and supper.

9.3.2.4 Supine (Recumbent) Hypertension

Patients with OH sometimes exhibit hypertension while lying down. This paradoxical hypertension is called supine hypertension (SH) or recumbent hypertension. The exact criteria for SH have not been defined. SH often goes undetected because BP is usually measured only in the seated position; therefore, the actual prevalence of this complication is not known. In an experiment where SH was defined as a systolic BP $\geq$ 150 mm Hg or diastolic BP $\geq$ 90 mm Hg in patients with OH, 65 of 117 (56 %) patients with severe autonomic failure like MSA and pure autonomic failure showed SH, despite normal seated and low upright BPs [42]. SH can be severe, and it complicates the treatment of OH. In particular, medications used for

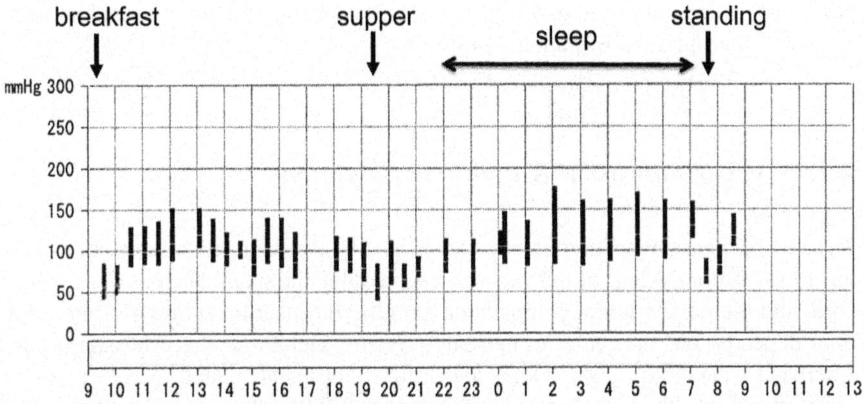

Fig. 9.2 The results of a 24-h ambulatory ECG and BP of an 85-year-old man with DLB are shown. They show OH and PPH after breakfast and supper together with SH in sleep. *OH* orthostatic hypotension, *PPH* postprandial hypotension, *SH* supine hypertension

the treatment of OH may worsen SH. Possible explanations of SH are impaired baroreflex buffering of the BP, inappropriate natriuresis, higher blood volume, and residual sympathetic tone acting on hypersensitive postsynaptic adrenoreceptors [42–45]. In our studies, the incidence of OH and SH in patients with DLB was 13/27 (48 %) and 4/27 (0.15 %) compared to 1/15 (0.07 %) and 1/15 (0.07 %) in patients with AD, respectively [41]. Figure 9.2 shows a 24-h ambulatory ECG and BP of an 85-year-old man with DLB. SH is shown during sleep.

9.3.3 *Urinary Autonomic Symptoms*

Normal urinary storage is dependent on the sacral autonomic reflex and is facilitated by several brain regions, including the pontine storage center, the hypothalamus, the cerebellum, the basal ganglia, and the frontal cortex [46]. Normal micturition is dependent on the spino-bulbo-spinal autonomic reflex, which is related to the midbrain periaqueductal gray matter and the pontine micturition center [46]. Bladder dysfunction can occur as a result of deficits in any of these regions. In PD, bladder dysfunction is related to altered dopamine-basal ganglia circuits [47]. This is likely the case in DLB, as well [48]. Urinary autonomic dysfunction includes both storage and voiding dysfunctions.

The symptoms of storage dysfunction are increased urinary frequency during the day and at night (nocturia), urgency, and urge incontinence. The symptoms of voiding dysfunction are difficulty of voiding, residual urine, and urinary retention. In patients with DLB, the frequencies of storage dysfunction symptoms are urgency in 93 % of patients, urge incontinence in 53 %, and overactive bladder in 92 % [49]. These symptoms tend to be much more severe than in PD patients [49]. On the other hand, the symptoms of voiding dysfunction characterized by residual urine are only found in 27 % of patients [48].

9.3.4 Gastrointestinal Autonomic Symptoms

The extrinsic gastrointestinal tract is innervated by the parasympathetic nerve from the dorsal motor nucleus of the vagus in the medulla, the sacral nucleus of the spinal cord, and the paravertebral sympathetic ganglia. Intrinsic innervation of the intestine depends on the enteric nervous system including the Meissner's and Auerbach's plexuses. Lewy bodies and Lewy neurites are found in both extrinsic and intrinsic intestinal innervation in PD and DLB [50]. In the gastrointestinal tract, one study showed a rostrocaudal gradient of decreasing Lewy body and Lewy neurite frequency and density, with the lower esophagus and submandibular gland showing the greatest involvement and the colon and rectum showing the lowest [2]. Lewy bodies and Lewy neurites play a significant role in esophageal dysmotility, delayed gastric emptying, and colonic dysfunction [27, 51].

Gastrointestinal autonomic dysfunction includes dysphagia, abdominal distention, fecal incontinence, and constipation. Aggravating factors are dehydration, immobility, a diet low in fiber, and medications such as diuretics, iron, antihypertensive, antipsychotics, anticholinergics, anticonvulsants, and opioids analgesics [51]. In patients with PD, PDD, and DLB, complications include gastric retention, fecal impaction, and paralytic ileus. As described in 9.3.1 case presentation, paralytic ileus can be an initial manifestation of DLB patients. Delayed gastric emptying slows the absorption of levodopa into the duodenum and reduces its bioavailability. Constipation is the most prominent gastrointestinal manifestation [52, 53] and is observed in 28–86 % of patients with DLB [27, 28, 52]. Figure 9.3 shows a chest CT scan of an 83-year-old woman with PDD. She was admitted to our hospital because of vomiting. The CT scan shows retention of foods in the lower esophagus.

9.3.5 Sudomotor Autonomic and Thermoregulatory Symptoms

Thermoregulatory and emotional sweating are controlled by several regions of the central nervous system including the hypothalamus, the limbic areas, and the brainstem, as well as the intermediolateral column of the spinal cord, in the sympathetic ganglia, and the postganglionic fibers to the sweat glands [51]. In DLB, sudomotor dysfunction is related to either central or peripheral lesions, according to the wide distribution of Lewy bodies and Lewy neurites [54]. Ikemura and colleagues reported that phosphorylated α-synuclein immunoreactivity was

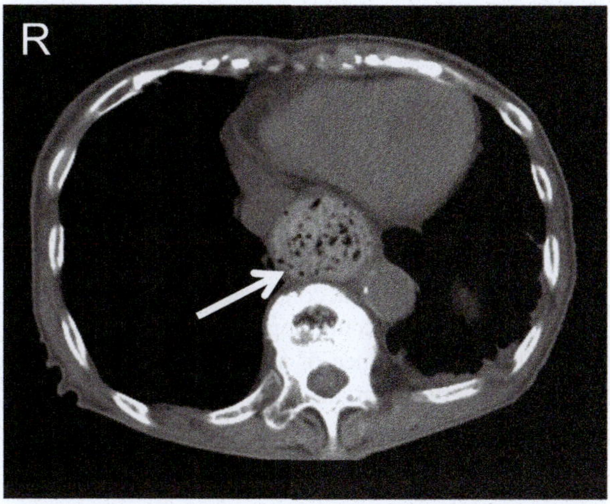

Fig. 9.3 A chest CT scan of an 83-year-old woman with PDD is shown. She was admitted to our hospital because of vomiting. The CT scan shows retention of foods in the lower esophagus

found in the skin from 20 of 85 autopsy-confirmed patients with DLB. These aggregates were localized to the blood vessels and arrector pili muscles together with what appeared to be eccrine glands [55]. Thermoregulatory dysfunction is caused by sudomotor dysfunction and skin vasomotor dysfunction.

Sweating symptoms include hyperhidrosis, hypohidrosis, or anhidrosis. Hypo- and anhidrosis are usually observed in the extremities, especially lower extremities. Hyperhidrosis is observed in the face, neck, and trunk of patients with DLB and is caused by compensatory mechanisms adjusting for the hypohidrosis and anhidrosis in the extremities [56]. Heat retention can also be observed in patients with Lewy body disease. A 71-year-old man with PD showed high fever (38–39 °C) in July, due to heat retention caused by anhidrosis below the trunk and lower limbs [57]. Slight fever was found in 72 % of autopsy-confirmed patients with DLB [27].

9.3.6 Sexual Dysfunction

The genital organs primarily share lumbosacral innervation with the lower urinary tract [46]. Sexual dysfunction includes erectile dysfunction, ejaculation difficulty, and change in libido [46]. Comprehensive assessment of sexual dysfunction in patients with DLB showed that change of libido was the most frequent symptom [58].

9.3.7 *Prodromal Symptoms*

In patients with DLB, some symptoms manifest prior to the onset of cognitive decline. Subjects with these symptoms have what is considered prodromal DLB. The DSM-5 has proposed the definition, "mild neurocognitive disorder due to Lewy bodies," which is roughly equivalent to prodromal DLB [59]. Symptoms of prodromal DLB are divided in three categories: cognitive impairment, behavioral/psychiatric phenomena, and physical symptoms [60]. Physical symptoms include parkinsonism, hyposmia, constipation, and OH. Constipation occurs approximately 9.2 years and OH occurs approximately 1.2 years prior to memory disturbance [28]. Thus, the presence of symptoms and signs associated with autonomic dysfunction is very important to differentiate DLB from other dementias even in the very early stage.

9.4 Autonomic Function Tests

9.4.1 *Tests for Orthostatic Dysregulation*

There are two kinds of head-up postural challenge tests, which can test for OH. One is the Schellong test and the other is a head-up tilt test. A head-up tilt test is performed using a tilt table. In both tests, each subject is in the supine position for 10 min. In the Schellong test, subjects then stand up by themselves. In the head-up tilt test, subjects are lifted in the head-up position at least 60° using a tilt table within 15 s of lift up (head-up tilt test). When a reduction of systolic BP of at least 20 mm Hg or diastolic BP of at least 10 mm Hg occurs within 3 min after the upright position, they are diagnosed with OH [29]. OH is found in 42–70 % of patients with DLB [7, 36, 37], and symptomatic OH is found in 31–50 % [7, 36–38] of patients.

9.4.2 *Heart Rate Variability*

Heart rate variability (HRV) is the variation in the time intervals between heartbeats. It is measured by the variation in the beat-to-beat interval using an ECG. HRV parameters include time-domain and frequency-domain variables [61]. Time-domain variables are (1) standardized deviation of all normal-to-normal (NN) (SDNN) intervals as an estimate of overall HRV, (2) root mean square successive differences of NN (RMSSD) intervals as an indicator of parasympathetic activity, and (3) percentage of consecutive RR intervals differing by more than 50 ms (pNN50) as an indicator of parasympathetic activity. Frequency-domain variables are the following: (1) High-frequency domain (HF, 0.15–0.4 Hz) reflects the respiratory sinus rhythm mediated by cardiac vagal control. (2) Low-frequency domain (LF, 0.04–0.15 Hz) is associated with both sympathetic and parasympathetic activity. (3) Very low frequency (VLF, <0.04 Hz) may involve thermoregulatory and peripheral vascular mechanisms. (4) Total spectral power (total power) shows the balance of NN intervals over the temporal segment and the global measure of HRV. (5) The LF/HF ratio may indicate sympathovagal balance [61].

In patients with dementia, reduced HL was observed in PDD, DLB, AD, VaD, and control patients, in that order. Reduced LF was observed in PDD, DLB, VaD, AD, and control patients, in that order [7]. In patients with DLB, almost all the parameters of HRV including SDNN, pNN50, RMSSD, VLF, LF, HF, and total power showed a significant decrease compared to those in patients with AD [61].

9.4.3 Valsalva Maneuver

The Valsalva maneuver can assess autonomic function in hemodynamics. It has been shown that findings from this maneuver are highly sensitive and reproducible for the assessment of arterial baroreflex [62]. In the Valsalva maneuver, patients are asked to exhale into a mouthpiece at an expiratory pressure of 40 mm Hg for 15 s. The maneuver generates a cascade of events involving baroreflexes, heart, and arterial vasoconstriction. It results in a stoppage of venous return, which causes a drop in BP, activation of baroreflex, reflex tachycardia, and peripheral vasoconstriction. BP and RR intervals are measured during the maneuver by tonometry, using a noninvasive BP monitoring system. The duration of the Valsalva maneuver is divided into four phases. Phase I is the inspiration phase. Phase II is the phase of blowing into the mouthpiece, with an increase in thoracic pressure to 40 mm Hg. Systolic BP decreases in early phase II because of reduced cardiac output, in turn decreasing venous return and stroke volume, despite tachycardia caused by the withdrawal of cardiovagal control. The decrease in systolic BP is arrested within 8 s at least. Late phase II is associated with an increase in BP, reflecting the activation of vasomotor sympathetic nerves. A transient fall in BP (phase III), lasting 1–2 s, occurs at the end of Valsalva maneuver, because of sudden drops in intrathoracic and abdominal pressures. Phase IV is the overshoot of BP due to the activation of cardiac sympathetic nerves. BP fell in early phase II, but increased in late phase II because of an increase in efferent sympathetic gain in a control subject (Fig. 9.4a). In a patient with DLB associated with autonomic failure, there is no increase in BP, and BP decreased in late phase II (Fig. 9.4b) [63]. Transient BP overshoot in phase IV is noted in the control subject, but not in the patient with DLB [63]. Changes in RR intervals are lacking in the patient with DLB as compared with the control subject [63].

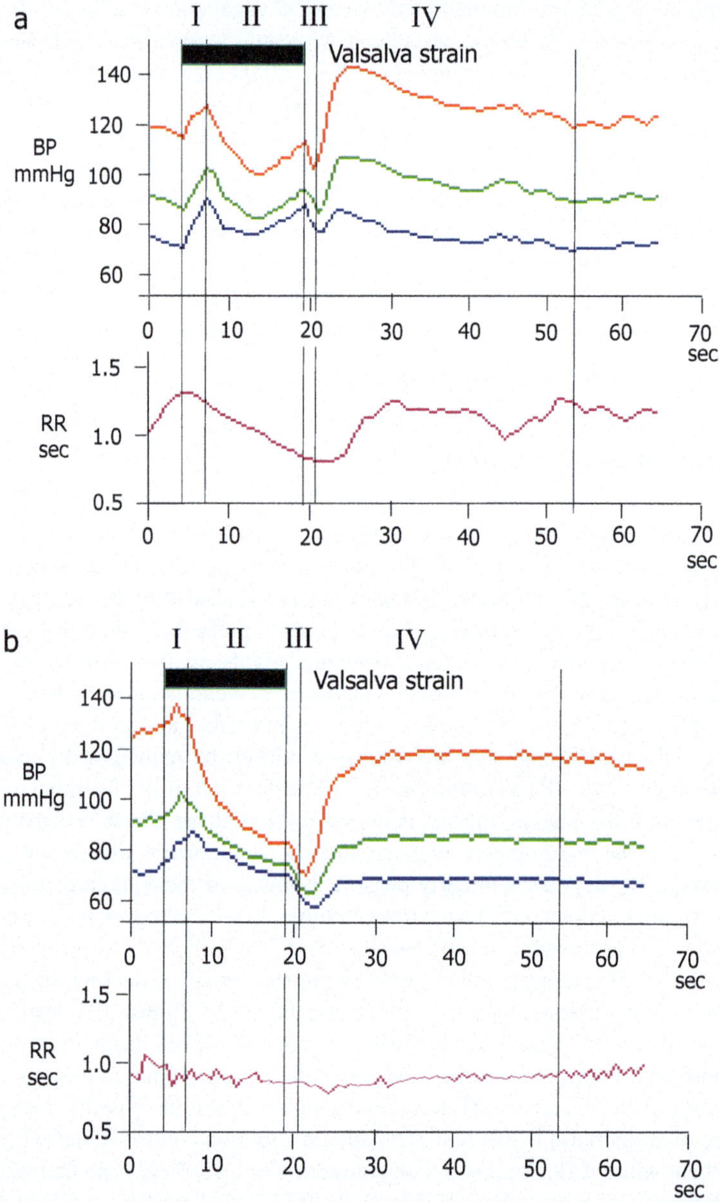

Fig. 9.4 The changes in BP and RR interval during Valsalva maneuver in a control subject (**a**) and a patient with DLB (**b**). The duration of the Valsalva maneuver is divided into four phases. Phase I is the inspiration phase. Phase II is the phase of blowing into the mouthpiece, with an increase in thoracic pressure to 40 mm Hg. Systolic BP decreases in early phase II because of reduced cardiac output, in turn decreasing venous return and stroke volume, despite tachycardia caused by the withdrawal of cardiovagal control. The decrease in systolic BP is arrested within 8 s at least. Late phase II is associated with an increase in BP, reflecting the activation of vasomotor sympathetic nerves. A transient fall in BP (phase III), lasting 1–2 s, occurs at the end of Valsalva maneuver, because of sudden drops in intrathoracic and abdominal pressures. Phase IV is the overshoot of BP

9.4.4 Carotid Sinus Massage Test

Carotid sinus syndrome (CSS) is characterized by exaggerated vagal responses, such as bradycardia and hypotension, to carotid sinus stimulation. The syndrome manifests clinically as dizziness, syncope, and falling. CSS testing is carried out after each subject is in the supine position for 10 min. Firm massage is applied over the right carotid sinus for five seconds. When subjects show a prolongation of an RR interval of more than three seconds or severe reduction of systolic BP, they are diagnosed with CSS. The prevalence of CSS was 31.5 % (12/38) in patients with DLB, 11.5 % (6/52) in AD, and 3.2 % (1/31) in control subjects [64].

9.4.5 Urodynamic Tests

Urodynamic tests consist of uroflowmetry, measurement of postvoid residuals, electromyography-cystometry, and pressure-flow analysis. In patients with DLB, detrusor over activity was found in 87.1 %, whereas postvoid residual was minimal. Neurogenic changes by the sphincter motor unit potential analysis were shown in 50 % [65].

9.4.6 Sudomotor/Skin Vasomotor Function Test

The sympathetic sweat response (SSwR), sympathetic skin response (SSR), and skin vasomotor reflex (SkVR) are autonomically controlled, homeostatic mechanisms. The SSwR is a transient rise of sweat secretion, the SSR is a transient change in skin potential, and the SkVR is a transient reduction of skin blood flow in the palm or sole, following a variety of internal or externally applied arousal stimuli. SSwR and SSR reflect emotional sweating, but are also evoked by nonemotional stimuli. SSwR is usually evoked with SkVR. Although the central pathways of SSwR, SSR, and SkVR have not yet been determined, the final afferent pathways are postganglionic sympathetic fibers. Therefore, SSwR, SSR, and SkVR tests are useful for the assessment of cutaneous autonomic function. SSR testing is easy to apply, but current procedures are not sufficiently reliable for diagnostic purposes

Fig. 9.4 (continued) due to the activation of cardiac sympathetic nerves. BP fell in early phase II, but increased in late phase II because of an increase in efferent sympathetic gain in a control subject (**a**). In a patient with DLB associated with autonomic failure, there is no increase in BP, and BP decreased in late phase II (**b**). Transient BP overshoot in phase IV is noted in the control subject, but not in the patient with DLB. Changes in RR intervals are lacking in the patient with DLB as compared with the control subject (Courtesy of Hisayoshi Oka, Jikei University School of Medicine, personal communication). I, phase I; II, phase II; III, phase III; IV, phase IV

and show imperfect correlations with both clinical features and other autonomic tests, in particular, sudomotor dysfunction. In one study, SSwR was found severely damaged in all patients with Lewy body disease compared to normal subjects, whereas SkVR was severely damaged in DLB and PDD, but not in PD [54]. Recently, it was reported that the amplitude of SSR was highly abnormal in patients with DLB at sensitivities of 85 % compared to patients with AD at sensitivity of 15 % [66].

9.4.7 Composite Autonomic Scoring Scale

The composite autonomic scoring scale (CASS) is an indicator of severity of sudomotor, cardiovagal, and adrenergic dysfunctions. This autonomic reflex screen consists of five components: (1) the quantitative sudomotor axon reflex test (QSART), which consists of one upper and three lower limb test sites; (2) orthostatic BP and heart rate response to head-up tilt; (3) heart rate response to deep breathing; (4) the Valsalva ratio; and (5) beat-to-beat BP measurements during the Valsalva maneuver [67]. In a study comparing scores, all the scores of CASS-sudomotor, CASS-cardiovagal, and CASS-adrenergic were highest in MSA patients, intermediate in DLB, and lowest in PD patients [68].

9.4.8 Pharmacological Pupil Function Test

Normal pupillary constriction is a balance between the parasympathetic (pupillary constriction) and sympathetic (pupillary dilatation) nervous systems. The pathway of pupillary constriction begins at the Edinger-Westphal nucleus. The fibers enter the superficial part of the oculomotor nerve and ultimately synapse at the ciliary ganglion. Postganglionic parasympathetic nerves travel forward to the ciliary muscle and iris sphincter. Sympathetic innervation begins at the hypothalamus where the neurons connect from higher centers, including the cortex. Postsynaptic neurons travel down through the brainstem and finally exit through the cervical sympathetic chain and the superior cervical ganglion. They synapse at the superior cervical ganglion, where third-order neurons travel through the carotid plexus and enter into the orbit through the first division of the trigeminal nerve [69]. A pharmacological pupil function test is a method to detect local or systemic autonomic dysfunction using denervation supersensitivity of pupils innervated by parasympathetic and sympathetic nerves. One study demonstrated that the mydriatic response to 0.5 % phenylephrine, a sympathetic agonist, was significantly greater in patients with DLB than in patients with AD and control subjects [70]. On the other hand, miotic response to 0.0625 % pilocarpine, a cholinergic agonist, was significantly greater in patients with DLB and AD than in control subjects, implying that a pharmacological pupil function test can differentiate DLB from AD [70].

9.4.9 Other Tests

The 24-h ambulatory ECG and BP tests are not autonomic tests, but rather useful methods to detect PPH or SH, as mentioned before (Sect. 9.3.2.3). MIBG cardiac scintigraphy and ventilatory response to hypercapnia are described in Chaps. 12 and 15, respectively.

References

1. Wakabayashi K, Mori F, Tanji K, et al. Involvement of the peripheral nervous system in synucleinopathies, tauopathies and other neurodegenerative proteinopathies of the brain. Acta Neuropathol. 2010;120(1):1–12.
2. Beach TD, Alder CH, Sue LI, et al. Multi-organ distribution of phosphorylated α-synuclein histopathology in subjects with Lewy body disorders. Acta Neuropathol. 2010;119 (6):689–702.
3. McKeith IG, Dickson DW, Lowe J, et al. Diagnosis and management of dementia with Lewy bodies: third report of the DLB Consortium. Neurology. 2005;65:1863–72.
4. Watanabe H, et al. Cardiac ^{123}I-meta-iodobenzylguanidine (MIBG) uptake in dementia with Lewy bodies: comparison with Alzheimer's disease. J Neurol Neurosurg Psychiatry. 2001;70:781–3.
5. Yoshita M, et al. A clinical role for[^{123}I-MIBG myocardial scintigraphy in the distinction between dementia of the Alzheimer's-type and dementia with Lewy bodies. J Neurol Neurosurg Psychiatry. 2001;71:583–8.
6. Orimo S, Amino T, Ito Y, et al. Cardiac sympathetic denervation precedes neuronal loss in the sympathetic ganglia in Lewy body disease. Acta Neuropathol (Berl). 2005;109:583–8.
7. Allan LM, Ballard CG, Allen J, et al. Autonomic dysfunction in dementia. J Neurol Neurosurg Psychiatry. 2007;78:671–7.
8. Benarroch EE. Central autonomic control. In: Robertson D, Bioggioni I, Burnstock G, Low PA, Paton JFR, editors. Primer on the autonomic nervous system. 3rd ed. London: Academic; 2012. p. 9–12.
9. Hamill RW, Schapiro RE, Vizzard MA. Peripheral autonomic nervous system. In: Robertson D, Bioggioni I, Burnstock G, Low PA, Paton JFR, editors. Primer on the autonomic nervous system. 3rd ed. London: Academic; 2012. p. 17–26.
10. Perneczky R, Diehl-Schmid J, Förstl H, et al. Urinary incontinence and its functional anatomy in frontotemporal lobar degenerations. Eur J Nucl Med Mol Imaging. 2008;35:605–10.
11. Chu CC, Tranel D, Damasio AR, et al. The autonomic-related cortex: pathology in Alzheimer's disease. Cereb Cortex. 1997;7:86–95.
12. Langston JW, Forno LS. The hypothalamus in Parkinson disease. Ann Neurol. 1978;3:129–33.
13. Wakabayashi K, Takahashi H. Neuropathology of autonomic nervous system in Parkinson's disease. Eur Neurol. 1997;38 Suppl 2:2–7.
14. Benarroch EE, Schmeichel AM, Low PA, et al. Involvement of medullary regions controlling sympathetic output in Lewy body disease. Brain. 2005;128:338–44.

15. Wakabayashi K, Takahashi H. The intermediolateral nucleus and Clarke's column in Parkinson's disease. Acta Neuropathol. 1997;94(3):287–9.
16. Bloch A, Probst A, Bissig H, et al. Alpha-synuclein pathology of the spinal and peripheral autonomic nervous system in neurologically unimpaired elderly subjects. Neuropathol Appl Neurobiol. 2006;32(3):284–95.
17. Kaufmann H, Nahm K, Purohit D, et al. Autonomic failure as the initial presentation of Parkinson disease and dementia with Lewy bodies. Neurology. 2004;63(6):1093–5.
18. Iwasaki Y, Yokokawa Y, Aiba I, et al. Autopsy findings in a case of dementia with Lewy bodies with marked autonomic failure and repetitive cardiopulmonary arrest. Clin Neurol. 2005;45(8):596–9.
19. Iwanaga K, Wakabayashi K, Yoshimoto M, et al. Lewy body-type degeneration in cardiac plexus in Parkinson's and incidental Lewy body diseases. Neurology. 1999;52:1269–71.
20. Braak H, de Vos RA, Bohl J, et al. Gastric α-synuclein immunoreactive inclusions in Meissner's and Auerbach's plexuses in cases staged for Parkinson's disease-related brain pathology. Neurosci Lett. 2006;396:67–72.
21. Orimo S, Uchihara T, Nakamura A, et al. Axonal α-synuclein aggregates herald centripetal degeneration of cardiac sympathetic nerve in Parkinson's disease. Brain. 2008;131:642–50.
22. Okada Y, Ito Y, Aida J, et al. Lewy bodies in the sinoatrial nodal ganglion: clinicopathological studies. Pathol Int. 2004;54:682–7.
23. Ghebremedhin E, Del Tredici K, Langston JW, et al. Diminished tyrosine hydroxylase immunoreactivity in the cardiac conduction system and myocardium in Parkinson's disease: an anatomical study. Acta Neuropathol. 2009;118:777–84.
24. Minguez-Castellanos A, Chamorro CE, Escamilla-Sevilla F, et al. Do α-synuclein aggregates in autonomic plexuses predate Lewy body disorders? A cohort study. Neurology. 2007;68:2012–18.
25. Navarro-Otano J, Gelpi E, Mestres CA, et al. Alpha-synuclein aggregates in epicardial fat tissue in living subjects without parkinsonism. Parkinsonism Relat Disord. 2013;19:27–31.
26. Gelpi E, Navarro-Otano J, Tolosa E, et al. Multiple organ involvement by alpha-synuclein pathology in Lewy body disorders. Mov Disord. 2014;29:1010–18.
27. Horimoto Y, Matsumoto M, Akatsu H, et al. Autonomic dysfunctions in dementia with Lewy bodies. J Neurol. 2003;250:530–3.
28. Fujishiro H, Iseki E, Nakamura S, et al. Dementia with Lewy bodies: early diagnostic challenges. Psychogeriatrics. 2013;13:128–38.
29. The Consensus statement of American Autonomic Society and the American Academy of Neurology: consensus statement on the definition of orthostatic hypotension, pure autonomic failure, and multiple system atrophy. Neurology. 1996;46:1470.
30. Perlmuter LC, Sarda G, Casavant V, et al. A review of the etiology, associated comorbidities, and treatment of orthostatic hypotension. Am J Ther. 2013;20:279–91.
31. Freeman R. Clinical practice: neurogenic orthostatic hypotension. N Engl J Med. 2008;358:615–24.
32. Robertson D. The pathophysiology and diagnosis of orthostatic hypotension. Clin Auton Res. 2008;18 Suppl 1:2–7.
33. Rosenbloom MH, Finley RR, Scheinman MM, et al. Donepezil associated bradyarrhythmia in a patient with dementia with Lewy bodies (DLB). Alzheimer Dis Assoc Disord. 2010;24 (2):209–11.
34. Kenny RA, Kalaria R, Ballard C. Neurocardiovascular instability in cognitive impairment and dementia. Ann N Y Acad Sci. 2002;977:183–95.
35. Heims HC, Critchley HD, Martin NH, et al. Cognitive functioning in orthostatic hypotension due to pure autonomic failure. Clin Auton Res. 2006;16:113–20.
36. Sonnesyn H, Nilsen DW, Rongve A, et al. High prevalence of orthostatic hypotension in mild dementia. Dement Geriatr Cogn Disord. 2009;28:307–13.
37. Bengtsson-Lindberg M, Larsson V, Minthon L, et al. Lack of orthostatic symptoms in dementia patients. Clin Auton Res. 2015;25(2):87–94.

38. Stubendorff K, Aarsland D, Minthon L, et al. The impact of autonomic dysfunction on survival in patients with dementia with Lewy bodies and Parkinson's disease with dementia. PLoS One. 2012;7, e45451.
39. Mathias CJ, Bannister SR. Postprandial hypotension in autonomic disorders. In: Mathias CJ, Bannister SR, editors. Autonomic failure. 4th ed. New York: Oxford University Press; 1999. p. 283–95.
40. Hoeldtke RD. Postprandial hypotension. In: Low PA, editor. Clinical autonomic disorders. 2nd ed. Philadelphia: Lippincott-Raven; 1997. p. 737–46.
41. Kanbe Y, Orimo S, Yasuda A, et al. Autonomic dysfunction and sleep problem in dementia with Lewy bodies. Jpn J Geriatr Psychiatry. 2014;25:1243–53.
42. Shannon J, Jordan J, Costa F, et al. The hypertension of autonomic failure and its treatment. Hypertension. 1997;30:1062–7.
43. Biaggioni I, Robertson RM. Hypertension in orthostatic hypotension and autonomic dysfunction. Cardiol Clin. 2002;20:291–301.
44. Lagi A, Rossi A, Cornelli A, et al. Postural hypotension in hypertensive patients. Blood Press. 2003;12:340–4.
45. Wilcox CS, Puritz R, Lightman SL, et al. Plasma volume regulation in patients with progressive autonomic failure during changes in salt intake and posture. J Lab Clin Med. 1984;104:331–9.
46. Sakakibara R, Uchiyama T, Yamanishi T, et al. Genitourinary dysfunction in Parkinson's disease. Mov Disord. 2010;1:2–12.
47. Winge K, Fowler CJ. Bladder dysfunction in Parkinsonism: mechanisms, prevalence, symptoms, and management. Mov Disord. 2006;21:737–45.
48. Sakakibara R, Ito T, Uchiyama T, et al. Lower urinary tract function in dementia of Lewy body type. J Neurol Neurosurg Psychiatry. 2005;76:729–32.
49. Ransmayr GN, Holliger S, Schletterer K, et al. Lower urinary tract symptoms in dementia with Lewy bodies, Parkinson's disease, and Alzheimer's disease. Neurology. 2008;70:299–303.
50. Wakabayashi K, Takahashi H, Ohama E, Takeda S, Ikuta F. Lewy bodies in the visceral autonomic nervous system in Parkinson's disease. Adv Neurol. 1993;60:609–12.
51. Idiaquez J, Roman GC. Autonomic dysfunction in neurodegenerative dementias. J Neurol Sci. 2011;305:22–7.
52. Allan LM, McKeith I, Ballard CG, et al. The prevalence of autonomic symptoms in dementia and their association with physical activity, activities of daily living and quality of life. Dement Geriatr Cogn Disord. 2006;22:230–7.
53. Idiaquez J, Benarroch EE, Rosales H, et al. Autonomic and cognitive dysfunction in Parkinson's disease. Clin Auton Res. 2007;17:93–8.
54. Akaogi Y, Asahina M, Yamanaka Y, et al. Sudomotor, skin vasomotor, and cardiovascular reflexes in 3 clinical forms of Lewy body disease. Neurology. 2009;7(73):59–65.
55. Ikemura M, Saito Y, Sengoku R, et al. Lewy body pathology involves cutaneous nerves. J Neuropathol Exp Neurol. 2008;67:945–53.
56. Schestatsky P, Valls-Solé J, Ehlers JA, et al. Hyperhidrosis in Parkinson's disease. Mov Disord. 2006;21:1744–8.
57. Hazama Y, Asou Y, Nakamura K, et al. Case of Parkinson disease with heat retention due to sweating dysfunction [Article in Japanese]. Rinsho Shinkeigaku. 2010;50(3):151–5.
58. Bae HJ, Cheon SM, Kim JW. Autonomic dysfunctions in parkinsonian disorders. J Mov Disord. 2009;2(2):72–7.
59. American Psychiatric Association. Diagnostic and statistical manual of mental disorders: DSM-5. 5th ed. Arlington: American Psychiatric Association; 2013.
60. Donaghy PC, McKeith IG. The clinical characteristics of dementia with Lewy bodies and a consideration of prodromal diagnosis. Alzheimers Res Ther. 2014;6:46.
61. Kasanuki K, Iseki E, Fujishiro H, et al. Impaired heart rate variability in patients with dementia with Lewy bodies: efficacy of electrocardiogram as a supporting diagnostic marker. Parkinsonism Relat Disord. 2015. doi:10.1016/j.parkreldis.2015.04.024.

62. Sandroni P. Clinical evaluation of autonomic disorders: primer on the autonomic nervous system. 3rd ed. London: Academic; 2012. p. 377–82.
63. Oka H, Morita M, Onouchi K, et al. Cardiovascular autonomic dysfunction in dementia with Lewy bodies and Parkinson's disease. J Neurol Sci. 2007;15(254):72–7.
64. Kenny RA, Shaw FE, O'Brien JT, et al. Carotid sinus syndrome is common in dementia with Lewy bodies and correlates with deep white matter lesions. J Neurol Neurosurg Psychiatry. 2004;75:966–71.
65. Tateno F, Sakakibara R, Ogata T, et al. Lower urinary tract function in dementia with Lewy bodies (DLB). Mov Disord. 2015;30(3):411–15.
66. Negami M, Maruta T, Takeda C, et al. Sympathetic skin response and heart rate variability as diagnostic tools for the differential diagnosis of Lewy body dementia and Alzheimer's disease: a diagnostic test study. BMJ Open. 2013;3(3):e001796.
67. Low PA. Composite autonomic scoring scale for laboratory quantification of generalized autonomic failure. Mayo Clin Proc. 1993;68:748–52.
68. Thaisetthawatkul P, Boeve BF, Benarroch EE, et al. Autonomic dysfunction in dementia with Lewy bodies. Neurology. 2004;62:1804–9.
69. Smith SA, Smith SE. Pupil function: tests and disorders. In: Mathias CJ, Bannister SR, editors. Autonomic failure. 4th ed. New York: Oxford University Press; 1999. p. 245–53.
70. Hanyu H, Hirao K, Shimizu S, et al. Phenylephrine and pilocarpine eye drop test for dementia with Lewy bodies and Alzheimer's disease. Neurosci Lett. 2007;414:174–7.

Part IV
Biological Markers

Chapter 10
CT, MRI, SPECT, and PET in DLB

Koji Kasanuki and Eizo Iseki

Abstract Neuroimaging has been used to diagnose dementia with Lewy bodies (DLB) for the past two decades. Undoubtedly, structural and functional neuroimaging should be considered strong diagnostic tools; however, there is still limited evidence regarding early diagnosis. In this chapter, we summarize the accepted findings on neuroimaging modalities (computed topography [CT], magnetic resonance imaging [MRI], single-photon emission computed tomography [SPECT], and positron emission tomography [PET]) in probable DLB. We also review the findings seen during the early stages of DLB. Lastly, we briefly discuss the usefulness of these imaging modalities for the early diagnosis of DLB.

Keywords Computed topography (CT) • Magnetic resonance imaging (MRI) • Single-photon emission computed tomography (SPECT) • Positron emission tomography (PET) • Amyloid imaging

Neuroimaging has been used to diagnose dementia with Lewy bodies (DLB) for the past two decades. Undoubtedly, structural and functional neuroimaging should be considered strong diagnostic tools; however, there is still limited evidence regarding early diagnosis. In this chapter, we summarize the accepted findings on neuroimaging modalities (computed topography [CT], magnetic resonance imaging

K. Kasanuki (✉)
Department of Neuroscience, Mayo Clinic, 4500 San Pablo Road, Jacksonville
FL 32224, USA

Juntendo Tokyo Koto Geriatric Medical Center PET/CT Dementia Research Center, 3-3-20 Shinsuna, Koto-ku, Tokyo 136-0075, Japan

Department of Psychiatry, Juntendo University School of Medicine, 2-1-1 Hongo, Bunkyo-ku, Tokyo 113-8421, Japan
e-mail: Kasanuki.Koji@mayo.edu

E. Iseki
Juntendo Tokyo Koto Geriatric Medical Center PET/CT Dementia Research Center, 3-3-20 Shinsuna, Koto-ku, Tokyo 136-0075, Japan

Department of Psychiatry, Juntendo University School of Medicine, 2-1-1 Hongo, Bunkyo-ku, Tokyo 113-8421, Japan

K. Kosaka (ed.), *Dementia with Lewy Bodies*, DOI 10.1007/978-4-431-55948-1_10

[MRI], single-photon emission computed tomography [SPECT], and positron emission tomography [PET]) in probable DLB. We will also review the findings seen during the early stages of DLB. Finally, we will briefly discuss the usefulness of these imaging modalities for the early diagnosis of DLB.

10.1 Structural Neuroimaging (CT and MRI)

On the CT and MRI scans of DLB subjects, medial temporal lobe atrophy (MTA) is relatively mild, compared to what is seen on the scans of patients who have Alzheimer's disease (AD) [1]. Additionally, overall brain atrophy is milder than other types of dementia [2]. Figures 10.1a, b represent the typical MRI findings of probable AD and DLB, respectively. As the disease progresses, concomitant AD pathologies including senile plaques and neurofibrillary tangles spread throughout

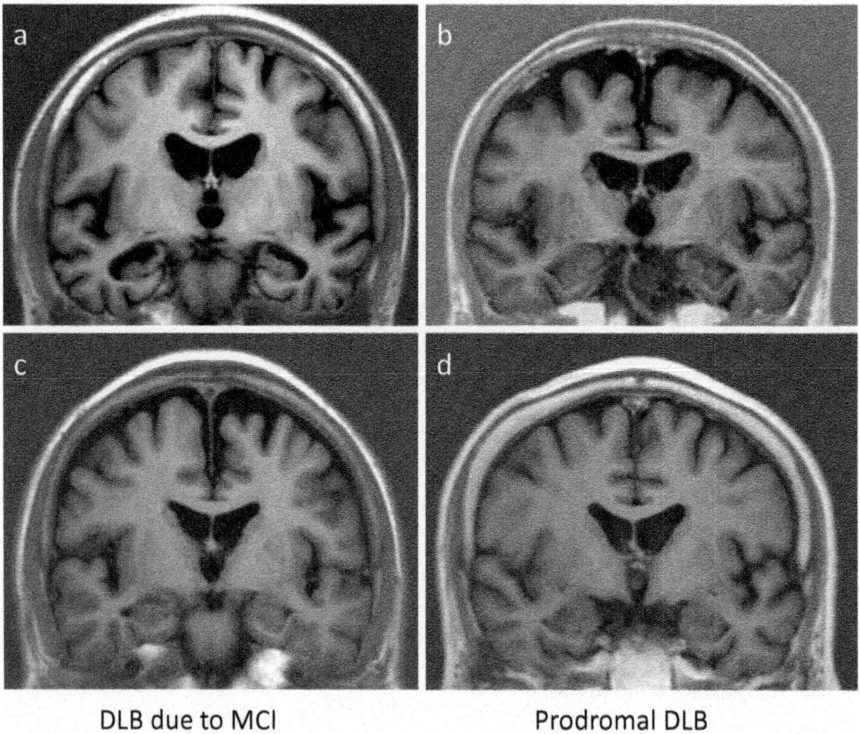

Fig. 10.1 (**a–d**) MRI findings of characteristic AD and DLB cases. (**a**) Probable AD case. Medial temporal lobe atrophy (MTA) is prominently evident bilaterally. (**b**) Probable DLB case. MTA is not severe as that seen in AD. (**c**) Case of MCI due to DLB. MTA is slightly milder than that in probable DLB. (**d**) Prodromal DLB case. MTA is minimal, and atrophy is almost within normal range for aging

the brain, causing neuronal loss in the medial temporal area, which is when MTA increases in severity.

Mild cognitive impairment (MCI) due to DLB has also been previously described [3–5]. Its neuropsychological features are focused on cognitive decline other than memory. The neuropsychological features of MCI affect the visuospatial and attention domains and are quite different from those seen on scans of patients who have typical AD [4]. As for the features identified from structural neuroimaging, during MCI the medial temporal lobe is preserved more than that seen in probable DLB (MCI due to DLB, Fig. 10.1c) [5]. Moreover, in the very early stage of the disease, recently called "prodromal stage of DLB" or "prodromal DLB" [6, 7], the medial temporal lobe is mostly preserved (Fig. 10.1d). The regional atrophic pattern and neuropathological correlates are discussed in the amyloid imaging section of this chapter.

Regarding cerebral microbleeds, which typically are associated with amyloid deposition and cerebral amyloid angiopathy and are detected as hypointense foci on T2* gradient-recalled echo MRI, a recent study from the Mayo Clinic showed similarity with AD; they used 3-tesla T2*-weighted gradient-recalled echo MRI, and the cerebral microbleed densities were highest in the occipital lobe both in DLB ($n=23$) and the age- and gender-matched probable AD group ($n=46$). The prevalence was 30 % in DLB and 24 % in AD, respectively. Compared with AD patients, DLB patients showed the smaller densities of microbleeds in the parietal and temporal lobes and the infratentorial regions [8]. Still, there is no established data on microbleed findings in MCI due to DLB or prodromal DLB.

10.2 Molecular and Functional Imaging (SPECT and PET)

10.2.1 Occipital Lobe Hypoperfusion/Hypometabolism

In this section, the characteristic findings of 18F-fluorodeoxyglucose positron emission tomography (FDG-PET) for cerebral metabolism in PET imaging, ^{99m}Tc-ethyl cysteinate dimer (ECD)-SPECT and N-isopropyl-p-123I-iodoamphetamine (IMP)-SPECT imaging for cerebral perfusion in SPECT imaging are described. Lastly, we briefly review the evidence for amyloid deposition finding in DLB. Currently, striatal dopamine transporter (DAT) imaging (e.g., FP-CIT SPECT) is the only neuroimaging tool accepted as the suggestive feature in the revised consensus criteria for DLB [9, 10]. Details of this tool would be described in another chapter. In addition to DAT ligands, several other representative radioligands for molecular and functional imaging are used to support the diagnosis of DLB, as shown in Table 10.1. In Japan, there is no functional cerebral neuroimaging modality approved by the Japanese Pharmaceutical and Medical Devices Agency (PMDA) for diagnosing DLB, other than FP-CIT SPECT.

Table 10.1 Representative radioligands for molecular and functional imaging (SPECT and PET)

SPECT	
Dopamine transporter loss	^{99m}Tc hexamethylpropyleneamine oxime
	N-Isopropyl-p-[123I]-iodoamphetamine
	^{99m}Tc-ethyl cysteinate dimer
Cerebral perfusion	^{99m}Tc hexamethylpropyleneamine oxime
	N-Isopropyl-p-[123I]-iodoamphetamine
	^{99m}Tc-ethyl cysteinate dimer
PET	
Metabolism	^{18}F-Fluorodeoxyglucose (FDG)
Amyloid deposition	Pittsburgh compound B (PIB)
Cholinergic pathway	N-[11C]Methylpiperidin-4-yl acetate and propionate
Dopaminergic pathway	18-Fluorodopa
	11C-Dihydrotetrabenazine

ECD-/IMP-SPECT and FDG-PET scans are helpful for the clinical diagnosis of DLB [11]. The characteristic occipital hypometabolism in DLB was first reported by Albin et al. [12]. Thereafter, to discriminate DLB from AD, Minoshima et al. clarified that the hypometabolism seen in the occipital lobe, especially in the primary visual cortex (PVC) detected by FDG-PET imaging, is a distinguishing finding in DLB subjects, and there is a high sensitivity and specificity (90 % and 80 %, respectively) [13]. In probable DLB, compared with the PVC, metabolism in the visual association cortex (VAC) is relatively preserved (Fig. 10.2a, b). However, the pathophysiological background of cerebral hypometabolism in the occipital lobe remains unclear. Neuropathologically, in DLB patients, the occipital lobe, which includes both the PVC and the VAC, is not a predominantly vulnerable area for Lewy pathology, such as Lewy bodies and Lewy neurites. Consequently, there is no severe cortical neuronal loss or occipital lobar atrophy. We previously reported that Lewy pathology in DLB brains does not occur in the neuronal cell bodies, including Lewy bodies (LBs), but it occurs in the axonal terminals, including Lewy neurites (LNs) initially [14], and secondary LBs may be formed by transneuronal degeneration in the regions where the degenerative axonal terminals are found [14, 15]. Hence, Lewy pathology in the occipital area may arise along with degeneration of the visuo-amygdaloid pathway [16, 17]. In fact, neuroanatomically, it is known that visual cortex has a connection with the amygdala, one of the most vulnerable areas for Lewy pathology, through the relay of the inferior temporal cortex [18].

A recent neuropathological survey showed that the levels of synaptic proteins such as synaptophysin and syntaxin and the choline acetyltransferase (ChAT) activity in PVC in DLB were significantly lower in those in AD and aged-control groups [19]. Moreover, the densities of LBs were correlated with these synaptic and ChAT changes, implying the association between molecular changes and functional neuroimaging in PVC [19].

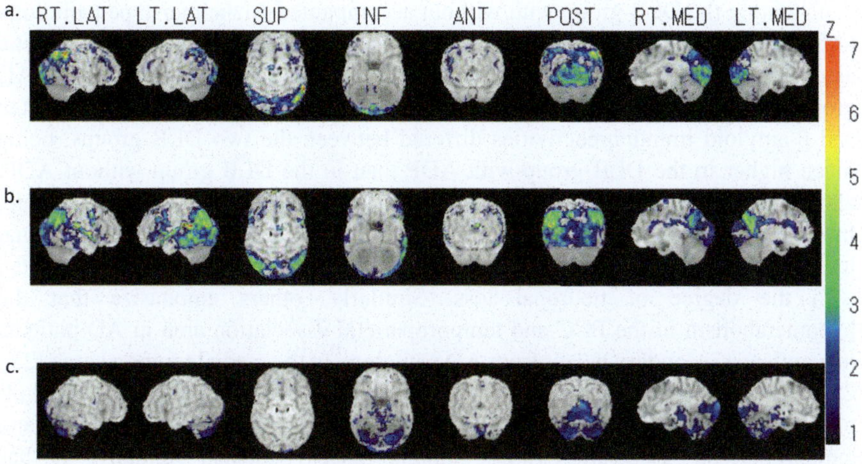

Fig. 10.2 (**a–c**) FDG-PET findings in DLB. Using three-dimensional stereotactic surface projection (3D-SSP) analysis with an age-matched normative database (77 normal healthy volunteers between 41 and 84 years of age [36 men and 41 women]), we evaluated the decrease in the regional cerebral metabolic rate of glucose for each patient. (**a**) Probable DLB. A case with cerebral hypometabolism with limited involvement of the primary visual and visual association area. Hypometabolism in the temporoparietal association area; pattern is almost preserved. In such cases, cognitive impairment is not prominent during the early stage of its clinical course. (**b**) Probable DLB. In addition to the primary visual and visual association area, these types of cases show cerebral hypometabolism in the posterior cingulate cortex, cuneus, precuneus, and temporoparietal association cortex. In such cases, cognitive impairment is prominent in the early stage of the clinical course. (**c**) DLB-MCI. In addition to primary visual and visual association area, cerebral hypometabolism is detected in the cerebellum

10.2.2 Other Involvement Areas

In addition to PVC, hypometabolism in the posterior cingulate cortex (PCC) and temporoparietal association area is the frequently accompanying finding in DLB patients [12, 20] (Fig. 10.2b). Minoshima et al. [13] indicated with multivariate analysis that there is a pathophysiological difference between FDG-PET hypometabolism in the temporoparietal association area and that in the occipital lobe area, especially in the PVC, in DLB patients. The detection of Lewy pathology in brains is essential for the pathological diagnosis of DLB. Previous studies, however, have shown that Lewy pathology and AD pathology mostly coexist in DLB brains [21, 22]. One of them reported that, among 42 autopsied DLB brains, about 80 % had a moderate to severe extent of concomitant AD pathology (National Institute on Aging (NIA) criteria: intermediate to high), and the remaining 20 % of brains had only mild AD pathology (NIA: low) [22]. Using postmortem DLB brains, we have previously performed the quantitative assessment regarding α-synuclein, tau, and β-amyloid immunoreactivities, in addition to neuronal number in the occipital, PCC, and temporoparietal association areas, and compared them among the DLB group with/without accompanied Alzheimer-type pathology (ADP) and the AD group [17]. As a result, in the PCC and temporoparietal association area, neuronal loss was milder in the DLB groups than in the AD group, although there were no differences between the two DLB groups. Both tau and β-amyloid immunoreactivities differed between the two DLB groups, being much higher in the DLB group with ADP than in the DLB group without ADP, although they were rather lower in the DLB group with ADP than in the AD group. In the DLB groups, tau and β-amyloid immunoreactivities participated in neuronal loss by multivariate analysis, and the severity of NFT pathology was correlated with the degree of neuronal loss. Similarly, others emphasize that the hypometabolism in the PCC and temporoparietal association area in AD patients may reflect a secondary defect from AD pathology in the medial temporal area [23–25]. These findings suggest that both primary and secondary effects of AD pathology might play an important role in the hypometabolism of the PCC and temporoparietal association areas among DLB patients. Actually, it has been accepted that the PCC is relatively spared from hypometabolism during DLB compared to AD, and so this has been recently called "cingulate island sign (CIS)" [26, 27]. It is intriguing that this characteristic sign is in accordance with our previous findings [17]. Originally, the relative preservation of cingulate cortex was reported by Japanese researchers using the quantitative analysis of FDG-PET data [28]. Its clinical value for differentiating DLB from AD has followed by Lim et al [27]. Through the neuropathological retrospective investigation, Graff-Radford et al. clarified that the CIS ratio did not correlate with amyloid burden, but did correlate with lower tau burden (Braak NFT staging). Then, they concluded that this findings indicate that the CIS in FDG-PET might be a surrogate marker for coexisting tau pathology in DLB [26]. In terms of the clinical relevance of hypometabolism in the temporoparietal and precuneus regions, we recently reported that visual and extracampine hallucinations were more frequently seen in a DLB subgroup with hypometabolism in these regions, than in a subgroup without hypometabolism in these regions [29].

10.2.3 SPECT/PET Findings in MCI Due to DLB and Prodromal DLB

Few studies have reported the functional imaging results in patients who have MCI due to DLB or prodromal DLB, including on ECD-/IMP-SPECT and FDG-PET scans. We previously reported that of 145 patients who were consulted in our memory clinic and had FDG-PET imaging, 25 patients revealed glucose hypometabolism in the PVC. Among these 25 cases, 12 cases (48 %) and 6 cases (24 %) fulfilled the criteria for probable DLB or possible DLB, respectively. Additionally, in these groups, the cognitive status ranged from MCI to dementia. In contrast, of 120 cases who did not exhibit PVC hypometabolism, the frequency of the subjects fulfilling probable and possible DLB was 5 % each [30]. In more than 3 years of follow-up studies on this cohort with PVC hypometabolism, we identified that the subgroup with hypometabolism in the parietal lobe and lateral occipital cortex at baseline converted to probable DLB [31]. Considering these results, it should be noted that glucose hypometabolism in the PVC is not only a common feature of DLB, but it is associated with the clinical features of DLB, regardless of cognitive status. Furthermore, as for CIS, we investigated whether this sign is evident not only when patients present with dementia but also when they present with MCI to differentiate between DLB and AD. As a result, MCI with both CIS and hypometabolism in the PVC led to a significantly high conversion to DLB, whereas MCI with hypometabolism in the PCC led to significantly high conversion to AD [32], supporting the value of CIS for early differentiation DLB from AD. To note, we have found that some cases with MCI due to DLB also presented with hypometabolism in the cerebellum, although its pathophysiological background is unclear (Fig. 10.2c).

10.2.4 Amyloid PET Imaging in DLB

Amyloid PET modality enables the detection of fibrillary amyloid-β in neuritic plaques found in human brains in vivo [33]. Regarding the association with AD-like cortical atrophy in LBD and amyloid deposition detected by [11C] Pittsburgh compound B, the accepted ligand of amyloid PET imaging, Shimada et al. investigated 15 LBD cases (8 with DLB and 7 with PDD), 14 AD cases, and 17 controls [34] and found 40 % of the LBD cases, and all of the AD cases showed amyloid positivity. Additionally, amyloid-positive LBD and AD revealed very similar patterns of cortical atrophy in the parahippocampal, lateral temporal, and parietal cortices areas. On the other hand, cases of LBD without amyloid positivity did not show any significant cortical atrophy. From their results, it is implied that upcoming therapies against amyloid may be effective for delaying AD-like atrophy in LBD subjects. Others have reported that the amyloid PET positivity is independent from CIS in FDG-PET [26].

According to a recent meta-analysis, the prevalence of amyloid positivity in clinically diagnosed subjects with dementia increases with both age and APO ε4 carrier status. In DLB, among 16 cases carrying APO ε4, the prevalence of amyloid positivity in the subjects over 60 and 80 years of age was 63 % and 83 %, respectively. In contrast, this positivity among 18 APO ε4 noncarriers over 60 and 80 years of age was 29 % and 54 %, respectively [35]. Thus, as indicated in AD, amyloid PET is more useful for diagnosing DLB in early-onset dementia subjects. Furthermore, both in AD and non-AD dementia, including DLB, amyloid positivity was associated with worse global cognition.

Our ultimate goals are to develop and establish a therapeutic strategy using disease-modifying drugs for DLB. To achieve this, it is essential to clarify the relationship between the available functional imaging tools (DAT imaging, MIBG scintigraphy, etc.) and correlate their findings with clinical relevance to provide a complete picture of the pathophysiology of DLB. Also, autopsy-confirmation studies are also warranted for proving these findings. The harmonization of these modalities would allow us to have a comprehensive understanding of this neurodegenerative disease.

References

1. Burton EJ, Barber R, Mukaetova-Ladinska EB, et al. Medial temporal lobe atrophy on MRI differentiates Alzheimer's disease from dementia with Lewy bodies and vascular cognitive impairment: a prospective study with pathological verification of diagnosis. Brain. 2009;132:195–203.
2. O'Brien J, Paling S, Barber R, et al. Progressive brain atrophy on serial MRI in dementia with Lewy bodies, AD and vascular dementia. Neurology. 2001;56:1386–8.
3. Boeve BF. Mild cognitive impairment associated with underlying Alzheimer's disease versus Lewy body disease. Parkinsonism Relat Disord. 2012;18:S41–4.
4. Ferman TJ, Smith GE, Kantarci K, et al. Nonamnestic mild cognitive impairment progresses to dementia with Lewy bodies. Neurology. 2013;81:2032–8.
5. Fujishiro H, Nakamura S, Kitazawa M, et al. Early detection of dementia with Lewy bodies in patients with amnestic mild cognitive impairment using ^{123}I-MIBG cardiac scintigraphy. J Neurol Sci. 2012;315:115–19.
6. Donaghy PC, O'Brien JT, Thomas AJ. Prodromal dementia with Lewy bodies. Psychol Med. 2015;45:259–68.
7. Fujishiro H, Nakamura S, Sato K, et al. Prodromal dementia with Lewy bodies. Geriatr Gerontol Int. 2015;15:817–26.
8. Gungor I, Sarro L, Graf-Radford J, et al. Frequency and topography of cerebral microbleeds in dementia with Lewy bodies compared to Alzheimer's disease. Parkinsonism Relat Disord. 2015;21:1–4.
9. McKeith IG, Dickson DW, Lowe J, et al. Diagnosis and management of dementia with Lewy bodies: third report of the DLB Consortium. Neurology. 2005;27:1863–72.
10. McKeith I, O'Brien J, Walker Z, et al. Sensitivity and specificity of dopamine transporter imaging with 123I-FP-CIT SPECT in dementia with Lewy bodies: a phase III, multicentre study. Lancet Neurol. 2007;6:305–13.
11. Mak E, Su L, Williams GB, et al. Neuroimaging characteristics of dementia with Lewy bodies. Alzheimers Res Ther. 2014;6:18–27.
12. Albin RL, Minoshima S, D'Amato CJ, et al. Fluorodeoxyglucose positron emission tomography in diffuse Lewy body disease. Neurology. 1996;47:462–8.
13. Minoshima S, Foster NL, Sima AA, et al. Alzheimer's disease versus dementia with Lewy bodies; cerebral metabolic distinction with autopsy confirmation. Ann Neurol. 2001;50:358–65.
14. Iseki E, Marui W, Kosaka K, et al. Degenerative terminals of the perforant pathway are human !-synuclein-immunoreactive in the hippocampus of patients with diffuse Lewy body disease. Neurosci Lett. 1998;258:81–4.
15. Katsuse O, Iseki E, Marui W, et al. Developmental stages of cortical Lewy bodies and their relation to axonal transport blockage in brains of patients with dementia with Lewy bodies. J Neurosci. 2003;211:29–35.
16. Yamamoto R, Iseki E, Murayama N, et al. Investigation of Lewy pathology in the visual pathway. J Neurosci. 2006;246:95–101.

17. Kasanuki K, Iseki E, Fujishiro H, et al. Neuropathological investigation of the hypometabolic regions on positron emission tomography with [18F] fluorodeoxyglucose in patients with dementia with Lewy bodies. J Neurol Sci. 2012;314:111–19.
18. Parent A. Carpenter's human neuroanatomy. 9th ed. Baltimore: Williams & Wilkins; 1996. p. 773–80.
19. Mukaetova-Ladinska EB, Andras A, Milne J, et al. Synaptic proteins and choline acetyltransferase loss in visual cortex in dementia with Lewy bodies. J Neuropathol Exp Neurol. 2013;72:53–60.
20. Ishii K, Imamura T, Sasaki M, et al. Regional cerebral glucose metabolism in dementia with Lewy bodies and Alzheimer's disease. Neurology. 1998;51:125–30.
21. Aarsland D, Perry R, Brown A, et al. Neuropathology of dementia in Parkinson's disease: a prospective, community-based study. Ann Neurol. 2005;58:773–6.
22. Fujishiro H, Ferman TJ, Boeve BF, et al. Validation of the neuropathologic criteria of the third consortium for dementia with Lewy bodies for prospectively diagnosed cases. J Neuropathol Exp Neurol. 2008;67:649–56.
23. Haxby JV, Grady CL, Koss E, et al. Longitudinal study of cerebral metabolic asymmetries and associated neuropsychological patterns in dementia of the Alzheimer type. Arch Neurol. 1990;47:977–80.
24. Mega MS, Chen SS, Thompson PM, et al. Mapping histology to metabolism: coregistration of stained whole-brain sections to premortem PET in Alzheimer's disease. Neuroimage. 1997;5:147–53.
25. Mosconi L, Pupi A, De Cristofaro MT, et al. Functional interactions of the entorhinal cortex: an 18F-FDG PET study on normal aging and Alzheimer's disease. J Nucl Med. 2004;45:382–92.
26. Graff-Radford J, Murray ME, Lowe VJ, et al. Dementia with Lewy bodies: basis of cingulate island sign. Neurology. 2014;26(83):801–9.
27. Lim SM, Katsifis A, Villemagne VL, et al. The 18F-FDG PET cingulate island sign and comparison to 123I-beta-CIT SPECT for diagnosis of dementia with Lewy bodies. J Nucl Med. 2009;50:1638–45.
28. Imamura T, Ishii K, Sasaki M, et al. Regional cerebral glucose metabolism in dementia with Lewy bodies and Alzheimer's disease: a comparative study using positron emission tomography. Neurosci Lett. 1997;235:49–52.
29. Chiba Y, Fujishiro H, Ota K, et al. Clinical profiles of dementia with Lewy bodies with and without Alzheimer's disease-like hypometabolism. Int J Geriatr Psychiatry. 2015;30:316–23.
30. Fujishiro H, Iseki E, Kasanuki K, et al. Glucose hypometabolism in primary visual cortex is commonly associated with clinical features of dementia with Lewy bodies regardless of cognitive conditions. Int J Geriatr Psychiatry. 2012;27:1138–46.
31. Fujishiro H, Iseki E, Kasanuki K, et al. A follow up study of non-demented patients with primary visual cortical hypometabolism: prodromal dementia with Lewy bodies. J Neurol Sci. 2013;15(334):48–54.
32. Daizo Kondo, Kazumi Ota, Koji Kasanuki, et al. Characteristics of mild cognitive impairment tending to convert into Alzheimer's disease or dementia with Lewy bodies: a follow-up study in a memory clinic. doi:http://dx.doi.org/10.1016/j.jns.2016.08.011.
33. Klunk WE, H E, Nordberg A, et al. Imaging brain amyloid in Alzheimer's disease with Pittsburgh compound-B. Ann Neurol. 2004;55(3):306–19.
34. Shimada H, Shinotoh H, Hirano S, et al. β-amyloid in lewy body disease is related to Alzheimer's disease-like atrophy. Mov Disord. 2013;28:169–75.
35. Ossenkoppele R, Jansen WJ, Rabinovici GD, et al. Prevalence of amyloid PET positivity in dementia syndromes: a meta-analysis. JAMA. 2015;19(313):1939–49.

Chapter 11
Dopamine Transporter Imaging

Louise Colledge, Tim Whitfield, and Zuzana Walker

Abstract Dementia with Lewy bodies (DLB) can be difficult to diagnose as it shares common features with both Alzheimer's disease (AD) and Parkinson's disease. Accurate differentiation from other types of dementia as well as early detection is essential to inform management and treatment. The use of biomarkers, particularly imaging, has greatly contributed to the accurate diagnosis of DLB. This chapter will give an overview of the contribution of dopaminergic imaging to (i) the diagnosis of DLB and (ii) a better understanding of the underlying pathology. It will concentrate on dopamine transporter imaging, at present the most extensively studied technique, and review the knowledge about its place in the differential diagnosis from AD and other types of dementia. It will also briefly review the methods used to assess dopamine transporter and how to interpret the scans. Apart from discussing differential diagnosis and the limitations, it will discuss some up to date correlations of imaging and various clinical features.

Keywords Dementia with Lewy bodies • Dopamine transporter • FP-CIT SPECT

11.1 Introduction

It is well know that dopamine dysfunction underpins Parkinson's disease (PD) and dementia with Lewy bodies (DLB). Differentiation between the dementias is known to be important as the prognosis and clinical course vary according to the underlying pathology. DLB is currently underdiagnosed in clinical settings [1], and the diagnosis is particularly challenging in the early stages of the disease as it shares many features with other dementias.

L. Colledge • T. Whitfield
North Essex Partnership University NHS Foundation Trust, Chelmsford, UK

Z. Walker (✉)
North Essex Partnership University NHS Foundation Trust, Chelmsford, UK

Division of Psychiatry, University College London, London, UK
e-mail: z.walker@ucl.ac.uk

K. Kosaka (ed.), *Dementia with Lewy Bodies*, DOI 10.1007/978-4-431-55948-1_11

Lewy body disease is characterised by profound dopaminergic loss; dopaminergic imaging can therefore help to differentiate DLB and Alzheimer's disease (AD). Clinical diagnosis is made on the basis of the patient's history, cognitive assessment and MRI or CT imaging. Unfortunately, relying on clinical assessment alone has led to suboptimal accuracy in diagnosis, particularly with the differentiation between DLB and AD in mild cases or patients with AD and motor symptoms. There has been increasing emphasis on identifying various biomarkers including imaging biomarkers to improve diagnostic accuracy.

In DLB there is accumulation of α-synuclein in the neuronal cytoplasm in the form of Lewy bodies and Lewy neurites. The affected neurones are found in the olfactory bulb, the dorsal motor nucleus of the vagal nerve, the peripheral autonomic nervous system, the brainstem, limbic and/or neocortical regions [2, 3].

Most, but not all, cases start with accumulation of α-synuclein in the brainstem which then spreads to other areas [4]. As a consequence, patients with DLB have severe nigrostriatal degeneration, leading to deficiency in dopamine in the striatum; this can be detected at different stages of the dopaminergic pathways. There are a number of ligands available to assess different targets along the dopamine pathway, including dopamine turnover, dopamine transporter (DaT), the vesicular monoamine transporter type 2 (VMAT2), and postsynaptic receptors. It has been shown that scans examining the dopaminergic pathway are abnormal in DLB but normal in AD with no difference compared to the control population [5].

11.2 Dopaminergic Pathways and Neuroimaging

The main dopaminergic pathways have important roles in cognition and behaviour. Dopaminergic neurones originate in the substantia nigra and ventral tegmental area. The nigrostriatal pathway connects the substantia nigra with the striatum and is mainly involved in movement. The mesocortical pathway connects to the prefrontal cortex and is involved in attention, initiative, planning, motivation, working memory and higher cortical functions. The mesolimbic pathway connects the nucleus accumbens and amygdala; it is involved in motivation, drive, reward and emotional behaviour [6].

At the nigrostriatal dopaminergic synapse, tyrosine is converted to L-DOPA by tyrosine hydroxylase. L-DOPA is then converted to dopamine. Dopamine is gathered by VMAT2 into vesicles and then released into the synaptic cleft. Dopamine binds to D1 and D2 receptors on the postsynaptic membrane. Some dopamine re-enters the presynaptic terminal via DaTs.

The nigrostriatal pathway is significantly affected in DLB. The loss of neurones within the nigrostriatal pathway cannot be visualised using structural imaging techniques (CT/MRI) in vivo but DaT can be visualised and used as a surrogate marker for neuronal degeneration.

DaT is a membrane-spanning protein which pumps dopamine back into presynaptic terminals of dopamine cells. It is therefore a reliable marker of the density of dopamine neurone synapses in most brain regions. DaT levels are high in the striatum and moderate in other cortical regions, including the anterior cingulate, orbitofrontal cortex and occipital lobes [7–9]. DaT can be visualised using radiolabeled ligands. A reduction in the uptake of the ligand corresponds to loss of dopaminergic neurones and can be visualised using single-photon emission computed tomography (SPECT) or positron emission tomography (PET) [10].

11.3 Methods of Scanning

Dopaminergic scanning uses SPECT or PET with a ligand (the active substance) labelled with a radionuclide (tracer). The radioactive ligand is administered intravenously and binds to specific targets along the nigrostriatal pathway.

Dopaminergic ligands can assess various targets: (i) dopamine turnover via amino acid decarboxylase activity with fluorodopa and PET; (ii) storage of dopamine in presynaptic vesicles (VMAT2) with, for example, dihydrotetrabenazine and PET; (iii) the presynaptic plasma membrane DaT using cocaine analogues and both SPECT or PET scanning; and (iv) the postsynaptic receptors. For example, D2-like receptors can be assessed with raclopride, desmethoxyfallypride and fallypride with PET and iodobenzamide (IBZM), iodobenzofuran and epidepride with SPECT (see Fig. 11.1).

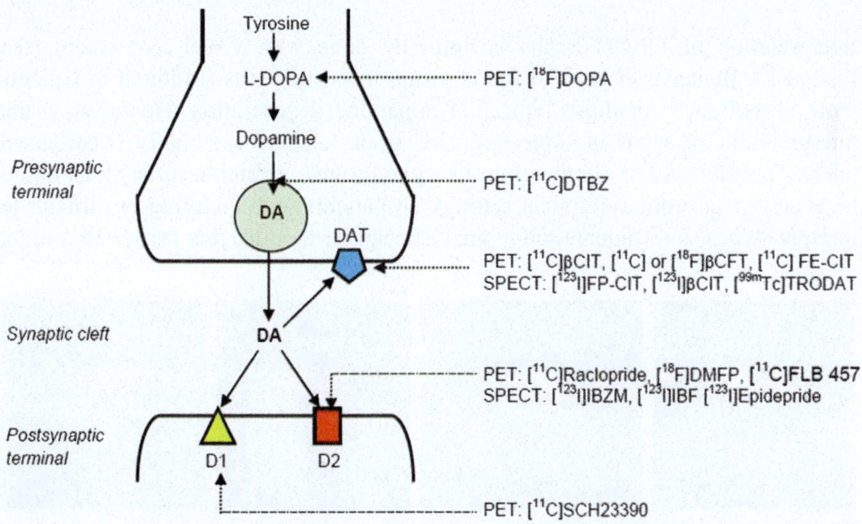

Fig. 11.1 Nigrostriatal dopaminergic synapse and targets of PET and SPECT ligands. Tyrosine is converted to L-DOPA by tyrosine hydroxylase. L-DOPA is then converted to dopamine, which is gathered into vesicles by vesicular monoamine transporter and from which it is released into the synaptic cleft. Dopamine binds to D1 and D2 receptors on the postsynaptic membrane. Some dopamine re-enters the presynaptic terminal via dopamine transporters (DaTs) (Reproduced with permission from Cambridge University Press [6])

The radionuclide attached to the ligand emits radiation which can be detected using PET or SPECT. SPECT uses gamma rays to provide 3D information from 2D images. For PET radionuclides emit positrons which travel a short distance before hitting an electron, producing a pair of photons moving in opposite directions. The detection of these photons enables production of 3D images. PET produces higher resolution images than SPECT. Manipulation of scanning parameters enables slices to be taken along any axis of the brain.

The active ligands are labelled by radionuclides with different half-lives. The most practical radionuclide is ^{123}Iodine which has a half-life of 13 h. Examples of ligands labelled with ^{123}Iodine include 2β-carbomethoxy-3β-(4-iodophenyl) tropane (β-CIT) and *n*-fluoropropyl-2β-carbomethoxy-3β-(4-iodophenyl)nortropane (FP-CIT).

The ligands used in PET scanning have shorter half-lives which pose more practical difficulties. SPECT scanning is more widely available and cheaper than PET. Ligands used with PET can be labelled with ^{18}Fluorine (half-life 110 min) or ^{11}Carbon (half-life 20 min).

The most researched ligand in DLB is FP-CIT which is used with SPECT. FP-CIT has high affinity and relatively good selectivity for DaT with the optimal scanning window being 3–6 h after injection of the ligand.

11.4 Interpretation of Dopaminergic Imaging

Interpretation of FP-CIT scans is normally done with visual assessment (see Fig. 11.2). Benamer et al. [11] found visual inspection was sufficient in patients with normal scans or those typical of dopamine degeneration. However, visual interpretation of scans is subjective, and trials tend to use highly experienced nuclear physicians and are therefore likely to provide greater accuracy than might be achieved in ordinary clinical settings. In patients with marginal or difficult to interpret scans, a semiquantitative analysis can be helpful; this can yield a more

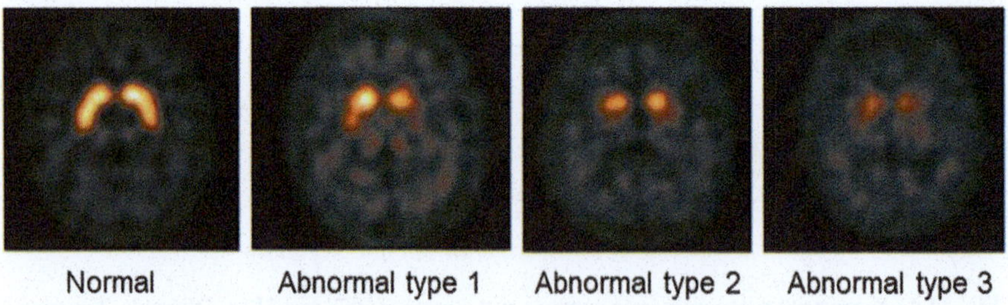

Fig. 11.2 Example of visual scan rating categories. Categories used here are normal (normal uptake in all regions); abnormal type 1 (asymmetric activity with one putamen showing reduced uptake); type 2 (absent activity in the putamen of both hemispheres); and type 3 (absent activity in the putamen of both hemispheres and greatly reduced in one or both caudate nuclei). Reproduced with permission from the Royal College of Psychiatrists [13]

objective interpretation of results. In clinical practice regions of interest with predefined templates of the striatum and nonspecific binding regions are commonly used. More recently semi-automated quantification tools have been developed, and there are several programmes able to quantify DaT studies. Söderland et al. [12] performed visual and semiquantitative analysis of FP-CIT scans. Although visual interpretation of scans provided good interobserver agreement (mean $k \pm SD$, 0.80 ± 0.05), this was improved as striatal binding ratios (0.86 ± 0.07), and caudate-to-putamen ratios (0.95 ± 0.04) were provided to the raters. The most experienced rater in the study made only minor changes in diagnosis after being provided with semiquantitative data in a small number of patients with more complex scans. Less experienced raters more frequently changed their diagnosis with additional information, and the updated diagnoses were in better agreement with the experienced rater. In clinical practice nuclear medicine physicians are likely to be less experienced than those used in research studies. This highlights that less experienced readers can perform as effectively as more experienced readers if provided with semiquantitative information.

11.5 Dopamine Transporter Imaging

Studies using DaT imaging have focused on a number of research questions. These include evaluating the accuracy of DLB diagnosis with and without the support of imaging and against autopsy diagnosis, imaging to monitor disease progression, comparison of dopaminergic imaging with other imaging techniques, evaluating the performance of different ligands and how imaging findings correlate with clinical symptoms and signs. We will discuss these in some detail below.

11.6 DLB Diagnosis Using Dopaminergic Imaging

11.6.1 DLB Compared to Normal and AD

The main studies comparing FP-CIT imaging in DLB and AD are summarised in Table 11.1.

Early single-centre studies showed good sensitivity and specificity for FP-CIT compared to clinical diagnosis. Walker et al. [14] scanned patients with DLB, AD, PD and controls using FP-CIT. Patients with DLB had reduced binding in both the posterior and anterior putamen and in the caudate nucleus when compared with AD and controls.

O'Brien et al. [15] extended a similar methodology to a larger cohort of 164 participants including PDD cases. As in Walker et al. [14], DLB subjects had significantly reduced FP-CIT binding in the caudate and anterior and posterior putamen compared to AD and controls. DaT loss in DLB was similar to PD, but

Table 11.1 Studies comparing DaT imaging results between DLB and AD

Paper	Ligand	Patients	Aim	Sensitivity of FP-CIT scan	Specificity of FP-CIT scan	Other information
Walker et al. [14]	FP-CIT	27 DLB	Distinguish DLB from AD	88 % in subsample with autopsy	100 % in subsample with autopsy	Lower striatal ligand uptake in DLB and PD compared to AD and controls
		17 AD				
		19 early PD				
		16 controls				
Ceravolo et al. [17]	FP-CIT	13 AD-P	To investigate DaT loss in AD patients with parkinsonism (AD-P) compared to DLB and controls	–	–	FP-CIT striatal uptake in patients with AD-P was similar to controls. DLB and PD had lower uptake in all striatal areas when compared to AD-P and controls
		15 DLB				
		20 PD				
		8 controls				
O'Brien et al. [15]	FP-CIT	23 DLB	To investigate DaT loss in DLB compared to AD, PD, PDD and controls	78 %	94 %	Striatal binding reduced in DLB, PD and PDD compared with AD and controls. Relatively greater caudate loss in DLB and PDD compared with PD
		36 PDD				
		34 AD				
		38 PD				
		33 controls				
McKeith et al. [18]	FP-CIT	151 DLB	Investigate the sensitivity and specificity of DaT against consensus diagnosis	78 %	90 %	Overall diagnostic accuracy 86 %. Positive predictive value 82 %. Negative predictive value 88 %
						Inter-reader agreement k = 0.87
		147 non-DLB dementia (mainly AD)				Possible DLB 38 % had an abnormal scan
Walker et al. [20]	FP-CIT	8 DLB	Determine sensitivity and specificity of DaT against autopsy	88 % visual rating	83 % visual rating	FP-CIT good sensitivity and very good specificity
		12 non-DLB		88 % semiquantitative	100 % semiquantitative	

O'Brien et al. [19]	FP-CIT	44 possible DLB	Accuracy of FP-CIT in diagnosis of possible DLB	63 %	100 %	12/19 cases of probable DLB at follow-up had abnormal baseline scan. 7/7 cases of AD at follow-up had normal scan
Walker et al. [13]	FP-CIT	114 possible DLB	To investigate whether performing a scan in patients with possible DLB would aid diagnosis	–	–	Use of the scans allowed the physicians to be more certain about their diagnosis. A positive scan was more likely to lead to a change in diagnosis

FP-CIT *n*-fluoropropyl-2β-carbomethoxy-3β-(4-iodophenyl)nortropane, *DLB* dementia with Lewy bodies, *AD* Alzheimer's disease, *PD* Parkinson's disease, *DaT* dopamine transporter, *PDD* Parkinson's disease dementia

with a less prominent caudate-putamen gradient. Patients with PDD had the greatest DaT loss in all striatal areas. The less pronounced caudate-putamen gradient in DLB was also observed by Walker et al. [16]. In that study the main emphasis was on comparison of DLB and PD cases.

Ceravolo et al. [17] examined patients with AD and extrapyramidal features using FP-CIT and compared them to patients with DLB and PD and controls. The AD patients showed similar results to control subjects in the putamen and caudate nucleus despite their extrapyramidal signs. There was, as expected, significant differences between DLB and AD in DaT binding across all the striatal areas.

McKeith et al. [18] completed a multicentre, multinational phase-III study using FP-CIT to examine 326 patients with diagnoses of probable or possible DLB and compared them to cases of non-DLB dementia. Clinical diagnosis was determined using consensus panel methodology (consensus of three independent clinical experts). The scans were visually rated by three nuclear medicine physicians as normal or abnormal. The mean sensitivity of FP-CIT imaging for a diagnosis of probable DLB was 78 % and mean specificity was 90 %. The mean overall diagnostic accuracy was 86 %, with 82 % for positive predictive value and 88 % for negative predictive value. Inter-reader agreement for rating scans was high ($k = 0.87$).

In a 1-year follow-up of the McKeith et al. [18] cohort, of the 44 patients given an initial diagnosis of possible DLB, 18 had no change in diagnosis, 19 converted to probable DLB and seven were diagnosed with AD. Of the 19 who converted to probable DLB, 12 had an abnormal scan at baseline and all seven patients that were assigned a diagnosis of AD at follow-up had a normal baseline scan. This indicated that FP-CIT result was able to point towards diagnosis at follow-up at a time when clinicians could only assign a possible DLB diagnosis [19].

The performance of the FP-CIT scan to facilitate an earlier diagnosis was further confirmed in a study with autopsy diagnosis. Walker et al. [20] found that reduced striatal uptake of FP-CIT had 88 % sensitivity and 100 % specificity when making a diagnosis of DLB compared to autopsy diagnosis (the gold standard). In comparison, an early clinical diagnosis without imaging had a sensitivity of 75 % and specificity of 42 %, indicating that the FP-CIT imaging facilitated a more accurate diagnosis. In an extension of this cohort, a modified analysis was used, whereby an abnormal scan was defined as uptake below 2 standard deviations of the mean of controls in the worse affected posterior putamen. Using this technique in the larger cohort showed the sensitivity of FP-CIT SPECT scan for diagnosing DLB to be 100 % and the specificity 92 % [21].

A recent phase-IV multinational study [13] randomised patients with possible DLB diagnoses (difficult to diagnose cases) to FP-CIT imaging or no imaging. Of the 170 patients, 114 were randomised to imaging and 56 were controls. Of the 114 patients with possible DLB, 43 % had an abnormal scan. More patients in the imaging group had a change to a more certain diagnosis (probable DLB or non-DLB) compared with controls at 24 weeks (71 % vs. 16 %). Interestingly, clinicians were much more likely to change the diagnosis if the scan was abnormal (82 %) than normal (46 %).

11.6.2 DLB Compared to PD and PDD

DLB, PD and PDD all feature nigrostriatal degeneration. However, there are subtle differences between PD/PDD and DLB on FP-CIT imaging, giving us some insight into the distribution of underlying pathology. However, in clinical practice FP-CIT imaging is never used for differential diagnosis between DLB and PD/PDD as this is always done on the basis of clinical and cognitive assessment.

Ransmayr et al. [22] showed DaT binding was lower in DLB patients compared to those with PD. The authors also showed that PD patients had a more asymmetrical uptake of β-CIT than DLB cases. O'Brien et al. [15] showed greater caudate involvement in DLB and PDD when compared to PD.

Walker et al. [16] compared both DLB and PD patients to controls. They found a difference in both groups in the binding in the caudate and putamen bilaterally relative to controls. The PD group had a more marked gradient of uptake than the DLB group. DLB showed a uniform decrease in the uptake of dopamine in the caudate and anterior and posterior putamen. PD patients had less severe loss in the caudate but increased loss in the putamen, particularly the posterior putamen contralateral to the most affected side. This resulted in marked asymmetry in posterior putaminal uptake compared to DLB and controls and fits with the clinical picture of more asymmetrical motor symptoms in PD than DLB.

Rossi et al. [23] investigated striatal DaT uptake in 30 patients with DLB and 30 with PDD using FP-CIT. They found that the striatal uptake of the DaT tracer was not significantly different between PDD and DLB.

Marquie et al. [8] used ^{11}C altropane (2β-carbomethoxy-3β(4-fluorophenyl)-n-(1-iodoprop-1-en-3-yl)), a PET ligand with a high selectivity for DaT, to measure striatal and extrastriatal DaT concentration across different diagnostic groups (DLB, PD and controls). They found that DaT concentrations in the putamen and caudate were similar in DLB and PD and significantly lower than in controls, independent of the presence of dementia. There were no significant differences in orbitofrontal and prefrontal regions between DLB, PD and controls suggesting these regions are not affected (see Table 11.2).

11.6.3 DLB Compared to Frontotemporal Dementia

Both frontotemporal dementia (FTD) and DLB may feature hallucinations and parkinsonism, and this could lead to diagnostic difficulties. The first study to observe changes in DaT uptake in patients with FTD was performed by Sedaghat et al. [24]. They observed that patients with FTD have a reduced striatal uptake of FP-CIT compared to controls using a semiquantitative method.

Morgan et al. [25] compared striatal DaT binding and found 33 % of patients with FTD, and 90 % of patients with DLB had an abnormal FP-CIT scan. All the

Table 11.2 Studies comparing DaT imaging results between DLB, PD and PDD

Paper	Ligand	Patients	Aim	Asymmetry	Gradient	Other info
Ransmayr et al. [22]	β-CIT	20 DLB 24 PD 10 controls	To compare loss of DaT in DLB vs. PD	Asymmetry more marked in PD than DLB	–	Striatal binding significantly lower in DLB and PD than controls
Walker et al. [16]	FP-CIT	21 DLB 19 PD 16 controls	Comparison of DaT uptake in DLB, PD and controls to assess asymmetry and gradient	PD > DLB	Caudate-putamen gradient PD > DLB	DLB and PD had lower binding in all striatal areas than controls. DLB had significantly lower binding in caudate nucleus compared to PD
O'Brien et al. [15]	FP-CIT	23 DLB 36 PDD 34 AD 38 PD 33 controls	To investigate DaT loss in DLB compared to AD, PD, PDD and controls and to evaluate gradient	–	FP-CIT uptake in DLB had a flatter rostrocaudal gradient than PD.	Greatest reduction of striatal FP-CIT uptake was seen in those with PDD
Rossi et al. [23]	FP-CIT and ECD SPECT	30 DLB 30 PDD 20 AD 10 controls	A comparison of FP-CIT and perfusion SPECT in DLB and PDD	No difference between DLB and PDD	No difference between DLB and PDD	Striatal uptake of FP-CIT was lower in DLB and PDD compared to controls
Marquie et al. [8]	^{11}C altropane PET	19 PD 10 DLB 17 controls	Comparison of DaT concentration in putamen, caudate, anterior cingulate, orbitofrontal and prefrontal regions in PD, DLB and controls	No difference between DLB and PD in caudate and putamen	-	-

β-CIT 2β-carbomethoxy-3β-(4-iodophenyl)tropane, *DLB* dementia with Lewy bodies, *PD* Parkinson's disease, *DaT* dopamine transporter, *FP-CIT* *n*-fluoropropyl-2β-carbomethoxy-3β-(4-iodophenyl)nortropane, *PDD* Parkinson's disease dementia, *AD* Alzheimer's disease, *ECD SPECT* 99mTc-ethyl cysteinate dimer single-photon emission computed tomography, *PET* positron emission tomography

Table 11.3 Studies comparing DaT imaging results between DLB and FTD

Paper	Ligand	Patients	Aim	Findings
Sedaghat et al. [24]	FP-CIT	7 FTD	To evaluate the dopaminergic status of the striatum in patients with FTD	Striatal uptake in FTD was reduced to 62 % (right) and 68 % (left) compared to controls
		7 controls		
Morgan et al. [25]	FP-CIT	12 FTD	To compare striatal DaT binding across groups by visually rating the caudate and putamen on scans	Scan was 90 % sensitive for DLB. 89 % specificity vs. AD but reduced to 67 % specificity vs. FTD
		10 DLB		
		9 AD		
Spehl et al. [26]	FP-CIT	13 FTD	To evaluate the role of FP-CIT in differentiating between FTD, DLB and AD	Using a semiquantitative analysis, 95 % of DLB cases were correctly discriminated
		12 DLB		
		9 AD		

FP-CIT n-fluoropropyl-2β-carbomethoxy-3β-(4-iodophenyl)nortropane, *FTD* frontotemporal dementia, *DLB* dementia with Lewy bodies, *DaT* dopamine transporter, *AD* Alzheimer's disease

DLB cases and some of the FTD cases had autopsy-confirmed diagnosis. This confirmed the findings of the earlier study by Sedaghat et al. [24] that some patients with FTD can have abnormal DaT uptake.

A more recent study by Spehl et al. [26] looked into the differentiation of FTD, DLB and AD. They used ^{18}F-FDG PET and FP-CIT and found 62 % of the FTD group had abnormal scans on visual assessment. On semiquantitative analysis, patients with FTD showed less severe reduction in uptake of FP-CIT than those with DLB. The difference was significant enough to separate FTD cases from DLB cases. FTD tends to occur in younger patients, and clinically the two conditions are fairly distinct and therefore the differential diagnosis should be made on clinical grounds. In conclusion, dopaminergic imaging has only limited use for separating DLB from FTD (see Table 11.3).

11.7 Correlation with Clinical Findings

Colloby et al. [27] repeated FP-CIT scans in patients with PD, PDD and DLB as well as controls after a 1-year interval. All the patient groups had a significant decline in DaT uptake in all striatal areas but the controls remained stable.

Roselli et al. [28] scanned 18 patients with DLB with FP-CIT SPECT comparing striatal DaT levels with the frequency and severity of neuropsychiatric symptoms. There was a significant inverse relationship between the uptake on FP-CIT uptake and the neuropsychiatric inventory (NPI) hallucination score. This remained significant after controlling for UPDRS and MMSE score, age, disease duration and education. No significant correlation was found between the striatal uptake and the MMSE or UPDRS score. When putaminal and caudate uptake were examined separately, they continued to correlate significantly with hallucination severity. Putaminal uptake was significantly correlated with UPDRS score. Caudate uptake showed significant correlation with NPI depression, apathy and delusion scores. Those results are in keeping with the concept that the dopaminergic mesocortical pathways form a circuit involved in reciprocal caudate-frontal and fronto-caudal projections, which are important for organisation, planning and attention. Difficulties in this area of the brain might lead to difficulties in filtering distractions and may lead to an increase in delusional behaviour.

David et al. [29] also found a correlation between apathy and FP-CIT uptake; however, in this study the correlation was between increased apathy and reduced uptake in bilateral putamen.

Another study that looked at the association between cognitive symptoms and dopaminergic activity was Marquie et al. [8]. They found that low caudate DaT levels and high anterior cingulate DaT levels were associated with greater impairment on cognitive testing in DLB. Lower concentration of caudate DaT was also associated with greater functional impairment and greater impairment of visuospatial skills.

Del Sole et al. [30] showed FP-CIT uptake is inversely correlated with the UPDRS score; showing the probability of an abnormal SPECT scan increases with the severity of EPSs in DLB. However, surprisingly eight of the 22 patients diagnosed clinically as DLB had a normal FP-CIT scan, raising the possibility that some of the cases had an alternative diagnosis.

11.8 Diagnosis of DLB with Dopaminergic Imaging Compared to Other Imaging Techniques

There have been several studies comparing FP-CIT with other ligands and imaging modalities.

Colloby et al. [31] compared 99mTc-exametazime perfusion SPECT and FP-CIT SPECT between DLB and AD. 99mTc-exametazime had a specificity of 67 % and sensitivity of 63 % for occipital lobe hypoperfusion. FP-CIT was superior with a sensitivity of 77 % and specificity of 88 %.

Comparison of β-CIT SPECT with FDG PET to differentiate between AD and DLB showed β-CIT to have greater accuracy, with 100 % sensitivity and specificity compared to 83 % and 93 %, respectively, for visual interpretation of FDG PET [32].

Treglia et al. [33] found that MIBG and FP-CIT had equally high sensitivity and specificity for differentiating DLB from non-DLB dementias. In contrast to FP-CIT, however, there are no studies of MIBG with autopsy-confirmed diagnosis.

11.9 Conclusion

Dopaminergic imaging, particularly FP-CIT, has been shown to be a useful adjunct to making a clinical diagnosis of DLB, particularly when the differential diagnosis is AD. There is now a rich body of research on DaT imaging with very consistent results that it facilitates an accurate clinical diagnosis in both possible and probable DLB. However, several types of dementia will give an abnormal FP-CIT scan, including several types of Parkinson's plus syndromes (progressive supranuclear palsy, corticobasal degeneration, multisystem atrophy), some FTD and Huntington's cases and cases with vascular pathology in basal ganglia. A positive result does not always indicate DLB but is strongly suggestive of DLB. Dopaminergic imaging should only be used in conjunction with a full clinical assessment to strengthen clinical suspicion of DLB. More recent studies have begun to explore the correlation between dopaminergic deficit and cognitive and psychiatric symptoms with some interesting results.

References

1. Nelson PT, Jicha GA, Kryscio RJ, et al. Low sensitivity in clinical diagnoses of dementia with Lewy bodies. J Neurol. 2010;257(3):359–66.
2. Donaghy PC, McKeith IG. The clinical characteristics of dementia with Lewy bodies and a consideration of prodromal diagnosis. Alzheimers Res Ther. 2014;6(4):46.
3. McKeith IG, Dickson DW, Lowe J, et al. Diagnosis and management of dementia with Lewy bodies – third report of the DLB consortium. Neurology. 2005;65(12):1863–72.
4. Braak H, Del Tredici K, Rub U, et al. Staging of brain pathology related to sporadic Parkinson's disease. Neurobiol Aging. 2003;24(2):197–211.
5. Tatsch K. Imaging of the dopaminergic system in differential diagnosis of dementia. Eur J Nucl Med Mol Imaging. 2008;35 Suppl 1:S51–7.
6. Walker Z, Rodda J. Dopaminergic imaging: clinical utility now and in the future. Int Psychogeriatr. 2011;23 Suppl 2:S32–40.
7. Lewis DA, Melchitzky DS, Sesack SR, et al. Dopamine transporter immunoreactivity in monkey cerebral cortex: regional, laminar, and ultrastructural localization. J Comp Neurol. 2001;432(1):119–36.
8. Marquie M, Locascio JJ, Rentz DM, et al. Striatal and extrastriatal dopamine transporter levels relate to cognition in Lewy body diseases: an (11)C altropane positron emission tomography study. Alzheimers Res Ther. 2014;6(5–8):52.
9. Sesack SR, Hawrylak VA, Matus C, et al. Dopamine axon varicosities in the prelimbic division of the rat prefrontal cortex exhibit sparse immunoreactivity for the dopamine transporter. J Neurosci. 1998;18(7):2697–708.
10. Colloby SJ, McParland S, O'Brien JT, et al. Neuropathological correlates of dopaminergic imaging in Alzheimer's disease and Lewy body dementias. Brain. 2012;135(Pt 9):2798–808.
11. Benamer TS, Patterson J, Grosset DG, et al. Accurate differentiation of parkinsonism and essential tremor using visual assessment of [123I]-FP-CIT SPECT imaging: the [123I]-FP-CIT study group. Mov Disord. 2000;15(3):503–10.
12. Soderlund TA, Dickson JC, Prvulovich E, et al. Value of semiquantitative analysis for clinical reporting of 123I-2-beta-carbomethoxy-3beta-(4-iodophenyl)-N-(3-fluoropropyl)nortropane SPECT studies. J Nucl Med. 2013;54(5):714–22.

13. Walker Z, Moreno E, Thomas A, et al. Clinical usefulness of dopamine transporter SPECT imaging with 123I-FP-CIT in patients with possible dementia with Lewy bodies: randomised study. Br J Psychiatry. 2015;206(2):145–52.
14. Walker Z, Costa DC, Walker RW, et al. Differentiation of dementia with Lewy bodies from Alzheimer's disease using a dopaminergic presynaptic ligand. J Neurol Neurosurg Psychiatry. 2002;73(2):134–40.
15. O'Brien JT, Colloby S, Fenwick J, et al. Dopamine transporter loss visualized with FP-CIT SPECT in the differential diagnosis of dementia with Lewy bodies. Arch Neurol. 2004;61 (6):919–25.
16. Walker Z, Costa DC, Walker RW, et al. Striatal dopamine transporter in dementia with Lewy bodies and Parkinson disease: a comparison. Neurology. 2004;62(9):1568–72.
17. Ceravolo R, Volterrani D, Gambaccini G, et al. Presynaptic nigro-striatal function in a group of Alzheimer's disease patients with parkinsonism: evidence from a dopamine transporter imaging study. J Neural Transm. 2004;111(8):1065–73.
18. McKeith I, O'Brien J, Walker Z, et al. Sensitivity and specificity of dopamine transporter imaging with (123)I-FP-CIT SPECT in dementia with Lewy bodies: a phase III, multicentre study. Lancet Neurol. 2007;6(4):305–13.
19. O'Brien JT, McKeith IG, Walker Z, et al. Diagnostic accuracy of I-123-FP-CIT SPECT in possible dementia with Lewy bodies. Br J Psychiatry. 2009;194(1):34–9.
20. Walker Z, Jaros E, Walker RW, et al. Dementia with Lewy bodies: a comparison of clinical diagnosis, FP-CIT single photon emission computed tomography imaging and autopsy. J Neurol Neurosurg Psychiatry. 2007;78(11):1176–81.
21. Walker RW, Walker Z. Dopamine transporter single photon emission computerized tomography in the diagnosis of dementia with Lewy bodies. Mov Disord. 2009;24 Suppl 2:S754–9.
22. Ransmayr G, Seppi K, Donnemiller E, et al. Striatal dopamine transporter function in dementia with Lewy bodies and Parkinson's disease. Eur J Nucl Med. 2001;28(10):1523–8.
23. Rossi C, Volterrani D, Nicoletti V, et al. "Parkinson-dementia" diseases: a comparison by double tracer SPECT studies. Parkinsonism Relat Disord. 2009;15(10):762–6.
24. Sedaghat F, Gotzamani-Psarrakou A, Dedousi E, et al. Evaluation of dopaminergic function in frontotemporal dementia using I-FP-CIT single photon emission computed tomography. Neurodegener Dis. 2007;4(5):382–5.
25. Morgan S, Kemp P, Booij J, et al. Differentiation of frontotemporal dementia from dementia with Lewy bodies using FP-CIT SPECT. J Neurol Neurosurg Psychiatry. 2012;83 (11):1063–70.
26. Spehl TS, Frings L, Hellwig S, et al. Role of semiquantitative assessment of regional binding potential in 123I-FP-CIT SPECT for the differentiation of frontotemporal dementia, dementia with Lewy bodies, and Alzheimer's dementia. Clin Nucl Med. 2015;40(1):e27–33.
27. Colloby SJ, Williams ED, Burn DJ, et al. Progression of dopaminergic degeneration in dementia with Lewy bodies and Parkinson's disease with and without dementia assessed using I-123-FP-CIT SPECT. Eur J Nucl Med Mol Imaging. 2005;32(10):1176–85.
28. Roselli F, Pisciotta NM, Perneczky R, et al. Severity of neuropsychiatric symptoms and dopamine transporter levels in dementia with Lewy bodies: a 123I-FP-CIT SPECT study. Mov Disord. 2009;24(14):2097–103.
29. David R, Koulibaly M, Benoit M, et al. Striatal dopamine transporter levels correlate with apathy in neurodegenerative diseases – A SPECT study with partial volume effect correction. Clin Neurol Neurosurg. 2008;110(1):19–24.
30. Del Sole A, Perini G, Lecchi M, et al. Correlation between I-123-FP-CIT brain SPECT and parkinsonism in dementia with Lewy bodies caveat for clinical use. Clin Nucl Med. 2015;40 (1):32–5.
31. Colloby SJ, Firbank MJ, Pakrasi SE, et al. A comparison of (99m)Tc-exametazime and (123)I-FP-CIT SPECT imaging in the differential diagnosis of Alzheimer's disease and dementia with Lewy bodies. Int Psychogeriatr. 2008;20(6):1124–40.

32. Lim SM, Katsifis A, Villemagne VL, et al. The 18F-FDG PET cingulate island sign and comparison to 123I-beta-CIT SPECT for diagnosis of dementia with Lewy bodies. J Nucl Med. 2009;50(10):1638–45.
33. Treglia G, Cason E, Cortelli P, et al. Iodine-123 metaiodobenzylguanidine scintigraphy and iodine-123 ioflupane single photon emission computed tomography in Lewy body diseases: complementary or alternative techniques? J Neuroimaging. 2014;24(2):149–54.

Chapter 12
^{123}I-Metaiodobenzylguanidine Myocardial Scintigraphy in Dementia with Lewy Bodies

Masahito Yamada, Mitsuhiro Yoshita, Miharu Samuraki, Junji Komatsu, and Kenichi Nakajima

Abstract Differential diagnosis of dementia with Lewy bodies (DLB) from Alzheimer's disease (AD) and other dementias is essential for better management. Metaiodobenzylguanidine (MIBG) is a physiological analogue of norepinephrine, and ^{123}I-MIBG myocardial scintigraphy has been used as a noninvasive tool for estimating myocardial sympathetic nerve damage due to various disorders such as heart and neurologic diseases. Degeneration of the cardiac sympathetic nerves is a neuropathological feature of Lewy body diseases including Parkinson's disease and DLB. Multiple single-center studies, including ours, reported very high sensitivity and specificity of ^{123}I-MIBG myocardial scintigraphy for the differential diagnosis of DLB from AD and other dementias; further, our first multicenter study of DLB with the standardized technique [1] substantiated the high diagnostic accuracy of ^{123}I-MIBG myocardial scintigraphy, which was comparable to that of ^{123}I-N-ω-fluoropropyl-2β-carbomethoxy-3β-(4-iodophenyl) nortropane (FP-CIT) SPECT multicenter study [2]. In the current version of the consensus diagnostic criteria for DLB [3], ^{123}I-FP-CIT SPECT was listed as one of the suggestive features of DLB, whereas ^{123}I-MIBG myocardial scintigraphy was listed as one of the supportive features. As ^{123}I-MIBG myocardial scintigraphy has been proved to have high diagnostic specificity, it is recommended to upgrade the abnormal MIBG myocardial scintigraphy to one of the suggestive features of DLB.

M. Yamada (✉) • M. Samuraki • J. Komatsu
Department of Neurology and Neurobiology of Aging, Kanazawa University Graduate School of Medical Sciences, 13-1 Takara-machi, Kanazawa 920-8640, Japan
e-mail: m-yamada@med.kanazawa-u.ac.jp

M. Yoshita
Department of Neurology and Neurobiology of Aging, Kanazawa University Graduate School of Medical Sciences, 13-1 Takara-machi, Kanazawa 920-8640, Japan

Department of Neurology, Hokuriku National Hospital, 5963 Nobusue, Nanto, Toyama 939-1893, Japan

K. Nakajima
Department of Nuclear Medicine, Kanazawa University Hospital, 13-1, Takara-machi, Kanazawa 920-8640, Japan

K. Kosaka (ed.), *Dementia with Lewy Bodies*, DOI 10.1007/978-4-431-55948-1_12

Keywords ^{123}I-Metaiodobenzylguanidine (MIBG) myocardial scintigraphy • Dementia with Lewy bodies • Alzheimer's disease • Differential diagnosis • Multicenter study

12.1 Introduction

Differential diagnosis of dementia with Lewy bodies (DLB) from Alzheimer's disease (AD) and other dementias is essential for better management, because patients with DLB present with various clinical features including fluctuating cognition, recurrent visual hallucination, parkinsonism, REM sleep behavior disorder (RBD), severe neuroleptic sensitivity, severe autonomic dysfunction, and depression [3]. The original consensus clinical diagnostic criteria [4] were reported with high specificity but low sensitivity when compared with neuropathological findings [5]. The most common misdiagnosis was AD [5, 6]. Currently, the revised version of the consensus diagnostic criteria has been widely used [3]. The inclusion of RBD as a suggestive feature of DLB in the revised criteria may have contributed to improvement of the diagnostic accuracy [7]. Further, low dopamine transporter (DAT) uptake in basal ganglia demonstrated by single-photon emission computed tomography (SPECT) or positron emission tomography (PET) imaging was also included as a suggestive feature of DLB [3], and the abnormal DAT findings by ^{123}I-N-ω-fluoropropyl-2β-carbomethoxy-3β-(4-iodophenyl) nortropane (FP-CIT) SPECT highly correlated with a clinical diagnosis of probable DLB [2].

Metaiodobenzylguanidine (MIBG) is a physiological analogue of norepinephrine (Fig. 12.1). As cardiac sympathetic nerve terminals uptake and release MIBG as shown in Fig. 12.2, density, distribution, and activity of cardiac sympathetic nerves can be evaluated with ^{123}I-MIBG, and ^{123}I-MIBG myocardial scintigraphy

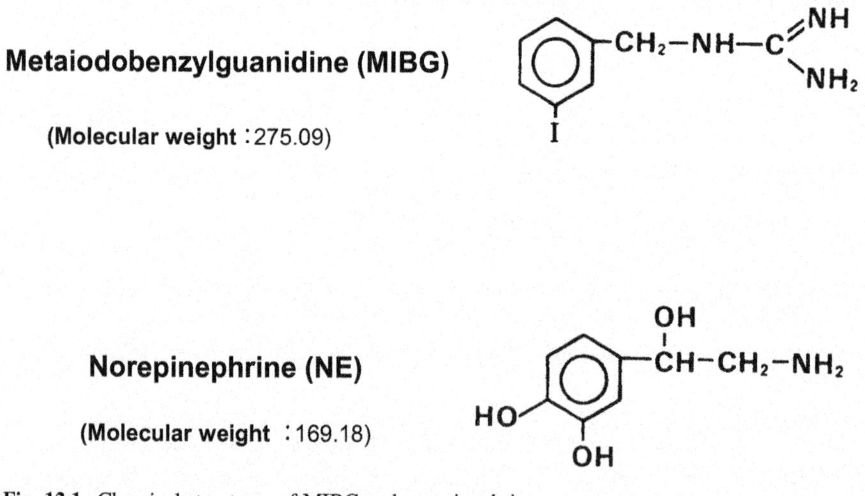

Fig. 12.1 Chemical structures of MIBG and norepinephrine

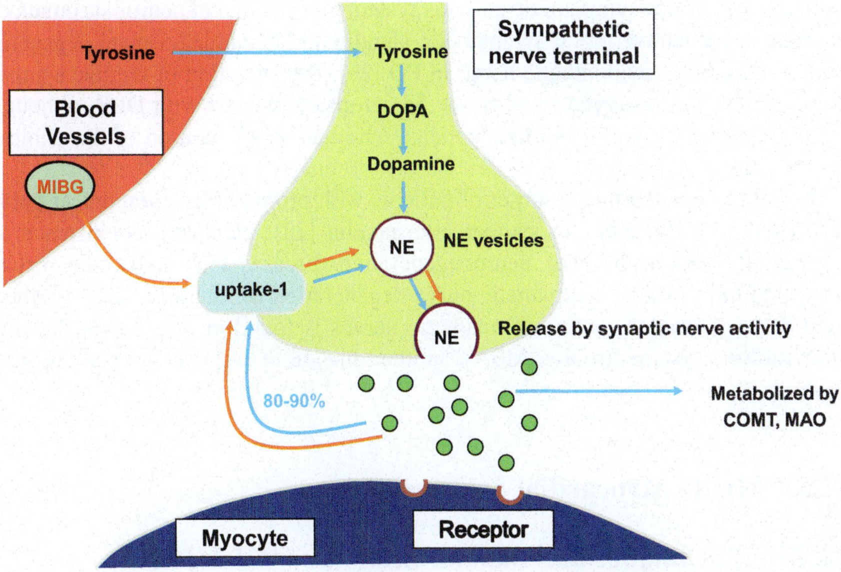

Fig. 12.2 Mechanism of MIBG accumulation in sympathetic nerve terminal. MIBG is uptaken to sympathetic nerve terminals via uptake-1, is transported to norepinephrine (NE) vesicles, and is released by exocytosis like NE by sympathetic nerve activity. MIBG does not bind to receptors on myocytes nor is metabolized by catechol-*O*-methyltransferase (COMT)/monoamine oxidase (MAO), which differs from NE. Pathways of MIBG and NE are shown with *arrows* of *red color* and *blue color*, respectively

has been used as a noninvasive tool for estimating myocardial sympathetic nerve damage due to various disorders such as heart and neurologic diseases [8–14]. Postganglionic sympathetic denervation is a common feature of Lewy body diseases (LBD) including dementia with Lewy bodies (DLB) and Parkinson's disease (PD). In this chapter, we describe about the value of ^{123}I-MIBG myocardial scintigraphy for the clinical diagnosis of DLB, indicating a significant contribution of this technique to increasing the diagnostic accuracy of DLB.

12.2 Degeneration of Cardiac Sympathetic Nerves in Lewy Body Diseases and Related Neurological Disorders

Peripheral as well as central autonomic nervous systems are involved in the disease process of LBD. Concerning postganglionic cardiac sympathetic nerves, Lewy body pathologies, including Lewy bodies and α-synuclein-positive neurites with loss of tyrosine hydroxylase-positive nerve fibers, are observed in the sympathetic ganglia, cardiac plexus, nerves of cardiac walls from patients with PD, incidental LBD (ILBD), and pure autonomic failure (PAF) [15–20]. The observations in PD and ILBD suggested that accumulations of α-synuclein aggregates in the distal axons of the cardiac sympathetic nervous system precede that of neuronal somata or neurites in the paravertebral sympathetic ganglia and herald centripetal degeneration of the cardiac sympathetic nerve in PD [20]. Degeneration of cardiac sympathetic nerves was observed in all of the 58 autopsied patients with DLB, although the degeneration was mild in four patients who had short duration of the clinical course [21].

It should be noted that a subset of patients with progressive supranuclear palsy (PSP) have Lewy bodies in sympathetic ganglia [22]; incidental coexistence or overlap of LBD with other neurodegenerative diseases than LBD may cause postganglionic cardiac sympathetic nerve degeneration as found in LBD. Further, mild degeneration of cardiac sympathetic nerves is found in a subset of patients with multiple system atrophy (MSA), another disease of α-synucleinopathies [23].

12.3 MIBG Myocardial Scintigraphy

12.3.1 Techniques and Standardization of ^{123}I-MIBG Myocardial Scintigraphy

A method for data acquisition of ^{123}I-MIBG myocardial scintigraphy was described elsewhere [24]. Briefly, after subjects have been in a supine position for 20 min, 111 MBq of ^{123}I-MIBG is injected intravenously. Anterior planar and SPECT images are obtained 20–30 min and 3–4 h after the injection as early and delayed images, respectively. On the anterior planar image, regions of interest (ROI) are set on the whole heart (H), including the left ventricle, and mediastinum (M) (Fig. 12.3), and the heart-to-mediastinum (H/M) uptake ratio is calculated as the index of cardiac MIBG uptake by dividing the count density of the ventricular ROI by that of the mediastinal ROI. The washout rate (WR) is calculated as the index of MIBG release as follows: WR (%) = 100 × (Ec − Dc)/Ec, where Ec is the early cardiac count density and Dc is the decay-corrected delayed cardiac count density (mediastinal counts are subtracted as backgrounds).

We developed software for semiautomatically measuring H/M ratio in ^{123}I-MIBG myocardial scintigraphy; using the semiautomatic method, the H/M ratio showed high reproducibility in both early and delayed imaging [25]. As different collimators and scinticameras are used for ^{123}I-MIBG myocardial scintigraphy in different institutions, standardization of the H/M ratio is necessary for correction of normal databases and for a multicenter study. For standardization of the H/M ratios, we developed the calibration phantom method which could be practically used for multicenter comparison of H/M ratios [1, 26]. To further standardize the H/M ratio with various camera-collimator combinations among institutions, a conversion coefficient for each camera-collimator system was created based on phantom studies; by using the reference H/M ratio and conversion coefficients for the system, H/M ratio in various conditions could be converted to the standard H/M ratios in a

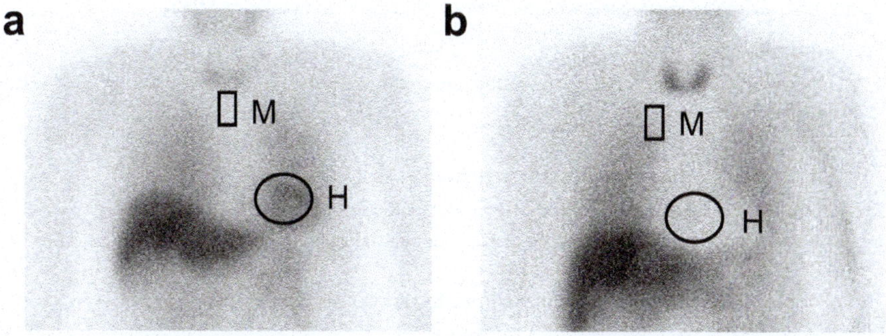

Fig. 12.3 Normal (**a**) and reduced (**b**) myocardial MIBG uptake in the anterior planar image of ^{123}I-MIBG myocardial scintigraphy. Regions of interest (ROI) are set on the heart (H) and mediastinum (M), and the H/M ratio is used to indicate the cardiac MIBG uptake

range of normal to low H/M ratios [27]. The standardized H/M ratio will be a good background to recommend universal use of MIBG study.

12.3.2 Diseases and Medicines That Influence Myocardial MIBG Uptake

Cardiac diseases, metabolic or endocrine diseases, and neurological diseases with postganglionic sympathetic nerve lesions are associated with reduction of the cardiac uptake of MIBG in ^{123}I-MIBG myocardial scintigraphy (Table 12.1). The neurological diseases include neuropathies involving autonomic nerves, such as diabetic neuropathy and amyloid neuropathy, as well as LBD, such as PD, DLB, and PAF. Besides DLB (see below), reduced MIBG uptake was reported in patients with PAF, PD, and familial amyloid polyneuropathy (FAP) and a subset of patients with PSP or MSA [12–14, 28–33]. In addition, marked reduction of cardiac MIBG uptake was reported with idiopathic RBD, and an association of Lewy body pathology was suggested [34]. Thus, when ^{123}I-MIBG myocardial scintigraphy is used for the diagnosis of LBD (PD, DLB, PAF, and RBD), cardiac diseases, metabolic or endocrine diseases, and the other neurological diseases with possible postganglionic sympathetic nerve lesions need to be excluded.

Further, it should be noted that some medicines interfere with biodistribution of ^{123}I-MIBG [35]. Several mechanisms of interaction were reported: (1) inhibition of uptake, (2) inhibition of active transport into vesicles, (3) competition for transport into vesicles, (4) depletion of content of storage vesicles, (5) calcium mediated, and (6) other possible unknown mechanisms [35]. List of medicines that are known to interact with MIBG is shown in Table 12.2; it is recommended to avoid or stop treatment with such medicines [33, 35].

Table 12.1 Diseases associated with reduction of the cardiac uptake of MIBG

1. Cardiac diseases
Congestive heart failure, cardiomyopathy, amyloidosis, ischemic heart disease, arrhythmias, transplanted hearts, etc.
2. Metabolic and endocrine diseases
Diabetes mellitus, pheochromocytoma, thyroid diseases, etc.
3. Neurological diseases with postganglionic sympathetic nerve lesions
a. Lewy body diseases: Parkinson's disease, dementia with Lewy bodies, pure autonomic failure, REM sleep behavior disorder, etc.
b. Peripheral neuropathies: diabetic neuropathy, amyloid neuropathy, etc.

Table 12.2 Medicines that are known to interact with MIBG

1. **Sympathomimetics and sympatholytics**: L-threo-DOPS, norepinephrine, dobutamine, dopamine, phenylephrine, phenylpropanolamine, salbutamol, selegiline, brimonidine, etc.
2. **Antidepressants**: amitriptyline, amoxapine, clomipramine, desipramine, imipramine, trazodone, mianserin, etc.
3. **Antipsychotics**: chlorpromazine, haloperidol, droperidol, clozapine, quetiapine, risperidone, etc.
4. **CNS stimulants**: cocaine, caffeine, amphetamine, etc.
5. **α- and β-Blockers**: labetalol, phenoxybenzamine, etc.
6. **Calcium channel blockers**: diltiazem, isradipine, nicardipine, nifedipine, nimodipine, verapamil, etc.

Cited from Refs. [33, 35]

12.4 Diagnostic Value of MIBG Myocardial Scintigraphy in DLB

12.4.1 Single-Center Studies

Since 2001, many single-center studies have reported usefulness of ^{123}I-MIBG myocardial scintigraphy to discriminate DLB from AD or other dementias since 2001 [36–45]. Our group investigated cardiac sympathetic denervation with MIBG scintigraphy in 37 patients with DLB (7 without parkinsonism and 30 with parkinsonism), 42 patients with AD, and 10 normal controls and found that, regardless of parkinsonism, delayed H/M ratio had a sensitivity of 100 %, a specificity of 100 %, and a positive predictive value of 100 % at a cutoff value of 1.68 in discrimination between DLB and AD (Fig. 12.4) [39]. In a systematic review and a meta-analysis [46], eight single-center studies were identified comprising a total of 346 patients with dementia (152 with DLB and 194 with other dementias); the pooled sensitivity of MIBG scintigraphy in detection of DLB was 98 % (95 % CI, 94–100 %); the pooled specificity of MIBG scintigraphy in differential diagnosis between DLB and other dementias was 94 % (95 % CI, 90–97 %). The data suggest that MIBG is an accurate test for differential diagnosis between DLB and other dementias.

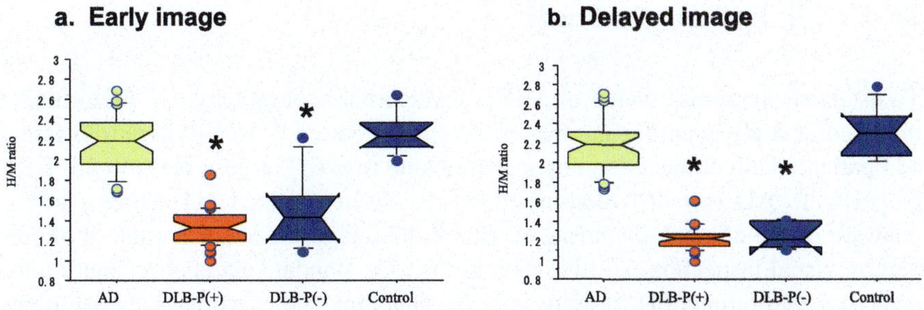

Fig. 12.4 Differential diagnosis of dementia with Lewy bodies (DLB) from Alzheimer's disease (AD) by ^{123}I-MIBG myocardial scintigraphy in a study at Kanazawa University Hospital [39]. H (heart)/M (mediastinum) ratios in early (**a**) and late images (**b**) are significantly lower in DLB with parkinsonism (DLB-P(+)) ($n = 37$) and DLB without parkinsonism (DLB-P(-)) ($n = 8$) compared with those in AD ($n = 42$) or healthy controls ($n = 10$). $*p < 0.0001$

Comparative value of MIBG myocardial scintigraphy with other diagnostic tools in distinguishing DLB from AD or other dementias has been investigated in several single-center studies. In a comparison between MIBG myocardial scintigraphy and brain perfusion SPECT with N-isopropyl-p-[^{123}I]iodoamphetamine (^{123}I-IMP) involving 19 patients with DLB and 39 patients with AD, brain perfusion SPECT failed to identify occipital hypoperfusion in five patients with DLB, while reduction of MIBG uptake was found in all the patients with DLB [41]. Some patients with probable or possible DLB showed no occipital hypoperfusion in ^{123}I-IMP SPECT, but showed low cardiac MIBG uptake [43]. Combination of brain FDG-PET with MIBG myocardial scintigraphy was useful in differentiation of DLB from AD [47]. Thus, MIBG myocardial scintigraphy would improve the sensitivity in detection of DLB in combination with brain perfusion SPECT or FDG-PET [48]. In patients with probable DLB (n = 28) studied by both ^{123}I-MIBG myocardial scintigraphy and ^{123}I-FP-CIT SPECT, cardiac MIBG uptake and FP-CIT binding in basal ganglia were reduced in parallel [49]. In differential diagnosis between DLB (n = 20) and other dementias (n = 11) using both ^{123}I-MIBG myocardial scintigraphy and ^{123}I-CIT-SPECT, the sensitivity and specificity were 90 % and 91 %, respectively, for MIBG, and were 90 % and 91 %, respectively, for FP-CIT; the same results confirmed the usefulness of both techniques in DLB diagnosis [50]. Compared with cerebrospinal fluid (CSF) tests, the diagnostic value of MIBG myocardial scintigraphy was superior to that of CSF markers including amyloid β 1–42, 181-phosphorylated tau [42], and α-synuclein [51].

Furthermore, subjects with mild cognitive impairment (MCI) and reduced cardiac uptake of MIBG were reported to later convert to probable DLB, suggesting that MIBG myocardial scintigraphy is useful for detection of DLB at MCI stage [52, 53].

12.4.2 A Multicenter Study

To establish diagnostic value of MIBG myocardial scintigraphy, we performed a multicenter study in ten Japanese sites, in which we used ^{123}I-MIBG scans to assess 133 patients with clinical diagnoses of probable (n = 61) or possible (n = 26) DLB or probable AD (n = 46) established by a consensus panel [1]. Three readers, unaware of the clinical diagnosis, classified the images as either normal or abnormal by visual inspection. All the institutions used standard acquisition conditions, and cross calibration of H/M ratios with the phantom studies among the institutions was performed as described elsewhere [26]. The H/M ratios were calculated using an automated region-of-interest-based system [25].

Individual values for the H/M ratio of ^{123}I-MIBG uptake and ROC analysis for discriminating probable DLB from probable AD groups are shown in Figs. 12.5 and 12.6, respectively. Using the H/M ratio calculated with the automated system, the sensitivity was 68.9 %, and the specificity was 89.1 % to differentiate probable DLB from probable AD at a cutoff value of 2.10 in both early and delayed images (Table 12.3). By visual assessment, the sensitivity and specificity were 68.9 % and

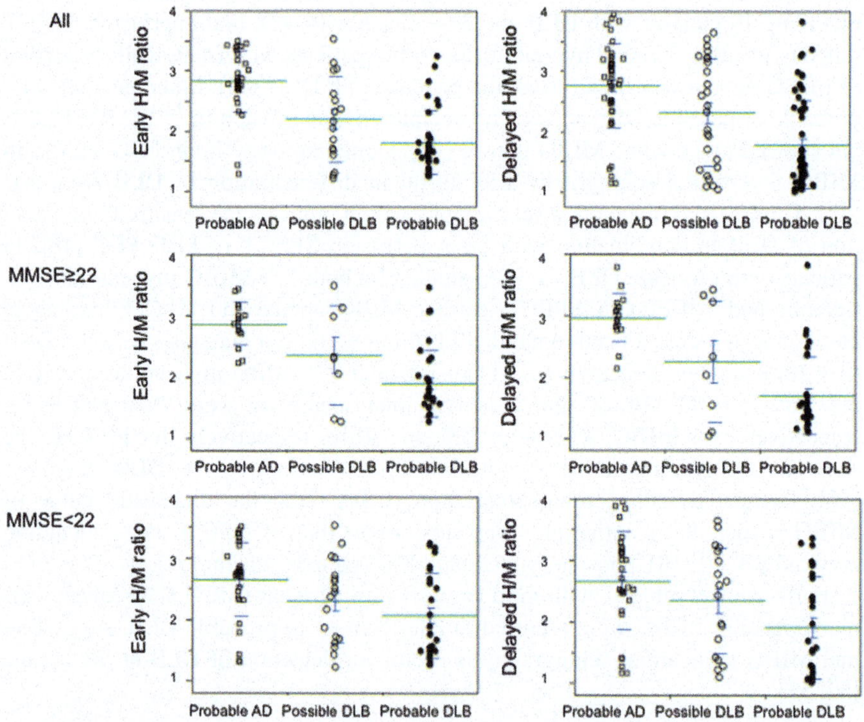

Fig. 12.5 Individual values for the H/M ratio of ^{123}I-MIBG uptake in a multicenter study [1]. Significant reductions in early and delayed H/M ratios were observed in probable DLB compared with probable AD group of all cases, mild dementia cases (MMSE ≥ 22), and moderate/severe dementia cases (MMSE ≤ 21) (see text). *Green lines* indicate the mean value of H/M ratio (*AD* Alzheimer's disease, *DLB* dementia with Lewy bodies)

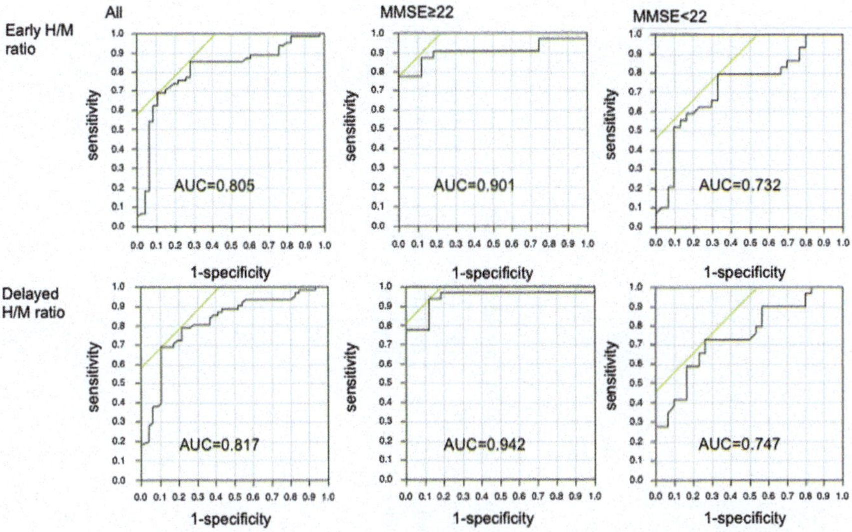

Fig. 12.6 ROC curves for the detection of probable DLB from probable AD based on H/M ratio of each group in a multicenter study with ^{123}I-MIBG myocardial scintigraphy [1]. The area under the ROC curve of the early H/M ratio was 0.805 ($p < 0.001$) for the all patients group, 0.901 ($p < 0.0001$) for the mild dementia group, and 0.732 ($p = 0.001$) for the moderate/severe dementia group, whereas that for the delayed H/M ratio was 0.817 ($p < 0.001$), 0.942 ($p < 0.0001$), and 0.747 ($p = 0.007$), respectively (*ROC* receiver operating characteristic, *AUC* area under the curve)

87.0 %, respectively. In a subpopulation of patients with mild dementia (MMSE $\geq$ 22, n = 47) (Figs. 12.5 and 12.6), the sensitivity and specificity were 77.4 % and 93.8 %, respectively, with the delayed H/M ratio. The moderate/severe dementia group, on the other hand, had a sensitivity of 59.6 % and a specificity of 83.3 % at a cutoff value of 2.10. No adverse events were noted during this study.

Our first multicenter study confirmed earlier single-site studies. The multicenter study using ^{123}I-FP-CIT SPECT showed mean sensitivity of 77.7 % for detecting clinical probable DLB, with specificity of 90.4 % for excluding non-DLB which was predominantly due to AD [2]. On the other hand, the recent clinicopathologic analyses showed that the DLB diagnostic criteria [3] had sensitivity of 85 % and specificity of 73 % for excluding non-DLB [7]. The sensitivity and specificity of ^{123}I-MIBG myocardial scintigraphy are comparable to those of ^{123}I-FP-CIT SPECT multicenter study [2], especially in mild dementia cases. The potential benefit in the diagnostic precision provided by ^{123}I-MIBG myocardial scintigraphy is therefore predominantly in the specificity of case detection, which could be increased from a mean of 73 to 89.1 %.

It is not clear why ^{123}I-MIBG myocardial scintigraphy showed lower sensitivity in the moderate to severe dementia group diagnosed with DLB by the consensus diagnostic criteria [3] compared with that in the mild dementia group. It was reported that extrapyramidal signs and hallucination occur frequently in AD cases

Table 12.3 Sensitivity and specificity of H/M ratio in differentiating between probable DLB and probable AD in a multicenter study [1]

	Sensitivity (95 % CI)	Specificity (95 % CI)	Accuracy (95 % CI)	PPV (95 % CI)	NPV (95 % CI)
Early H/M ratio (cutoff, 2.10)	68.9 (57.2–80.5)	89.1 (80.1–98.1)	77.6 (69.7–85.5)	89.4 (80.5–98.2)	68.3 (56.6–80.1)
Delayed H/M ratio (cutoff, 2.10)	68.9 (57.2–80.5)	89.1 (80.1–98.1)	77.6 (69.7–85.5)	89.4 (80.5–98.2)	68.3 (56.6–80.1)

PPV positive predictive value, *NPV* negative predictive value

with faster cognitive decline [54]. In neuropathological examination at autopsy, extrapyramidal symptoms in AD were reported to be correlated with neuronal loss in substantia nigra, and tau as well as α-synuclein pathologies correlated with the neuronal loss in substantia nigra [55]. The subclinical comorbid pathologies may exist in patients with dementia [56]. Clinical diagnosis in moderate to severe dementia cases by the diagnostic criteria may be influenced by these factors.

12.5 Conclusions

Our first multicenter study of DLB with the standardized technique [1] substantiated the high diagnostic accuracy of ^{123}I-MIBG myocardial scintigraphy, which was comparable to that of ^{123}I-FP-CIT SPECT multicenter study [2]. Neuropathologically, reduction of cardiac MIBG uptake reflects Lewy body pathology and degeneration of postganglionic cardiac sympathetic nerves in LBD; on the other hand, decreased FP-CIT binding in basal ganglia reflects degeneration of the nigrostriatal pathway. In the current version of the consensus diagnostic criteria for DLB [3], ^{123}I-FP-CIT SPECT was listed as one of the suggestive features of DLB, whereas ^{123}I-MIBG myocardial scintigraphy was listed as one of the supportive features. As ^{123}I-MIBG myocardial scintigraphy has been proved to have high diagnostic specificity, it is recommended to upgrade the abnormal MIBG myocardial scintigraphy to one of the suggestive features of DLB.

Acknowledgments The study was supported by the grant of Japan Foundation for Neuroscience and Mental Health (to M. Yamada). The funder had no role in preparation of the manuscript. The authors thank Ms. Etsuko Tsujiguchi for her secretarial assistance.

References

1. Yoshita M, Arai H, Arai T, et al. Diagnostic accuracy of ^{123}I-meta-iodobenzylguanidine myocardial scintigraphy in dementia with Lewy bodies: a multicenter study. PLoS One. 2015;10:e0120540.
2. McKeith I, O'Brien J, Walker Z, et al. Sensitivity and specificity of dopamine transporter imaging with 123I-FP-CIT SPECT in dementia with Lewy bodies: a phase III, multicentre study. Lancet Neurol. 2007;6:305–13.
3. McKeith I, Dickson DW, Lowe J, et al. Diagnosis and management of dementia with Lewy bodies: third report of the DLB consortium. Neurology. 2005;65:1863–72.
4. McKeith IG, Galasko D, Kosaka K, et al. Consensus guidelines for the clinical and pathologic diagnosis of dementia with Lewy bodies (DLB): report of the consortium on DLB international workshop. Neurology. 1996;47:1113–24.
5. Lopez OL, Becker JT, Kaufer DI, et al. Research evaluation and prospective diagnosis of dementia with Lewy bodies. Arch Neurol. 2002;59:43–6.
6. McKeith IG, Ballard CG, Perry RH, et al. Prospective validation of consensus criteria for the diagnosis of dementia with Lewy bodies. Neurology. 2000;54:1050–8.

7. Ferman TJ, Boeve BF, Smith GE, et al. Inclusion of RBD improves the diagnostic classification of dementia with Lewy bodies. Neurology. 2011;77:875–82.
8. Kline RC, Swanson DP, Wieland DM, et al. Myocardial imaging in man with I-123 meta-iodobenzylguanidine. J Nucl Med. 1981;22:129–32.
9. Dae MW, O'Connell JW, Botvinick EH, et al. Scintigraphic assessment of regional cardiac adrenergic innervation. Circulation. 1989;79:634–44.
10. Glowniak JV, Turner FE, Gray LL, et al. Iodine-123 metaiodobenzylguanidine imaging of the heart in idiopathic congestive cardiomyopathy and cardiac transplants. J Nucl Med. 1989;30:1182–91.
11. Nakajima K, Bunko H, Taki J, et al. Quantitative analysis of ^{123}I-meta-iodobenzylguanidine (MIBG) uptake in hypertrophic cardiomyopathy. Am Heart J. 1990;119:1329–37.
12. Hakusui S, Yasuda T, Yanagi T, et al. A radiological analysis of heart sympathetic functions with *meta*-[^{123}I]iodobenzylguanidine in neurological patients with autonomic failure. J Auton Nerv Syst. 1994;49:81–4.
13. Iwasa K, Nakajima K, Yoshikawa H, et al. Decreased myocardial ^{123}I-MIBG uptake in Parkinson's disease. Acta Neurol Scand. 1998;97:303–6.
14. Yoshita M. Differentiation of idiopathic Parkinson's disease from striatonigral degeneration and progressive supranuclear palsy using iodine-123 meta-iodobenzylguanidine myocardial scintigraphy. J Neurol Sci. 1998;155:60–7.
15. Wakabayashi K, Takahashi H. Neuropathology of autonomic nervous system in Parkinson's disease. Eur Neurol. 1997;38 Suppl 2:2–7.
16. Iwanaga K, Wakabayashi K, Yoshimoto M, et al. Lewy body-type degeneration in cardiac plexus in Parkinson's and incidental Lewy body diseases. Neurology. 1999;52:1269–71.
17. Orimo S, Ozawa E, Oka T, et al. Different histopathology accounting for a decrease in myocardial MIBG uptake in PD and MSA. Neurology. 2001;57:1140–1.
18. Orimo S, Oka T, Miura H, et al. Sympathetic cardiac denervation in Parkinson's disease and pure autonomic failure but not in multiple system atrophy. J Neurol Neurosurg Psychiatry. 2002;73:776–7.
19. Mitsui J, Saito Y, Momose T, et al. Pathology of the sympathetic nervous system corresponding to the decreased cardiac uptake in ^{123}I-metaiodobenzylguanidine (MIBG) scintigraphy in a patient with Parkinson disease. J Neurol Sci. 2006;243:101–4.
20. Orimo S, Uchihara T, Nakamura A, et al. Axonal α-synuclein aggregates herald centripetal degeneration of cardiac sympathetic nerve in Parkinson's disease. Brain. 2008;131:642–50.
21. Orimo S, Nakamura A, Uchihara T, et al. Relationship among degeneration of the cardiac sympathetic nerve, clinical features and neuropathological findings in dementia with Lewy bodies. Neuropathology. 2012;32 Suppl:62.
22. Mori H, Oda M, Komori T, et al. Lewy bodies in progressive supranuclear palsy. Acta Neuropathol. 2002;104:273–8.
23. Orimo S, Kanazawa T, Nakamura A, et al. Degeneration of cardiac sympathetic nerve can occur in multiple system atrophy. Acta Neuropathol. 2007;113:81–6.
24. Nakajima K, Yoshita M, Matsuo S, et al. Iodine-123-MIBG sympathetic imaging in Lewy-body diseases and related movement disorders. Q J Nucl Med Mol Imaging. 2008;52:378–87.
25. Okuda K, Nakajima K, Hosoya T, et al. Semi-automated algorithm for calculating heart-to-mediastinum ratio in cardiac Iodine-123 MIBG imaging. J Nucl Cardiol. 2011;18:82–9.
26. Nakajima K, Okuda K, Matsuo S, et al. Standardization of metaiodobenzylguanidine heart to mediastinum ratio using a calibration phantom: effects of correction on normal databases and a multicentre study. Eur J Nucl Med Mol Imaging. 2012;39:113–19.
27. Nakajima K, Okuda K, Yoshimura M, et al. Multicenter cross-calibration of I-123 metaiodobenzylguanidine heart-to-mediastinum ratios to overcome camera-collimator variations. J Nucl Cardiol. 2014;21:970–8.
28. Hirayama M, Hakusui S, Koike Y, et al. A scintigraphical qualitative analysis of peripheral vascular sympathetic function with meta-[^{123}I]iodobenzylguanidine in neurological patients with autonomic failure. J Auton Nerv Syst. 1995;53:230–4.

29. Yoshida M, Fukumoto Y, Kuroda Y, et al. Sympathetic denervation of myocardium demonstrated by ^{123}I-MIBG scintigraphy in pure progressive autonomic failure. Eur Neurol. 1997;38:291–6.
30. Yoshita M, Hayashi M, Hirai S. Decreased myocardial accumulation of ^{123}I-meta-iodobenzyl guanidine in Parkinson's disease. Nucl Med Commun. 1998;19:137–42.
31. Orimo S, Ozawa E, Nakade S, et al. ^{123}I-metaiodobenzylguanidine myocardial scintigraphy in Parkinson's disease. J Neurol Neurosurg Psychiatry. 1999;67:189–94.
32. Goldstein DS, Holmes C, Li ST, et al. Cardiac sympathetic denervation in Parkinson disease. Ann Intern Med. 2000;133:338–47.
33. Yoshita M. Value of MIBG in the differential diagnosis of neurodegenerative disorders. In: Dierckx RAJO, Otte A, de Vries EFJ, van Waarde A, Leenders KL, editors. PET and SPECT in neurology. New York/Berlin/Heidelberg: Springer; 2014. p. 437–49.
34. Miyamoto T, Miyamoto M, Inoue Y, et al. Reduced cardiac 123I-MIBG scintigraphy in idiopathic REM sleep behavior disorder. Neurology. 2006;67:2236–8.
35. Solanki KK, Bomanji J, Moyes J, et al. A pharmacological guide to medicines which interfere with the biodistribution of radiolabelled meta-iodobenzylguanidine (MIBG). Nucl Med Commun. 1992;13:513–21.
36. Yoshita M, Taki J, Yamada M. A clinical role for [^{123}I]MIBG myocardial scintigraphy in the distinction between dementia of the Alzheimer's-type and dementia with Lewy bodies. J Neurol Neurosurg Psychiatry. 2001;71:583–8.
37. Watanabe H, Ieda T, Katayama T, et al. Cardiac ^{123}I-meta-iodobenzylguanidine (MIBG) uptake in dementia with Lewy bodies: comparison with Alzheimer's disease. J Neurol Neurosurg Psychiatry. 2001;70:781–3.
38. Oide T, Tokuda T, Momose M, et al. Usefulness of [^{123}I]metaiodobenzylguanidine ([^{123}I] MIBG) myocardial scintigraphy in differentiating between Alzheimer's disease and dementia with Lewy bodies. Intern Med. 2003;42:686–90.
39. Yoshita M, Taki J, Yokoyama K, et al. Value of ^{123}I-MIBG radioactivity in the differential diagnosis of DLB from AD. Neurology. 2006;66:1850–4.
40. Hanyu H, Shimizu S, Hirao K, et al. The role of ^{123}I-metaiodobenzylguanidine myocardial scintigraphy in the diagnosis of Lewy body disease in patients with dementia in a memory clinic. Dement Geriatr Cogn Disord. 2006;22:379–84.
41. Hanyu H, Shimizu S, Hirao K, et al. Comparative value of brain perfusion SPECT and [^{123}I] MIBG myocardial scintigraphy in distinguishing between dementia with Lewy bodies and Alzheimer's disease. Eur J Nucl Med Mol Imaging. 2006;33:248–53.
42. Wada-Isoe K, Kitayama M, Nakaso K, et al. Diagnostic markers for diagnosing dementia with Lewy bodies: CSF and MIBG cardiac scintigraphy study. J Neurol Sci. 2007;260:33–7.
43. Inui Y, Toyama H, Manabe Y, et al. Evaluation of probable or possible dementia with lewy bodies using ^{123}I-IMP brain perfusion SPECT, ^{123}I-MIBG, and 99mTc-MIBI myocardial SPECT. J Nucl Med. 2007;48:1641–50.
44. Estorch M, Camacho V, Paredes P, et al. Cardiac ^{123}I-metaiodobenzylguanidine imaging allows early identification of dementia with Lewy bodies during life. Eur J Nucl Med Mol Imaging. 2008;35:1636–41.
45. Novellino F, Bagnato A, Salsone M, et al. Myocardial ^{123}I-MIBG scintigraphy for differentiation of Lewy bodies disease from FTD. Neurobiol Aging. 2010;31:1903–11.
46. Treglia G, Cason E. Diagnostic performance of myocardial innervation imaging using MIBG scintigraphy in differential diagnosis between dementia with lewy bodies and other dementias: a systematic review and a meta-analysis. J Neuroimaging. 2012;22:111–17.
47. Schmidt SL, Correa PL, Tolentino JC, et al. Value of combining activated brain FDG-PET and cardiac MIBG for the differential diagnosis of dementia: differentiation of dementia with Lewy bodies and Alzheimer disease when the diagnoses based on clinical and neuroimaging criteria are difficult. Clin Nucl Med. 2008;33:398–401.

48. Sakamoto F, Shiraishi S, Yoshida M, et al. Diagnosis of dementia with Lewy bodies: diagnostic performance of combined ^{123}I-IMP brain perfusion SPECT and ^{123}I-MIBG myocardial scintigraphy. Ann Nucl Med. 2014;28:203–11.
49. Camacho V, Marquié M, Lleó A, et al. Cardiac sympathetic impairment parallels nigrostriatal degeneration in probable dementia with Lewy bodies. Q J Nucl Med Mol Imaging. 2011;55:476–83.
50. Treglia G, Cason E, Cortelli P, et al. Iodine-123 metaiodobenzylguanidine scintigraphy and iodine-123 ioflupane single photon emission computed tomography in Lewy body diseases: complementary or alternative techniques? J Neuroimaging. 2014;24:149–54.
51. Noguchi-Shinohara M, Tokuda T, Yoshita M, et al. CSF α-synuclein levels in dementia with Lewy bodies and Alzheimer's disease. Brain Res. 2009;28:1–6.
52. Fujishiro H, Nakamura S, Kitazawa M, et al. Early detection of dementia with Lewy bodies in patients with amnestic mild cognitive impairment using ^{123}I-MIBG cardiac scintigraphy. J Neurol Sci. 2012;315:115–19.
53. Oda H, Ishii K, Terashima A, et al. Myocardial scintigraphy may predict the conversion to probable dementia with Lewy bodies. Neurology. 2013;81:1741–5.
54. Chui HC, Lyness SA, Sobel E, et al. Extrapyramidal signs and psychiatric symptoms predict faster cognitive decline in Alzheimer's disease. Arch Neurol. 1994;51:676–81.
55. Attems J, Quass M, Jellinger KA. Tau and α-synuclein brainstem pathology in Alzheimer disease: relation with extrapyramidal signs. Acta Neuropathol. 2007;113:53–62.
56. White L. Brain lesions at autopsy in older Japanese-American men as related to cognitive impairment and dementia in the final years of life: a summary report from the Honolulu-Asia aging study. J Alzheimers Dis. 2009;18:713–25.

Chapter 13
Alpha-Synuclein in Cerebrospinal Fluid

Takahiko Tokuda, Ryotaro Ishii, Harutsugu Tatebe, Takashi Kasai, and Omar M.A. El-Agnaf

Abstract The current status of biochemical biomarker candidates for dementia with Lewy bodies (DLB) and synucleinopathy has been previously discussed. The majority of the studies on biochemical biomarkers were cross-sectional, retrospective, and tested with pathologically unproven subjects. α-Synuclein (A-syn) plays a pivotal role both in the development of the disease and propagation of the pathology in Parkinson's disease (PD). Levels of total A-syn in cerebrospinal fluid (CSF) can discriminate PD from controls or tauopathies as groups. However, it is hard to diagnose an individual patient according to the level of CSF A-syn alone. The CSF total A-syn could also be useful as a surrogate biomarker for PD for monitoring the severity of the disease. CSF levels of A-syn oligomers could be a promising biomarker for the diagnosis of PD and are reported to correlate with motor and cognitive scores in PD, also suggesting their possible ability as a biomarker to monitor disease severity. With regard to the diagnosis of DLB, some studies, including two meta-analyses, demonstrated significantly lower CSF levels of total A-syn in DLB patients compared to AD patients. However, the sensitivity and specificity as well as diagnostic ability of CSF total A-syn remain to be elucidated. Whether CSF A-syn oligomers are useful or not for the diagnosis of DLB has not been examined. To study plasma levels of total and oligomeric A-syn, it is essential to eliminate the interference from heterophilic antibodies that have a significant impact on the assays of plasma A-syn, despite never being considered in any of the studies reported so far.

T. Tokuda (✉)
Department of Molecular Pathobiology of Brain Diseases, Kyoto Prefectural University of Medicine, Kajii-cho 465, Kamigyo-ku, Kyoto 602-8566, Japan

Department of Neurology, Kyoto Prefectural University of Medicine, Kajii-cho 465, Kamigyo-ku, Kyoto 602-8566, Japan
e-mail: ttokuda@koto.kpu-m.ac.jp

R. Ishii • H. Tatebe • T. Kasai
Department of Neurology, Kyoto Prefectural University of Medicine, Kajii-cho 465, Kamigyo-ku, Kyoto 602-8566, Japan

O.M.A. El-Agnaf
College of Science, Engineering and Technology, HBKU, P.O.Box: 5825, Education City, Doha, Qatar

K. Kosaka (ed.), *Dementia with Lewy Bodies*, DOI 10.1007/978-4-431-55948-1_13

For future studies developing biochemical biomarkers for DLB and synucleinopathy, it will be necessary to not only validate the already reported candidates and translate them to clinical practice but also to identify novel biomarkers that are more closely associated with the underlying pathophysiologies, including certain oligomers or protofibrils of A-syn that are specifically relevant to neurotoxicity and/or prion-like propagation of the diseases. To accomplish these goals, a large, prospective, and longitudinal cohort study carried out using standardized diagnostic criteria and stringent protocols with quality-controlled methods will definitely be needed.

Keywords Dementia with Lewy bodies • Biochemical biomarker • Cerebrospinal fluid • α-Synuclein • Oligomer

13.1 Introduction

Dementia with Lewy bodies (DLB) is clinically characterized by fluctuating cognitive decline, visual hallucinations, delusions, and parkinsonism and is acknowledged as the second most common form of neurodegenerative dementia after Alzheimer's disease (AD) [1, 2]. A key pathological feature of DLB is the widespread deposition of α-synuclein (A-syn), a major filamentous component of Lewy bodies and Lewy neurites [3]. Differentiating DLB from AD is important, although the consensus criteria for the clinical diagnosis of DLB [4] are not sensitive despite the high specificity [5]. There is considerable overlap of clinical manifestations as well as neuropathology between patients with DLB and AD, which could lead to an inaccurate antemortem diagnosis [5]. For these reasons, development of biomarkers is urgently needed to make a correct diagnosis of DLB in the early or even prodromal stage of the disease and to monitor disease progression and efficacy of therapeutic interventions. Diagnostic biomarkers in cerebrospinal fluid (CSF) have been explored to determine the etiology of dementia in patients. The usefulness of the CSF levels of amyloid-β (Aβ) and tau as diagnostic and surrogate biomarkers has been widely approved in AD [6] and has also been used in clinical trials for patients with AD [7, 8]. In this chapter, biochemical biomarkers, mainly CSF A-syn species, for the diagnosis of DLB, Parkinson's disease (PD), and other synucleinopathies, will be discussed.

13.2 Basic Concepts of Biomarkers for Neurodegenerative Diseases

"Biomarker" was defined by the Biomarkers Definitions Working Group (NIH) as "a characteristic that is objectively measured and evaluated as an indicator of normal biological processes, pathogenic processes, or pharmacological responses to a therapeutic intervention" [9]. This definition implies that biomarkers can be used for different purposes, for example: (1) to make a correct and differential diagnosis (diagnostic biomarkers), (2) to monitor disease severity (surrogate biomarkers), (3) to predict disease progression (predictive biomarkers), and (4) as tools for therapeutic optimization and monitoring of the disease (surrogate biomarkers). In addition, the definition includes several modalities of biomarkers such as neuroimaging evaluation (see previous chapters) and biochemical assays [10]. In this chapter, we will focus on biochemical biomarkers for DLB and PD including CSF A-syn.

13.2.1 Current Status of Imaging and Biochemical Biomarkers in the Diagnosis of Synucleinopathy

Regarding the present status of imaging and biochemical biomarkers for PD, Mollenhauer and Zhang stated that the most mature biomarkers currently used to support the diagnosis of PD are derived from functional neuroimaging [11]. However, they pointed out the limitations of neuroimaging because current functional neuroimaging such as dopamine transporter imaging only reflects changes in the integrity of dopaminergic terminals and is not indicative of the underlying neuropathological processes. They therefore proposed that biochemical markers reflecting the pathophysiology of PD are also needed as diagnostic, surrogate, and predictive biomarkers. They also emphasized that in the discovery of biochemical biomarkers, functional neuroimaging could be the gold standard used to define patients because neuroimaging can be substituted for pathological diagnosis.

13.2.2 Characteristics of Ideal Biomarkers (Diagnostic Biomarkers)

What are the important characteristics of diagnostic biomarkers for neurodegenerative diseases? In AD research, the ideal diagnostic biomarker should be: (1) able to detect a fundamental feature of Alzheimer's neuropathology, (2) validated in neuropathologically confirmed AD cases, (3) precise and able to detect AD early in its course and distinguish it from other dementias, (4) reliable, (5) noninvasive, (6) simple to perform, and (7) inexpensive [12]. The recommended steps in the process of establishing a biomarker were also proposed and describe that there should be at least two independent studies that specify the biomarker's sensitivity and specificity and that sensitivity and specificity should be no less than 80 % [12]. These criteria should also be applied to biomarkers for other neurodegenerative diseases including PD and DLB.

13.3 Significance of A-syn in the Pathogenesis of Synucleinopathy

13.3.1 Molecular Characteristics of A-syn

A-syn is a 140-residue (~14 kDa) neuronal protein that is highly expressed in the brain [13]. It is a member of a conserved family of proteins that also includes β-synuclein and γ-synuclein [14]. The A-syn protein is intrinsically unfolded, which means that in the purified form at neutral pH, it lacks an ordered secondary or tertiary structure. A-syn has no endoplasmic reticulum (ER) signal peptide and was thought at first to be an exclusively intracellular protein [13, 15]. However, this notion has been revised because A-syn is detected in blood plasma and CSF [16, 17]. Furthermore, A-syn is secreted into the culture medium of neuronal cells [17–20]. The mechanism of A-syn release has not been fully elucidated, but data point toward a non-classic, secretory pathway that involves vesicle trafficking but is independent of the ER-Golgi apparatus [21].

The exact function of A-syn remains to be established. Under physiological conditions, A-syn is enriched at neuronal presynaptic terminals. Thus, A-syn is assumed to play a role in the regulation of synaptic vesicle release and to provide a stabilizing effect on complexes of SNARE (soluble NSF attachment protein [SNAP] receptors) family proteins [22–25].

13.3.2 Pivotal Role of A-syn in the Pathogenesis of PD and Synucleinopathy

The importance of A-syn in the pathogenesis of PD was first suggested by the identification of missense mutations in the gene encoding A-syn (*SNCA*) in families with autosomal dominant forms of PD (A53T, A30P, E46K, G51D, H50Q) [26–30]. The identification of the first mutation led to the discovery that A-syn is the main component of Lewy bodies in PD and DLB and glial cytoplasmic inclusions of multiple system atrophy (MSA) [3, 31, 32].

Not only those missense mutations but triplications and duplications of *SNCA* have been identified in patients with familial PD [33–35]. A family with *SNCA* triplication showed early-onset parkinsonism and dementia resembling the phenotype of DLB, whereas the phenotype of patients with *SNCA* duplication was typical for idiopathic PD and did not show signs of dementia [34, 35]. These findings indicate that there is a clear gene dosage effect of *SNCA*, implying that an increase in the production of wild-type A-syn without mutation directly aggravates the disease phenotypes.

Further evidence has been derived from two independent genome-wide association studies of sporadic PD patients from different ethnic groups. These studies identified polymorphisms in *SNCA* as the strongest risk factor for development of sporadic PD [36, 37]. The effects of these genetic variations on the protein have not been fully elucidated; however, some polymorphisms may be associated with increased expression of A-syn protein [38, 39].

13.4 Significance and Usefulness of A-syn as a Biomarker for Synucleinopathy

13.4.1 Total A-syn in Human CSF Examined in Studies Mainly Targeted to PD

The importance of expression levels of A-syn in the pathogenesis of PD and other synucleinopathies has been widely recognized, and thus, considerable attention has been paid to protein levels of A-syn in the brain and CSF of patients with PD. At first, A-syn was thought to exist only as a cytoplasmic protein [13, 15]. However, El-Agnaf et al. found that cultured neuronal cells normally secrete A-syn, and they also identified A-syn in normal human CSF and plasma [17].

Tokuda et al. first quantified levels of A-syn in human CSF with an originally developed enzyme-linked immunosorbent assay (ELISA) specific to A-syn [40]. They showed that the levels of CSF total A-syn, which consists mainly of monomeric A-syn, in PD patients are significantly lower than those in age-matched controls. Following this first study, decreases in the CSF level of total A-syn in PD and other synucleinopathies have been reproduced by many groups [41–49]. However, discrepant reports have shown similar CSF levels of total A-syn among PD, other synucleinopathies, and controls [50–52]. Such discrepancy has been attributed to confounding factors such as [53]: (1) blood contamination causing hemolysis of red blood cells (RBCs) that contain abundant A-syn [42]; (2) large variance in the examined cohort of both PD and controls; (3) inconsistency in handling and storage of CSF samples; (4) different assay procedures, including standard peptides for ELISAs and employed antibodies that detect different A-syn species; and (5) interference by heterophilic antibodies (HAs) [54]. When those confounding factors are well controlled, it is generally thought that the CSF levels of A-syn are lower in patients with PD and MSA compared to controls and those with tauopathies [42, 43, 49]. However, there is a large overlap in CSF levels of total A-syn between groups of patients with synucleinopathy and controls. Thus, it could be currently acknowledged that CSF total A-syn can discriminate PD from controls or patients with tauopathies as groups, but it is hard to diagnose an individual patient only by measuring the value of A-syn. Recently, two meta-analyses were conducted to determine whether CSF total A-syn can discriminate PD from other neurodegenerative diseases [55, 56]. Both studies reported a significantly lower mean concentration of CSF total A-syn in PD patients compared to normal/neurological controls. One of those studies determined the sensitivity and specificity of CSF A-syn, and additionally, summary receiver operating characteristic (SROC) curves were plotted to count the area under the curve (AUC) for evaluation of the overall performance of the diagnostic test accuracy. The sensitivity of CSF total A-syn in the diagnosis of PD was high (0.88, 95 % confidence interval; 0.84–0.91), but the specificity was low (0.40, 95 % confidence interval; 0.35–0.45). Furthermore, the corresponding SROC had an AUC of 0.73 (SE = 0.05), indicating a medium diagnostic value [56].

It has been widely known that A-syn and tau interact dynamically and synergistically to promote mutual aggregation. In one study, CSF levels of A-syn and total tau (t-tau) were measured in 721 patients with a synucleinopathy including PD, DLB, or MSA and a tauopathy such as AD or PSP (progressive supranuclear palsy). A combination of CSF total A-syn and t-tau values provided the most accurate discrimination of synucleinopathy from the other neurological disorders [43]. In another study, lower t-tau/total A-syn and phosphorylated tau (p-tau)/total A-syn ratios discriminated PD from DLB, FTD (frontotemporal dementia), and AD [44]. Furthermore, one recent study from the Parkinson's Progression Markers Initiative (PPMI) data set reported that CSF levels of total A-syn were strongly correlated with measures of CSF t-tau in both a PD cohort and healthy controls [57]. Using multivariate linear regression analysis with adjustment for confounders, A-syn was significantly associated with both the unified Parkinson's disease rating scale (UPDRS) part III motor score and the Hoehn and Yahr stage of the patients. This study also demonstrated that lower levels of CSF Aβ1-42 and p-tau181 (tau phosphorylated at the threonine residue at position 181) were significantly associated with the postural instability-gait disturbance motor phenotype [57]. This phenotype progresses more quickly along both motor and nonmotor trajectories and has a poorer prognosis compared with the tremor-dominant phenotype [58–62]. Thus, these data suggest that CSF A-syn could be useful as a surrogate biomarker for monitoring disease severity, and CSF Aβ1-42 and p-tau could be predictive biomarkers of poorer prognosis in PD patients.

13.4.2 A-syn Oligomers in Human CSF

The fundamental problem with using CSF total A-syn as a diagnostic biomarker for PD is that it is not a real pathogenic molecule but rather a natural protein released from neuronal cells [17]. From the viewpoint of pathogenic molecules, soluble oligomers of A-syn have been attracting a great deal of attention. Regarding point mutations in *SNCA*, the common biochemical mechanism is not an increase in A-syn fibrils but an increase in A-syn oligomers [63] (Fig. 13.1a). On the other hand, it was recently recognized that A-syn pathology gradually progresses in PD brain from certain regions to adjacent regions just like brain lesions caused by pathological prion proteins (Fig. 13.1b). Furthermore, it was reported that A-syn aggregates, such as Lewy bodies, emerged in grafted neurons in the brains of PD patients who had undergone implantation of fetal mesencephalic tissue, suggesting host-to-graft propagation of A-syn pathology [64, 65] (Fig. 13.1c). The molecular

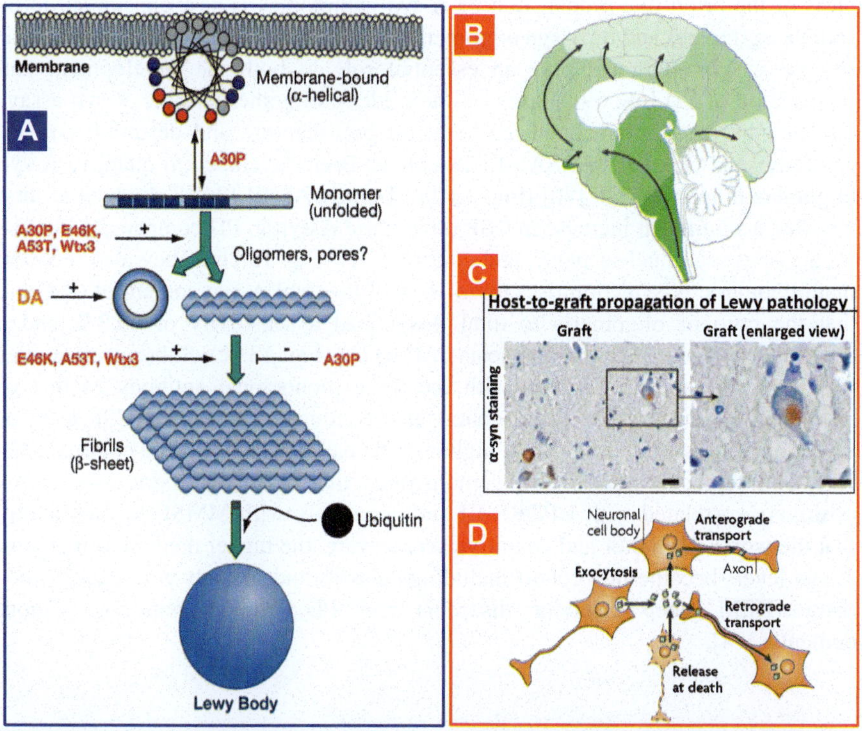

The common mechanism of the pathological mutations of *SNCA* is an increase in α-syn oligomers, not an increase in fibril formation.

Soluble aggregates and/or oligomers of A-syn are considered as the molecular basis of the prion-like propagation.

Fig. 13.1 Extracellular soluble A-syn oligomers play an important role in both the development and progression of PD. (**a**) The cascade of A-syn aggregation. The A53T mutation promotes the formation of fibrillar A-syn species, but the A30P mutation does not. The A30P mutation slows the rate of fibril accumulation but strongly promotes the formation of oligomeric species. Thus, the common mechanism of the pathological mutations of *SNCA* (*point mutations such as A53T*, *A30P*, *E46K*, *and triplication*) is an increase in A-syn oligomers, not an increase in fibril formation (From [63] (Cookson MR. Annu Rev Biochem. 2005;74:29–52)). (**b**) Illustration of prion-like propagation of A-syn pathologies that spread spatiotemporally in PD brain during disease progression. A-syn pathologies (Lewy neurites and Lewy bodies) are suggested to first appear in the dorsal motor nucleus of the vagal nerve in the brain stem and anterior olfactory structures (*darkest green*) and then to spread stereotypically to finally occupy large parts of the brain (From [67] (Brundin P, et al. Nat Rev Mol Cell Biol. 2010;11:301–7)). (**c**) Prion-like propagation of A-syn pathologies to grafted neurons in PD brain. A-syn-positive Lewy bodies were found in grafted dopaminergic neurons in a patient with PD who had undergone implantation of fetal mesencephalic tissue into the putamen 12 years before death. Classic Lewy bodies in the grafts are immunoreactive for A-syn (From [64] (Li JY, et al. Nat Med. 2008;14:501–3)). (**d**) The proposed molecular basis of prion-like propagation shown in (**b**) and (**c**). Intracellular soluble A-syn oligomers/aggregates can be released from neurons by exocytosis or cell death. The aggregates are taken up by adjacent neuronal cell bodies, for example, and are either retained in the cell soma (local spread of pathology) or transported anterogradely by axons. Alternatively, they are taken up by axon terminals and transported retrogradely to the cell soma. The protein aggregates can spread between brain regions by axonal transport. Those soluble aggregates and/or oligomers of A-syn are considered to be the molecular basis of the prion-like propagation observed in (**b**) and (**c**) (From [67] (Brundin P, et al. Nat Rev Mol Cell Biol. 2010;11:301–7))

basis of the prion-like propagation of A-syn pathologies is now considered to be soluble aggregates and/or A-syn oligomers [66, 67] (Fig. 13.1d). Thus, extracellular soluble A-syn oligomers play an essential role in both the development and progression of PD [68, 69]. Based on these ideas, oligomer-specific A-syn assays that use the same monoclonal antibody for both capture and detection (single-antibody sandwich ELISA: SAS-ELISA) have been developed to quantify A-syn oligomers in human CSF [70] (Fig. 13.2a). Using SAS-ELISA, Tokuda et al. first reported a significant increase in CSF oligomeric A-syn in PD compared with AD, progressive supranuclear palsy, and controls [71] (Fig. 13.2b). They also reported that oligomeric A-syn comprises up to 10 % of the total A-syn content of CSF and that the ratio of oligomeric to total A-syn had a sensitivity of 89.3 % and a specificity of 90.6 % for the diagnosis of PD [71] (Fig. 13.2c). Subsequent studies that used similar SAS-ELISAs with the same monoclonal antibody as that of Tokuda et al. in an independent cohort also demonstrated that the CSF level of A-syn oligomers was significantly higher in PD patients compared to controls [72–74]. One of those studies also demonstrated that CSF oligomeric A-syn was positively correlated with UPDRS-III and negatively with MMSE in such a way that the worse the motor and cognitive scores were, the higher the CSF oligomeric A-syn levels became in a cohort including controls and patients with iRBD (idiopathic REM sleep behavior disorder) and PD patients with or without dementia [74].

13.4.3 Other A-syn Species in Human CSF: Phosphorylated A-syn

Most of the A-syn in Lewy bodies is phosphorylated at the serine residue at position 129 (Ser129) (p129-A-syn) [75–79]. The phosphorylation of S129 alters the propensity of A-syn to aggregate [75, 80, 81].

The usefulness of CSF p129-A-syn levels as a diagnostic and/or surrogate biomarker for synucleinopathy has been investigated. In a large cohort (~600 samples) of patients with PD, MSA, and controls, CSF levels of p129-A-syn showed a positive correlation with the severity of PD symptoms, and the combination of CSF total A-syn (lower in PD) and p129-A-syn (higher in PD) improved discrimination between PD and other forms of parkinsonism [82]. However, a large cohort study (more than 300 subjects) that investigated the longitudinal relationship between CSF levels of p129-A-syn and UPDRS scores in PD patients reported discrepant results [83]. This study showed that the relationship between the levels of CSF p129-A-syn and disease severity may depend on the disease stage of PD in which lower p129-A-syn levels were correlated with a worse clinical condition at early stages but with a better condition at later stages. This observation would make it difficult to use CSF p129-A-syn as a surrogate biomarker for monitoring the disease severity of PD.

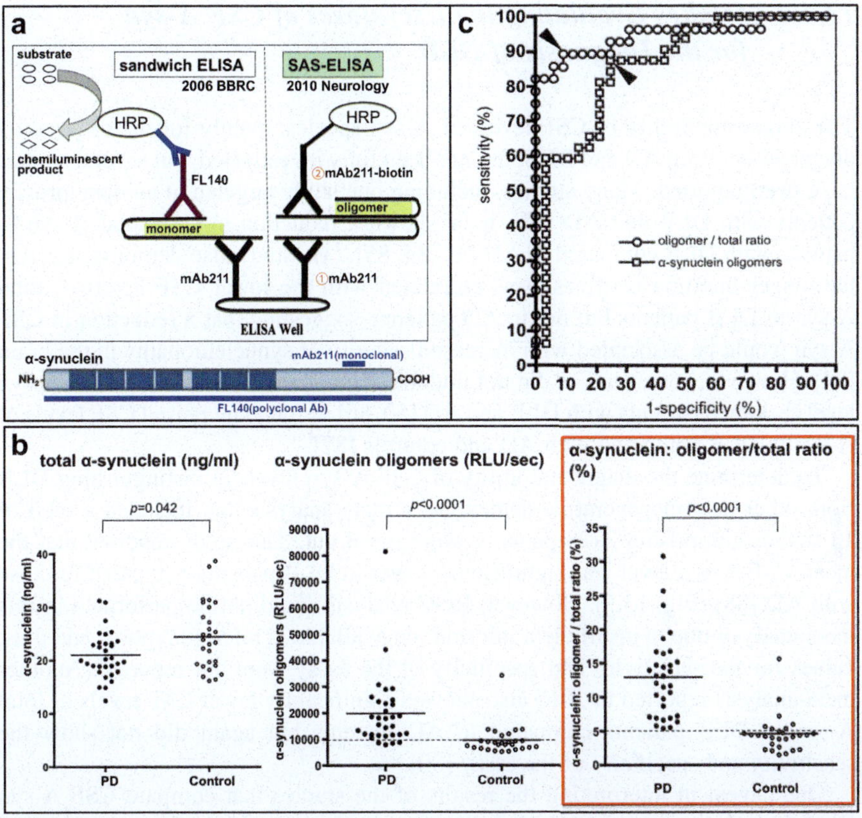

Fig. 13.2 Specific ELISA for α-synuclein (A-syn) oligomers and quantification of A-syn oligomers in PD and controls [70, 71]. (**a**) The method of single-antibody sandwich ELISA (SAS-ELISA) and usual sandwich ELISA for the quantification of total A-syn and A-syn oligomers, respectively, in human CSF. The SAS-ELISA uses a well-characterized single monoclonal antibody both for capture and detection of antigens. This type of ELISA cannot detect A-syn monomers because the capture antibody occupies the only antibody-binding site available on monomers. Meanwhile, the SAS-ELISA can theoretically detect A-syn oligomers because multiple antibody-binding sites are exposed on the surface of the three-dimensional structure of the oligomers. (**b**) Individual values of the measured level of total A-syn (*left*), A-syn oligomers (*middle; RLU* = relative luminescence units), and the ratio of A-syn oligomers to total A-syn (C; oligomer/total ratio, %) in CSF from patients with PD (*solid circles*) and controls (*open circles*). Each bar represents the mean value. Dashed lines in the middle and right subfigures indicate respective cutoff values that yield the most reliable sensitivity and specificity with ROC curves (9950 RLU/s for the levels of CSF A-syn oligomers; 6.165 % for the ratio of A-syn oligomers to total A-syn in CSF). (**c**) ROC curves for the levels of CSF A-syn oligomers (*open squares*) and the ratio of A-syn oligomers to total A-syn in CSF (*open circles*) for discrimination of PD from controls. Over a range of cutoff points, the *arrowhead* indicates a cutoff value that yields the most appropriate sensitivity and specificity

13.4.4 *Studies Evaluating the Usefulness of CSF A-syn for the Diagnosis of DLB*

The diagnostic ability of CSF levels of A-syn species, mainly for the differential diagnosis between AD and DLB, has not been fully investigated, but several studies have been reported. Many studies, including one study targeted at autopsy-proven patients with DLB and AD [43], have shown a reduction in CSF total A-syn in patients with DLB compared to AD [41, 84, 85]. One study also demonstrated that the longer duration of illness was correlated with the lower CSF levels of total A-syn in DLB patients but not in AD patients, suggesting that a reduction in CSF A-syn would be associated with increased severity of synucleinopathy in the brain [84]. However, some studies did not find any significant differences in CSF A-syn levels between patients with DLB and AD [50, 86] or found increased CSF levels of A-syn in DLB compared with AD and controls [87].

To determine the diagnostic utility of CSF A-syn levels in distinguishing DLB from other neurodegenerative dementias, a meta-analysis that included a total of 13 studies comprising 2728 patients was carried out. This study reported that the mean CSF A-syn level was significantly lower in DLB patients compared to those with AD [88] (Fig. 13.3). However, ROC analysis could not be performed in this meta-analysis due to insufficient information available in referred reports, and thus, values for the sensitivity and specificity of the assay were not reported. Another meta-analysis reported in 2015 also showed significantly lower CSF levels of total A-syn in DLB patients compared to AD patients but again did not show the sensitivity and specificity of the assay [89].

One caveat in interpreting the results of the studies that compare CSF A-syn levels between patients with DLB and AD cannot be ignored: there is a subgroup of AD patients with additional Lewy body pathology [90–92]. In the ADNI (Alzheimer's Disease Neuroimaging Initiative) cohort, there is a clear bimodal

	DLB			AD				Mean Difference
Study or Subgroup	Mean	SD	Total	Mean	SD	Total	Weight	IV, Random, 95% CI
Kasuga 2010	8.2	4.2	34	12.2	5.8	31	0.7%	-4.00 [-6.48, -1.52]
Mollenhauer 2008	3.8	3.3	38	6.2	4.2	13	0.7%	-2.40 [-4.91, 0.11]
Mollenhauer 2011a	1.42	1.26	55	1.85	1.47	62	12.2%	-0.43 [-0.92, 0.06]
Mollenhauer 2011c	0.3	0.2	13	0.8	0.9	21	15.9%	-0.50 [-0.90, -0.10]
Noguchi-Shinohara 2009	44.7	24.9	16	49.3	44.5	21	0.0%	-4.60 [-27.21, 18.01]
Parnetti 2008	18.1	16	32	34.8	54	48	0.0%	-16.70 [-32.95, -0.45]
Spies 2009	38	29	40	37	36.1	131	0.0%	1.00 [-9.91, 11.91]
Tateno 2011	0.0976	0.0581	6	0.1841	0.0711	9	36.6%	-0.09 [-0.15, -0.02]
Wennstrom 2012	0.378	0.166	18	0.464	0.233	26	33.9%	-0.09 [-0.20, 0.03]
Total (95% CI)			252			362	100.0%	-0.24 [-0.45, -0.03]

Heterogeneity: $Tau^2 = 0.03$; $Chi^2 = 22.66$, df = 8 (P = 0.004); $I^2 = 65\%$
Test for overall effect: Z = 2.24 (P = 0.02)

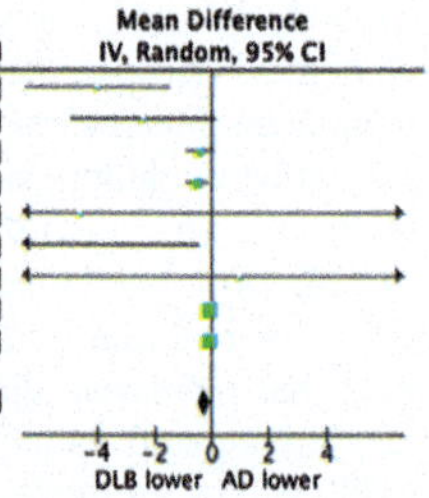

Fig. 13.3 Forest plot of the included studies in meta-analysis comparing mean CSF total A-syn concentrations of DLB vs. AD patients. A meta-analysis was carried out to determine the diagnostic utility of CSF total A-syn analysis in distinguishing DLB from other neurodegenerative dementias including DLB. A total of 13 studies that included 2728 patients were included in the final review, and 7 out of 13 studies (1301 patients) were included in the meta-analysis. The mean CSF total A-syn concentration was significantly lower in DLB patients compared to those with AD (weighted mean difference −0.24; 95 % confidence interval, −0.45, −0.03; $p = 0.02$) (From [88] (Lim X, et al. Parkinsonism Relat Disord. 2013;19:851–8))

distribution of CSF A-syn levels in relationship to t-tau; subjects with abnormally increased t-tau values had high levels of total A-syn, and there were no subjects with elevated levels of CSF A-syn among those with normal t-tau values [93]. Furthermore, a positive correlation was generally noted between CSF total A-syn and p-tau181, but there were some cases with high p-tau181 levels accompanied by low A-syn levels in the ADNI cohort. This result suggests that a mismatch between the measured CSF level of A-syn and the expected levels of A-syn from the levels of CSF p-tau181 would be observed in AD cases with concomitant Lewy body pathology [93].

13.4.5 Measurement of A-syn Species in Human Blood (Plasma/Serum) and Confounding Factors

An ideal biomarker should be noninvasive (such as a blood test) or only moderately invasive (such as CSF biomarkers). Thus, blood tests quantifying A-syn have been reported for the diagnosis of DLB and other synucleinopathies, but their results were inconsistent. Several studies showed significantly higher levels of plasma total A-syn [70, 94, 95] or plasma p129-A-syn [96] in patients with PD. By contrast, some studies found that plasma levels of total A-syn were significantly lower in PD compared to controls [97], as in DLB compared to AD and controls [98]. Other studies found comparable levels of plasma total A-syn among controls, PD, and AD [72, 99]. Those discrepant results are considered to be due to certain confounding factors as mentioned above (see Sect. 13.4.1).

Previous studies emphasized that hemolysis is an important confounding factor that provides a strong positive signal in A-syn ELISAs [42, 57] because greater than 99 % of A-syn in blood resides in RBCs [100]. However, a considerable number of samples with high levels of hemoglobin (Hb) in the study showed average or less than average levels of CSF A-syn [42]. Ishii et al. also reported that there was not a significant relationship between the levels of Hb and CSF or plasma A-syn [54]. Instead of hemolysis, it has been reported that interference from HAs is an important and prevailing confounding factor in ELISAs [101–104]. Recently, Ishii et al. demonstrated that plasma A-syn levels were significantly lower in PD than in controls only under the condition in which HA interference was eliminated. HAs are human antibodies capable of binding to animal immunoglobulins and may possibly interfere with the reaction between animal-derived antibodies and the analyte, which is part of all immunoassays [101–104]. HA interference is known to be more prominent in blood samples than in CSF samples; HAs were found in up to 40 % of human serum samples, and assay interference from HAs occurs in as many as 15 % of serum samples despite highly depending on the specific assay setup [102, 104]. There have been two studies describing HA interference in Aβ ELISA; HA generally affects micro-quantitative ELISA more strongly in plasma than in CSF and produces false positive rather than false negative signals

[104, 105]. These findings suggest that HA is an important confounding factor that can generally affect ELISAs that measure very small amounts of antigens and is not limited to the A-syn ELISAs. It should be concluded that HA interference, rather than contamination with RBCs and hemolysis, is a major confounder in some A-syn ELISAs. Eliminating HA interference in A-syn ELISAs is indispensable, although none of the previous studies, other than that of Ishii et al. which examined plasma A-syn with ELISAs, were adjusted for HA interference.

13.5 Other Potential Biomarkers for DLB

There are many reports on CSF biomarkers other than A-syn species for the diagnosis of DLB and synucleinopathy [refer to reviews: 106–109].

13.5.1 AD-Related Biomarkers for Diagnosis and Prediction of Prognosis in DLB and PD

As a diagnostic biomarker, CSF levels of Aβ1-42 are usually decreased in patients with DLB compared to non-demented controls [110]. A meta-analysis of 50 studies demonstrated that Aβ1-42 was moderately lower in AD compared to DLB [111]. Calculation of the Aβ1-42/Aβ1-40 ratio could be promising for the differentiation of AD from DLB [112]. Nevertheless, most studies could not determine exact cutoff scores valuable to distinguish AD and DLB in clinical practice [113–115], including a meta-analysis [111]. The oxidized isoform of Aβ1-40 (Aβ1-40^{ox}) has been shown to be increased in DLB patients compared to patients with PD with dementia (PDD) and non-demented disease controls [116] and has recently also been shown in autopsy-proven AD and DLB [117].

One important prospective cohort study demonstrated that lower baseline CSF Aβ1-42 (≤192 pg/mL), but neither t-tau nor p-tau181, was associated with a more rapid cognitive decline within a 2-year period of follow-up in patients with PD [118]. These results are consistent with previous research showing that AD pathology contributes to cognitive impairment in PD [119–122]. The CSF level of Aβ1-42 may provide clinically useful prognostic information as a prognostic biomarker for cognitive impairment in PD.

In DLB, levels of CSF tau protein are lower compared to AD [113] and higher compared to PD and PDD [123]. Some CSF studies have revealed better specificity for the discrimination of AD when using p-tau181 as a diagnostic biomarker rather than total tau protein [124]. A meta-analysis of 16 studies that included 909 AD patients and 265 DLB patients showed that there was a significant ($p < 0.001$) difference between CSF p-tau181 levels in AD (71–136 pg/mL) and DLB (34.5–76.6 pg/mL) [125]. From these findings, quantification of p-tau species in CSF may serve as a specific biomarker to discriminate AD from DLB [124, 126].

13.5.2 PD-Related Biomarkers Other Than A-syn Species for the Diagnosis of DLB

Neurosin, a brain-rich serine protease, can cleave A-syn and thereby may play a major role in the pathomechanisms of diseases associated with A-syn pathology [127–129]. Neurosin was decreased in CSF from patients with synucleinopathy compared with healthy controls and patients with AD. The lowest levels have been found in patients with DLB, thereby offering a potential diagnostic biomarker for DLB [130].

13.5.3 Other Potential CSF/Blood Biomarkers for the Diagnosis of DLB and PDD

Reduced CSF levels of metabolites such as homovanillic acid (HVA), 5-hydroxyindoleacetic acid (5-HIAA), and 3-methoxy-4-hydroxyphenylethyleneglycol (MHPG) have been reported in DLB compared with AD [131]. Especially MHPG, in combination with the levels of t-tau, p-tau, and Aβ1-42, could increase the sensitivity and specificity of discriminating DLB from AD [132].

With regard to blood biomarkers, it has been reported that serum levels of heart-type fatty acid-binding proteins (FABPs) are distinctly elevated in DLB [133–135], despite lower levels of these proteins that were reported in the brains of AD patients [135]. One study using a multiplex immunoassay that can quantify more than 100 plasma proteins simultaneously identified epidermal growth factor (EGF) as a predictive biomarker of cognitive impairment in patients with PD [136]. In this study, low levels of plasma EGF were not only correlated with poor cognitive test scores at baseline but also predicted an eightfold greater risk of cognitive decline to dementia for those with intact baseline cognition during follow-up period with a median time-to-conversion of 14 months.

13.6 Conclusions and Future Prospective

Recent remarkable advance in functional neuroimaging such as dopamine transporter scans and MIBG scintigraphy have brought us clinically useful imaging biomarkers for the diagnosis of DLB and synucleinopathy. However, those imaging biomarkers have limitations, as mentioned above (see Sect. 13.2.1). Consequently, biochemical biomarkers that are useful for early diagnosis and appropriate management of DLB in clinical practice are also urgently needed.

This chapter has introduced the studies reported so far and discussed the current status of biochemical biomarker candidates for DLB (Table 13.1), but the majority

Table 13.1 Summary of reported candidates of biochemical biomarkers for the diagnosis of DLB and differential diagnosis between DLB and AD and surrogate biomarkers for PD

	CSF biomarkers	Plasma/serum biomarkers
DLB	A-syn↓	Heart-type FABPs↑
	(A-syn oligomers? ↑in PD)	EGF↓
	Neurosin↓	
	Oxidized Aβ1-40↑	
	HVA, 5-HIAA, MHPG↓	
DLB vs. AD	Aβ1-42 (AD < DLB)	Heart-type FABPs (AD < DLB)
		t-tau, p-tau (AD > DLB)
PD	A-syn (to monitor disease severity)	EGF (to predict cognitive decline)
	Aβ1-42, p-tau (to predict prognosis)	
	A-syn oligomers (to predict prognosis)	

DLB dementia with Lewy bodies, *A-syn* α-synuclein, *PD* Parkinson's disease, *FABPs* fatty acid-binding proteins, *EGF* epidermal growth factor, *HVA* homovanillic acid, *5-HIAA* 5-hydroxyindoleacetic acid, *MHPG* 3-methoxy-4-hydroxyphenylethyleneglycol, *AD* Alzheimer's disease, *t-tau* total tau, *p-tau* phosphorylated tau

of the studies discussed here were cross-sectional, retrospective, and investigated pathologically unproven subjects. In addition, those studies have other considerable caveats including heterogeneity of examined subjects (both patients and controls) as well as a lack of standardization of sample collection and handling, sample processing, and assay procedures, making them impossible for providing reference values and diagnostic cutoff values that can be globally used. After taking those limitations and caveats into consideration, the summary points of this chapter are as follows:

- The purpose of biomarkers can be typically classified as diagnostic, disease-monitoring, predictive, or effect measurement.
- There are important requirements for the ideal diagnostic biomarker, including (1) the ability to reflect fundamental disease process, (2) validation in pathologically confirmed patients, and (3) precision with high sensitivity and specificity.
- A-syn plays a pivotal role both in the development of the disease and propagation of the pathology in the brain in PD and other synucleinopathies.
- CSF levels of total A-syn can discriminate PD from controls or tauopathies as groups. However, it is hard to diagnose an individual patient only with CSF A-syn. The PPMI data set suggested the CSF total A-syn could be useful for monitoring disease severity as a surrogate biomarker for PD.
- CSF levels of A-syn oligomers could be a promising biomarker for the diagnosis of PD. The CSF levels of A-syn oligomers are reported to correlate with motor and cognitive scores in PD, suggesting its possibility as a biomarker to monitor disease severity.
- With regard to the diagnosis of DLB, some studies including two meta-analyses demonstrated significantly lower CSF levels of total A-syn in DLB patients compared to AD patients. However, the sensitivity and specificity as well as

diagnostic ability of CSF total A-syn still remain to be elucidated. Whether CSF A-syn oligomers are useful or not for the diagnosis of DLB has not been examined.

- To study plasma/serum levels of total and oligomeric A-syn, it is essential to eliminate interference from heterophilic antibodies, which have a significant impact on the assays of plasma/serum A-syn despite never being considered in any of the studies reported so far that determined plasma/serum levels of A-syn.
- The higher levels of Aβ1-42 and Aβ1-40^{ox} as well as lower levels of p-tau181 and neurosin in CSF from patients with DLB compared to those from AD patients would be useful for the differential diagnosis of these two diseases.

For the future perspective of biomarkers for DLB and synucleinopathy, it will be necessary to accomplish the following two objectives: (A) validation of already-reported candidates and translation of them to clinical practice and (B) identification of novel biomarkers that are more closely associated with the specific disease process of the diseases. For objective (A), the candidate CSF biomarkers include total A-syn, A-syn oligomers, p129-A-syn, and AD-related biomarkers, whereas the candidate plasma biomarkers are A-syn oligomers, EGF, and so on. For objective (B), the most important thing is to identify the true culprit species of A-syn, namely, certain oligomers or protofibrils of A-syn that are specifically relevant to the development (neurotoxicity) and/or progress (prion-like propagation in the brain) of an individual synucleinopathy, including DLB, PDD, PD, and MSA. To accomplish these objectives, future studies should ideally fulfill the following conditions [7, 8, 11, 88]:

1. A large, prospective, multicenter, and longitudinal cohort design
2. Inclusion of patients with DLB and other synucleinopathies and at-risk subjects diagnosed with standardized criteria (pathological or neuroimaging criteria)
3. Simultaneous quantification of multiple biomarkers in the CSF and/or blood by using strictly standardized protocols including quality controls of biomarker assays [53]
4. A long-term follow-up period with serial determinations of the biological markers
5. Final pathological confirmation by examination of the brains and bodies of patients

References

1. McKeith IG, Galasko D, Kosaka K, et al. Consensus guidelines for the clinical and pathologic diagnosis of dementia with Lewy bodies (DLB): report of the consortium on DLB international workshop. Neurology. 1996;47:1113–24. doi:10.1212/WNL.47.5.1113.
2. Vann Jones SA, O'Brien JT. The prevalence and incidence of dementia with Lewy bodies: a systematic review of population and clinical studies. Psychol Med. 2014;44:673–83. doi:10.1017/S0033291713000494.

3. Spillantini MG, Schmidt ML, Lee VM, et al. α-synuclein in Lewy bodies. Nature. 1997;388:839–40.
4. McKeith IG, Dickson DW, Lowe J, et al. Consortium on DLB. Diagnosis and management of dementia with Lewy bodies: third report of the DLB Consortium. Neurology. 2005;65:1863–72. doi:10.1212/01.wnl.0000187889.17253.b1.
5. Aarsland D, Kurz M, Beyer M, et al. Early discriminatory diagnosis of dementia with Lewy bodies: the emerging role of CSF and imaging biomarkers. Dement Geriatr Cogn Disord. 2008;25:195–205. doi:10.1159/000113417.
6. Sunderland T, Linker G, Mirza N, et al. Decreased β-amyloid1-42 and increased tau levels in cerebrospinal fluid of patients with Alzheimer disease. JAMA. 2003;289:2094–103. doi:10.1001/jama.289.16.2094.
7. Ahmed RM, Paterson RW, Warren JD, et al. Biomarkers in dementia: clinical utility and new directions. J Neurol Neurosurg Psychiatry. 2014;85:1426–34. doi:10.1136/jnnp-2014-307662.
8. Lleó A, Cavedo E, Parnetti L, et al. Cerebrospinal fluid biomarkers in trials for Alzheimer and Parkinson diseases. Nat Rev Neurol. 2015;11:41–55. doi:10.1038/nrneurol.2014.232.
9. Biomarkers Definitions Working Group. Biomarkers and surrogate endpoints: preferred definitions and conceptual framework. Clin Pharmacol Ther. 2001;69:89–95. doi:10.1067/mcp.2001.113989.
10. Shi M, Huber BR, Zhang J. Biomarkers for cognitive impairment in Parkinson disease. Brain Pathol. 2010;20:660–71. doi:10.1111/j.1750-3639.2009.00370.x.
11. Mollenhauer B, Zhang J. Biochemical premotor biomarkers for Parkinson's disease. Mov Disord. 2012;27:644–50. doi:10.1002/mds.24956.
12. Consensus report of the Working Group on: "Molecular and Biochemical Markers of Alzheimer's Disease". The Ronald and Nancy Reagan Research Institute of the Alzheimer's Association and the National Institute on Aging Working Group. Neurobiol Aging. 1998;19:109–16. doi:10.1016/S0197-4580(98)00020-0.
13. Jakes R, Spillantini MG, Goedert M. Identification of two distinct synucleins from human brain. FEBS Lett. 1994;345:27–32. doi:10.1016/0014-5793(94)00395-5.
14. Uéda K, Fukushima H, Masliah E, et al. Molecular cloning of cDNA encoding an unrecognized component of amyloid in Alzheimer disease. Proc Natl Acad Sci U S A. 1993;90:11282–6.
15. Iwai A, Masliah E, Yoshimoto M, et al. The precursor protein of non-Aβ component of Alzheimer's disease amyloid is a presynaptic protein of the central nervous system. Neuron. 1995;14:467–75. doi:10.1016/0896-6273(95)90302-X.
16. Borghi R, Marchese R, Negro A, et al. Full length α-synuclein is present in cerebrospinal fluid from Parkinson's disease and normal subjects. Neurosci Lett. 2000;287:65–7. doi:10.1016/S0304-3940(00)01153-8.
17. El-Agnaf OM, Salem SA, Paleologou KE, et al. α-Synuclein implicated in Parkinson's disease is present in extracellular biological fluids, including human plasma. FASEB J. 2003;17:1945–7. doi:10.1096/fj.03-0098fje.
18. Sung JY, Park SM, Lee CH, et al. Proteolytic cleavage of extracellular secreted α-synuclein via matrix metalloproteinases. J Biol Chem. 2005;280:25216–24. doi:10.1074/jbc.M503341200.
19. Lee HJ, Patel S, Lee SJ. Intravesicular localization and exocytosis of α-synuclein and its aggregates. J Neurosci. 2005;25:6016–24. doi:10.1523/JNEUROSCI.0692-05.2005.
20. Emmanouilidou E, Melachroinou K, Roumeliotis T, et al. Cell-produced α-synuclein is secreted in a calcium-dependent manner by exosomes and impacts neuronal survival. J Neurosci. 2010;30:6838–51. doi:10.1523/JNEUROSCI.5699-09.2010.
21. Vekrellis K, Xilouri M, Emmanouilidou E, et al. Pathological roles of α-synuclein in neurological disorders. Lancet Neurol. 2011;10:1015–25. doi:10.1016/S1474-4422(11)70213-7.

22. Abeliovich A, Schmitz Y, Fariñas I, et al. Mice lacking α-synuclein display functional deficits in the nigrostriatal dopamine system. Neuron. 2000;25:239–52. doi:10.1016/S0896-6273(00)80886-7.
23. Chandra S, Gallardo G, Fernández-Chacón R, et al. α-synuclein cooperates with CSPα in preventing neurodegeneration. Cell. 2005;123:383–96. doi:10.1016/j.cell.2005.09.028.
24. Larsen KE, Schmitz Y, Troyer MD, et al. α-Synuclein overexpression in PC12 and chromaffin cells impairs catecholamine release by interfering with a late step in exocytosis. J Neurosci. 2006;26:11915–22. doi:10.1523/JNEUROSCI.3821-06.2006.
25. Burré J, Sharma M, Tsetsenis T, et al. α-Synuclein promotes SNARE-complex assembly in vivo and in vitro. Science. 2010;329(5999):1663–7. doi:10.1126/science.1195227.
26. Polymeropoulos MH, Lavedan C, Leroy E, et al. Mutation in the α-synuclein gene identified in families with Parkinson's disease. Science. 1997;276:2045–7. doi:10.1126/science.276.5321.2045.
27. Krüger R, Kuhn W, Müller T, et al. Ala30Pro mutation in the gene encoding α-synuclein in Parkinson's disease. Nat Genet. 1998;18:106–8. doi:10.1038/ng0298-106.
28. Zarranz JJ, Alegre J, Gómez-Esteban JC, et al. The new mutation, E46K, of α-synuclein causes Parkinson and Lewy body dementia. Ann Neurol. 2004;55:164–73. doi:10.1002/ana.10795.
29. Lesage S, Anheim M, Letournel F, et al. French Parkinson's Disease Genetics Study Group: G51D α-synuclein mutation causes a novel parkinsonian-pyramidal syndrome. Ann Neurol. 2013;73:459–71. doi:10.1002/ana.23894.
30. Proukakis C, Dudzik CG, Brier T, et al. A novel α-synuclein missense mutation in Parkinson disease. Neurology. 2013;80:1062–4. doi:10.1212/WNL.0b013e31828727ba.
31. Baba M, Nakajo S, Tu PH, et al. Aggregation of α-synuclein in Lewy bodies of sporadic Parkinson's disease and dementia with Lewy bodies. Am J Pathol. 1998;152:879–84.
32. Gai WP, Power JH, Blumbergs PC, et al. Multiple-system atrophy: a new α-synuclein disease? Lancet. 1998;352:547–8. doi:10.1016/S0140-6736(05)79256-4.
33. Singleton AB, Farrer M, Johnson J, et al. α-Synuclein locus triplication causes Parkinson's disease. Science. 2003;302:841. doi:10.1126/science.1090278.
34. Chartier-Harlin MC, Kachergus J, Roumier C, et al. α-Synuclein locus duplication as a cause of familial Parkinson's disease. Lancet. 2004;364:1167–9. doi:10.1016/S0140-6736(04)17103-1.
35. Ibáñez P, Bonnet AM, Débarges B, et al. Causal relation between α-synuclein gene duplication and familial Parkinson's disease. Lancet. 2004;364:1169–71. doi:10.1016/S0140-6736(04)17104-3.
36. Satake W, Nakabayashi Y, Mizuta I, et al. Genome-wide association study identifies common variants at four loci as genetic risk factors for Parkinson's disease. Nat Genet. 2009;41:1303–7. doi:10.1038/ng.485.
37. Simón-Sánchez J, Schulte C, Bras JM, et al. Genome-wide association study reveals genetic risk underlying Parkinson's disease. Nat Genet. 2009;41:1308–12. doi:10.1038/ng.487.
38. Fuchs J, Tichopad A, Golub Y, Munz M, et al. Genetic variability in the SNCA gene influences α-synuclein levels in the blood and brain. FASEB J. 2008;22:1327–34. doi:10.1096/fj.07-9348com.
39. Mata IF, Shi M, Agarwal P, et al. SNCA variant associated with Parkinson disease and plasma α-synuclein level. Arch Neurol. 2010;67:1350–6. doi:10.1001/archneurol.2010.279.
40. Tokuda T, Salem SA, Allsop D, et al. Decreased α-synuclein in cerebrospinal fluid of aged individuals and subjects with Parkinson's disease. Biochem Biophys Res Commun. 2006;349:162–6. doi:10.1016/j.bbrc.2006.08.024.
41. Mollenhauer B, Cullen V, Kahn I, et al. Direct quantification of CSF α-synuclein by ELISA and first cross-sectional study in patients with neurodegeneration. Exp Neurol. 2008;213:315–25. doi:10.1016/j.expneurol.2008.06.004.
42. Hong Z, Shi M, Chung KA, et al. DJ-1 and α-synuclein in human cerebrospinal fluid as biomarkers of Parkinson's disease. Brain. 2010;133:713–26. doi:10.1093/brain/awq008.

43. Mollenhauer B, Locascio JJ, Schulz-Schaeffer W, et al. α-Synuclein and tau concentrations in cerebrospinal fluid of patients presenting with parkinsonism: a cohort study. Lancet Neurol. 2011;10:230–40. doi:10.1016/S1474-4422(11)70014-X.
44. Parnetti L, Chiasserini D, Bellomo G, et al. Cerebrospinal fluid Tau/α-synuclein ratio in Parkinson's disease and degenerative dementias. Mov Disord. 2011;26:1428–35. doi:10.1002/mds.23670.
45. Shi M, Bradner J, Hancock AM, et al. Cerebrospinal fluid biomarkers for Parkinson disease diagnosis and progression. Ann Neurol. 2011;69:570–80. doi:10.1002/ana.22311.
46. Tateno F, Sakakibara R, Kawai T, et al. α-Synuclein in the cerebrospinal fluid differentiates synucleinopathies (Parkinson disease, dementia with Lewy bodies, multiple system atrophy) from Alzheimer disease. Alzheimer Dis Assoc Disord. 2012;26:213–6. doi:10.1097/WAD.0b013e31823899cc.
47. Wennström M, Londos E, Minthon L, et al. Altered CSF orexin and α-synuclein levels in dementia patients. J Alzheimers Dis. 2012;29:125–32. doi:10.3233/JAD-2012-111655.
48. Mollenhauer B, Trautmann E, Taylor P, et al. Total CSF α-synuclein is lower in de novo Parkinson patients than in healthy subjects. Neurosci Lett. 2013;532:44–8. doi:10.1016/j.neulet.2012.11.004.
49. Parnetti L, Castrioto A, Chiasserini D, et al. Cerebrospinal fluid biomarkers in Parkinson disease. Nat Rev Neurol. 2013;9:131–40. doi:10.1038/nrneurol.2013.10.
50. Ohrfelt A, Grognet P, Andreasen N, et al. Cerebrospinal fluid α-synuclein in neurodegenerative disorders-a marker of synapse loss? Neurosci Lett. 2009;450:332–5. doi:10.1016/j.neulet.2008.11.015.
51. Reesink FE, Lemstra AW, van Dijk KD, et al. CSF α-synuclein does not discriminate dementia with Lewy bodies from Alzheimer's disease. J Alzheimers Dis. 2010;22:87–95. doi:10.3233/JAD-2010-100186.
52. Aerts MB, Esselink RA, Abdo WF, et al. CSF α-synuclein does not differentiate between parkinsonian disorders. Neurobiol Aging. 2012;33:430.e1–3. doi:10.1016/j.neurobiolaging.2010.12.001.
53. Mollenhauer B, El-Agnaf OM, Marcus K, et al. Quantification of α-synuclein in cerebrospinal fluid as a biomarker candidate: review of the literature and considerations for future studies. Biomark Med. 2010;4:683–99. doi:10.2217/bmm.10.90.
54. Ishii R, Tokuda T, Tatebe H, et al. Decrease in plasma levels of α-synuclein is evident in patients with Parkinson's disease after elimination of heterophilic antibody interference. PLoS One. 2015;10, e0123162. doi:10.1371/journal.pone.0123162.
55. Sako W, Murakami N, Izumi Y, et al. Reduced α-synuclein in cerebrospinal fluid in synucleinopathies: evidence from a meta-analysis. Mov Disord. 2014;29:1599–605. doi:10.1002/mds.26036.
56. Gao L, Tang H, Nie K, et al. Cerebrospinal fluid α-synuclein as a biomarker for Parkinson's disease diagnosis: a systematic review and meta-analysis. Int J Neurosci. 2014. doi:10.3109/00207454.2014.961454.
57. Kang JH, Irwin DJ, Chen-Plotkin AS, et al.; Parkinson's progression markers initiative. Association of cerebrospinal fluid β-amyloid 1–42, T-tau, P-tau181, and α-synuclein levels with clinical features of drug-naive patients with early Parkinson disease. JAMA Neurol. 2013;70:1277–87. doi:10.1001/jamaneurol.2013.3861.
58. Zetusky WJ, Jankovic J, Pirozzolo FJ. The heterogeneity of Parkinson's disease: clinical and prognostic implications. Neurology. 1985;35:522–6. doi:10.1212/WNL.35.4.522.
59. Jankovic J, McDermott M, Carter J, et al. Variable expression of Parkinson's disease: a baseline analysis of the DATATOP cohort: The Parkinson Study Group. Neurology. 1990;40:1529–34. doi:10.1212/WNL.40.10.1529.
60. Burn DJ, Rowan EN, Allan LM, et al. Motor subtype and cognitive decline in Parkinson's disease, Parkinson's disease with dementia, and dementia with Lewy bodies. J Neurol Neurosurg Psychiatry. 2006;77:585–9. doi:10.1136/jnnp.2005.081711.

61. Alves G, Larsen JP, Emre M, et al. Changes in motor subtype and risk for incident dementia in Parkinson's disease. Mov Disord. 2006;21:1123–30. doi:10.1002/mds.20897.
62. Williams-Gray CH, Foltynie T, Brayne CE, et al. Evolution of cognitive dysfunction in an incident Parkinson's disease cohort. Brain. 2007;130:1787–98. doi:10.1093/brain/awm111.
63. Cookson MR. The biochemistry of Parkinson's disease. Annu Rev Biochem. 2005;74:29–52. doi:10.1146/annurev.biochem.74.082803.133400.
64. Li JY, Englund E, Holton JL, et al. Lewy bodies in grafted neurons in subjects with Parkinson's disease suggest host-to-graft disease propagation. Nat Med. 2008;14:501–3. doi:10.1038/nm1746.
65. Kordower JH, Chu Y, Hauser RA, et al. Lewy body-like pathology in long-term embryonic nigral transplants in Parkinson's disease. Nat Med. 2008;14:504–6. doi:10.1038/nm1747.
66. Olanow CW, Prusiner SB. Is Parkinson's disease a prion disorder? Proc Natl Acad Sci U S A. 2009;106:12571–2. doi:10.1073/pnas.0906759106.
67. Brundin P, Melki R, Kopito R. Prion-like transmission of protein aggregates in neurodegenerative diseases. Nat Rev Mol Cell Biol. 2010;11:301–7. doi:10.1038/nrm2873.
68. Irwin DJ, Lee VM, Trojanowski JQ. Parkinson's disease dementia: convergence of α-synuclein, tau and amyloid-β pathologies. Nat Rev Neurosci. 2013;14:626–36. doi:10.1038/nrn3549.
69. Lee HJ, Bae EJ, Lee SJ. Extracellular α-synuclein – a novel and crucial factor in Lewy body diseases. Nat Rev Neurol. 2014;10:92–8. doi:10.1038/nrneurol.2013.275.
70. El-Agnaf OM, Salem SA, Paleologou KE, et al. Detection of oligomeric forms of α-synuclein protein in human plasma as a potential biomarker for Parkinson's disease. FASEB J. 2006;20:419–25. doi:10.1096/fj.03-1449com.
71. Tokuda T, Qureshi MM, Ardah MT, et al. Detection of elevated levels of α-synuclein oligomers in CSF from patients with Parkinson disease. Neurology. 2010;75:1766–72. doi:10.1212/WNL.0b013e3181fd613b.
72. Park MJ, Cheon SM, Bae HR, et al. Elevated levels of α-synuclein oligomer in the cerebrospinal fluid of drug-naïve patients with Parkinson's disease. J Clin Neurol. 2011;7:215–22. doi:10.3988/jcn.2011.7.4.215.
73. Parnetti L, Farotti L, Eusebi P, et al. Differential role of CSF alpha-synuclein species, tau, and Aβ42 in Parkinson's Disease. Front Aging Neurosci. 2014;6:53. doi:10.3389/fnagi.2014.00053.
74. Compta Y, Valente T, Saura J, et al. Correlates of cerebrospinal fluid levels of oligomeric- and total-α-synuclein in premotor, motor and dementia stages of Parkinson's disease. J Neurol. 2015;262:294–306. doi:10.1007/s00415-014-7560-z.
75. Fujiwara H, Hasegawa M, Dohmae N, et al. α-Synuclein is phosphorylated in synucleinopathy lesions. Nat Cell Biol. 2002;4:160–4. doi:10.1038/ncb748.
76. Saito Y, Kawashima A, Ruberu NN, et al. Accumulation of phosphorylated α-synuclein in aging human brain. J Neuropathol Exp Neurol. 2003;62:644–54.
77. Anderson JP, Walker DE, Goldstein JM, et al. Phosphorylation of Ser-129 is the dominant pathological modification of α-synuclein in familial and sporadic Lewy body disease. J Biol Chem. 2006;281:29739–52. doi:10.1074/jbc.M600933200.
78. Covy JP, Yuan W, Waxman EA, et al. Clinical and pathological characteristics of patients with leucine-rich repeat kinase-2 mutations. Mov Disord. 2009;24:32–9. doi:10.1002/mds.22096.
79. Walker DG, Lue LF, Adler CH, et al.; Arizona Parkinson disease consortium. Changes in properties of serine 129 phosphorylated α-synuclein with progression of Lewy-type histopathology in human brains. Exp Neurol. 2013;240:190–204. doi:10.1016/j.expneurol.2012.11.020.
80. Chen L, Feany MB. α-Synuclein phosphorylation controls neurotoxicity and inclusion formation in a Drosophila model of Parkinson disease. Nat Neurosci. 2005;8:657–63. doi:10.1038/nn1443.

81. Gorbatyuk OS, Li S, Sullivan LF, et al. The phosphorylation state of Ser-129 in human α-synuclein determines neurodegeneration in a rat model of Parkinson disease. Proc Natl Acad Sci U S A. 2008;105:763–8. doi:10.1073/pnas.0711053105.
82. Wang Y, Shi M, Chung KA, et al. Phosphorylated α-synuclein in Parkinson's disease. Sci Transl Med. 2012;4:121ra20. doi:10.1126/scitranslmed.3002566.
83. Stewart T, Sossi V, Aasly JO, et al. Phosphorylated α-synuclein in Parkinson's disease: correlation depends on disease severity. Acta Neuropathol Commun. 2015;3:7. doi:10.1186/s40478-015-0185-3.
84. Noguchi-Shinohara M, Tokuda T, Yoshita M, et al. CSF α-synuclein levels in dementia with Lewy bodies and Alzheimer's disease. Brain Res. 2009;1251:1–6. doi:10.1016/j.brainres.2008.11.055.
85. Kasuga K, Tokutake T, Ishikawa A, et al. Differential levels of α-synuclein, β-amyloid42 and tau in CSF between patients with dementia with Lewy bodies and Alzheimer's disease. J Neurol Neurosurg Psychiatry. 2010;81:608–10. doi:10.1136/jnnp.2009.197483.
86. Spies PE, Melis RJ, Sjögren MJ, et al. Cerebrospinal fluid α-synuclein does not discriminate between dementia disorders. J Alzheimers Dis. 2009;16:363–9. doi:10.3233/JAD-2009-0955.
87. Kapaki E, Paraskevas GP, Emmanouilidou E, et al. The diagnostic value of CSF α-synuclein in the differential diagnosis of dementia with Lewy bodies vs. normal subjects and patients with Alzheimer's disease. PLoS One. 2013;8, e81654. doi:10.1371/journal.pone.0081654.
88. Lim X, Yeo JM, Green A, et al. The diagnostic utility of cerebrospinal fluid α-synuclein analysis in dementia with Lewy bodies – a systematic review and meta-analysis. Parkinsonism Relat Disord. 2013;19:851–8. doi:10.1016/j.parkreldis.2013.06.008.
89. Wang ZY, Han ZM, Liu QF, et al. Use of CSF α-synuclein in the differential diagnosis between Alzheimer's disease and other neurodegenerative disorders. Int Psychogeriatr. 2015. doi:10.1017/S1041610215000447.
90. Lippa CF, Fujiwara H, Mann DM, et al. Lewy bodies contain altered alpha-synuclein in brains of many familial Alzheimer's disease patients with mutations in presenilin and amyloid precursor protein genes. Am J Pathol. 1998;153:1365–70. doi:10.1016/S0002-9440(10)65722-7.
91. Hamilton RL. Lewy bodies in Alzheimer's disease: a neuropathological review of 145 cases using α-synuclein immunohistochemistry. Brain Pathol. 2000;10:378–84. doi:10.1111/j.1750-3639.2000.tb00269.x.
92. Nelson PT, Alafuzoff I, Bigio EH, et al. Correlation of Alzheimer disease neuropathologic changes with cognitive status: a review of the literature. J Neuropathol Exp Neurol. 2012;71:362–81. doi:10.1097/NEN.0b013e31825018f7.
93. Toledo JB, Korff A, Shaw LM, et al. CSF α-synuclein improves diagnostic and prognostic performance of CSF tau and Aβ in Alzheimer's disease. Acta Neuropathol. 2013;126:683–97. doi:10.1007/s00401-013-1148-z.
94. Lee PH, Lee G, Park HJ, et al. The plasma α-synuclein levels in patients with Parkinson's disease and multiple system atrophy. J Neural Transm. 2006;113:1435–9. doi:10.1007/s00702-005-0427-9.
95. Duran R, Barrero FJ, Morales B, et al. Plasma α-synuclein in patients with Parkinson's disease with and without treatment. Mov Disord. 2010;25:489–93. doi:10.1002/mds.22928.
96. Foulds PG, Mitchell JD, Parker A, et al. Phosphorylated α-synuclein can be detected in blood plasma and is potentially a useful biomarker for Parkinson's disease. FASEB J. 2011;25:4127–37. doi:10.1096/fj.10-179192.
97. Li QX, Mok SS, Laughton KM, et al. Plasma α-synuclein is decreased in subjects with Parkinson's disease. Exp Neurol. 2007;204:583–8. doi:10.1016/j.expneurol.2006.12.006.
98. Laske C, Fallgatter AJ, Stransky E, et al. Decreased α-synuclein serum levels in patients with Lewy body dementia compared to Alzheimer's disease patients and control subjects. Dement Geriatr Cogn Disord. 2011;31:413–6. doi:10.1159/000329763.

99. Shi M, Furay AR, Sossi V, et al. DJ-1 and αSYN in LRRK2 CSF do not correlate with striatal dopaminergic function. Neurobiol Aging. 2012;33:836.e5–7. doi:10.1016/j.neurobiolaging.2011.09.015.
100. Barbour R, Kling K, Anderson JP, et al. Red blood cells are the major source of alpha-synuclein in blood. Neurodegener Dis. 2008;5:55–9. doi:10.1159/000112832.
101. Kricka LJ. Human anti-animal antibody interferences in immunological assays. Clin Chem. 1999;45:942–56.
102. Levinson SS, Miller JJ. Towards a better understanding of heterophile (and the like) antibody interference with modern immunoassays. Clin Chim Acta. 2002;325:1–15. doi:10.1016/S0009-8981(02)00275-9.
103. Preissner CM, O'Kane DJ, Singh RJ, et al. Phantoms in the assay tube: heterophile antibody interferences in serum thyroglobulin assays. J Clin Endocrinol Metab. 2003;88:3069–74. doi:10.1210/jc.2003-030122.
104. Sehlin D, Söllvander S, Paulie S, et al. Interference from heterophilic antibodies in amyloid-β oligomer ELISAs. J Alzheimers Dis. 2010;21:1295–301. doi:10.3233/JAD-2010-100609.
105. Tamaoka A, Fukushima T, Sawamura N, et al. Amyloid β protein in plasma from patients with sporadic Alzheimer's disease. J Neurol Sci. 1996;141:65–8. doi:10.1016/0022-510X(96)00143-8.
106. Sinha N, Firbank M, O'Brien JT. Biomarkers in dementia with Lewy bodies: a review. Int J Geriatr Psychiatry. 2012;27:443–53. doi:10.1002/gps.2749.
107. Warr L, Walker Z. Identification of biomarkers in Lewy-body disorders. Q J Nucl Med Mol Imaging. 2012;56:39–54.
108. Donaghy PC, McKeith IG. The clinical characteristics of dementia with Lewy bodies and a consideration of prodromal diagnosis. Alzheimers Res Ther. 2014;6:46. doi:10.1186/alzrt274.
109. Schade S, Mollenhauer B. Biomarkers in biological fluids for dementia with Lewy bodies. Alzheimers Res Ther. 2014;6:72. doi:10.1186/s13195-014-0072-3.
110. Kanemaru K, Kameda N, Yamanouchi H. Decreased CSF amyloid β42 and normal tau levels in dementia with Lewy bodies. Neurology. 2000;54:1875–6. doi:10.1212/WNL.54.9.1875.
111. Tang W, Huang Q, Wang Y, et al. Assessment of CSF Aβ42 as an aid to discriminating Alzheimer's disease from other dementias and mild cognitive impairment: a meta-analysis of 50 studies. J Neurol Sci. 2014;345:26–36. doi:10.1016/j.jns.2014.07.015.
112. Nutu M, Zetterberg H, Londos E, et al. Evaluation of the cerebrospinal fluid amyloid-β1-42/amyloid-β1-40 ratio measured by alpha-LISA to distinguish Alzheimer's disease from other dementia disorders. Dement Geriatr Cogn Disord. 2013;36(1–2):99–110. doi:10.1159/000353442.
113. Clark CM, Xie S, Chittams J, et al. Cerebrospinal fluid tau and β-amyloid: how well do these biomarkers reflect autopsy-confirmed dementia diagnoses? Arch Neurol. 2003;60:1696–702. doi:10.1001/archneur.60.12.1696.
114. Vanderstichele H, De Vreese K, Blennow K, et al. Analytical performance and clinical utility of the INNOTEST PHOSPHO-TAU181P assay for discrimination between Alzheimer's disease and dementia with Lewy bodies. Clin Chem Lab Med. 2006;44:1472–80. doi:10.1515/CCLM.2006.258.
115. Mollenhauer B, Bibl M, Wiltfang J, et al. Total tau protein, phosphorylated tau (181p) protein, β-amyloid(1–42), and β-amyloid(1–40) in cerebrospinal fluid of patients with dementia with Lewy bodies. Clin Chem Lab Med. 2006;44:192–5. doi:10.1515/CCLM.2006.035.
116. Bibl M, Mollenhauer B, Lewczuk P, et al. Validation of amyloid-β peptides in CSF diagnosis of neurodegenerative dementias. Mol Psychiatry. 2007;12:671–80. doi:10.1038/sj.mp.4001967.
117. Mollenhauer B, Esselmann H, Trenkwalder C, et al. CSF amyloid-β peptides in neuropathologically diagnosed dementia with Lewy bodies and Alzheimer's disease. J Alzheimers Dis. 2011;24:383–91. doi:10.3233/JAD-2011-101551.
118. Siderowf A, Xie SX, Hurtig H, et al. CSF amyloid β 1–42 predicts cognitive decline in Parkinson disease. Neurology. 2010;75:1055–61. doi:10.1212/WNL.0b013e3181f39a78.

119. Jendroska K, Kashiwagi M, Sassoon J, et al. Amyloid beta-peptide and its relationship with dementia in Lewy body disease. J Neural Transm Suppl. 1997;51:137–44. doi:10.1093/brain/awl063.
120. Edison P, Rowe CC, Rinne JO, et al. Amyloid load in Parkinson's disease dementia and Lewy body dementia measured with [11C]PIB positron emission tomography. J Neurol Neurosurg Psychiatry. 2008;79:1331–8. doi:10.1136/jnnp.2007.127878.
121. Gomperts SN, Rentz DM, Moran E, et al. Imaging amyloid deposition in Lewy body diseases. Neurology. 2008;71:903–10. doi:10.1212/01.wnl.0000326146.60732.d6.
122. Slaets S, Le Bastard N, Theuns J, et al. Amyloid pathology influences Aβ1-42 cerebrospinal fluid levels in dementia with lewy bodies. J Alzheimers Dis. 2013;35:137–46. doi:10.3233/JAD-122176.
123. Mollenhauer B, Cepek L, Bibl M, et al. Tau protein, Aβ42 and S-100B protein in cerebrospinal fluid of patients with dementia with Lewy bodies. Dement Geriatr Cogn Disord. 2005;19:164–70. doi:10.1159/000083178.
124. Parnetti L, Lanari A, Amici S, et al. CSF phosphorylated tau is a possible marker for discriminating Alzheimer's disease from dementia with Lewy bodies: Phospho-Tau International Study Group. Neurol Sci. 2001;22:77–8. doi:10.1007/s100720170055.
125. Tang W, Huang Q, Yao YY, et al. Does CSF p-tau181 help to discriminate Alzheimer's disease from other dementias and mild cognitive impairment? A meta-analysis of the literature. J Neural Transm. 2014;121:1541–53. doi:10.1007/s00702-014-1226-y.
126. Hampel H, Goernitz A, Buerger K. Advances in the development of biomarkers for Alzheimer's disease: from CSF total tau and Aβ(1–42) proteins to phosphorylated tau protein. Brain Res Bull. 2003;61:243–53. doi:10.1016/S0361-9230(03)00087-X.
127. Iwata A, Maruyama M, Akagi T, et al. Alpha-synuclein degradation by serine protease neurosin: implication for pathogenesis of synucleinopathies. Hum Mol Genet. 2003;12:2625–35. doi:10.1093/hmg/ddg283.
128. Kasai T, Tokuda T, Yamaguchi N, et al. Cleavage of normal and pathological forms of α-synuclein by neurosin in vitro. Neurosci Lett. 2008;436:52–6. doi:10.1016/j.neulet.2008.02.057.
129. Tatebe H, Watanabe Y, Kasai T, et al. Extracellular neurosin degrades α-synuclein in cultured cells. Neurosci Res. 2010;67:341–6. doi:10.1016/j.neures.2010.04.008.
130. Wennström M, Surova Y, Hall S, et al. Low CSF levels of both α-synuclein and the α-synuclein cleaving enzyme neurosin in patients with synucleinopathy. PLoS One. 2013;8, e53250. doi:10.1371/journal.pone.0053250.
131. Aerts MB, Esselink RA, Claassen JA, et al. CSF tau, Aβ42, and MHPG differentiate dementia with Lewy bodies from Alzheimer's disease. J Alzheimers Dis. 2011;27:377–84. doi:10.3233/JAD-2011-110482.
132. Herbert MK, Aerts MB, Kuiperij HB, et al. Addition of MHPG to Alzheimer's disease biomarkers improves differentiation of dementia with Lewy bodies from Alzheimer's disease but not other dementias. Alzheimers Dement. 2014;10:448–55.e2. doi:10.1016/j.jalz.2013.05.1775.
133. Steinacker P, Mollenhauer B, Bibl M, et al. Heart fatty acid binding protein as a potential diagnostic marker for neurodegenerative diseases. Neurosci Lett. 2004;370:36–9. doi:10.1016/j.neulet.2004.07.061.
134. Mollenhauer B, Steinacker P, Bahn E, et al. Serum heart-type fatty acid-binding protein and cerebrospinal fluid tau: marker candidates for dementia with Lewy bodies. Neurodegener Dis. 2007;4:366–75. doi:10.1159/000105157.
135. Cheon MS, Kim SH, Fountoulakis M, et al. Heart type fatty acid binding protein (H-FABP) is decreased in brains of patients with Down syndrome and Alzheimer's disease. J Neural Transm Suppl. 2003;67:225–34. doi:10.1007/978-3-7091-6721-2_20.
136. Chen-Plotkin AS, Hu WT, Siderowf A, et al. Plasma epidermal growth factor levels predict cognitive decline in Parkinson disease. Ann Neurol. 2011;69:655–63. doi:10.1002/ana.22271.

Chapter 14
Electroencephalography in DLB

Mieko Tanaka, Toshimitsu Musha, Yohei Kobayashi, Haruyasu Matsuzaki, and Yukio Kosugi

Abstract The authors have developed a technology called neuronal activity topography (NAT), using which a pair of markers is obtained by spectral analysis of the electroencephalogram (EEG) of a subject, when he or she is in an awake, resting state with eyes closed, to determine minute differences in his or her brain activity. The markers provide a numerical index indicating the degree to which the subject resembles the average patterns of certain brain disorders. NAT images obtained from a group of patients with dementia with Lewy bodies (DLB) displayed such average features as the presence of slow-wave activity in the temporoparietal lobes in the occipital region and diffuse alpha, both of which were found to be more pronounced compared to a group of patients with Alzheimer's disease. The tendencies agree with features observed by EEG visual inspection. Using this technology, it was possible to distinguish between cognitively normal subjects and DLB patients with 95 % accuracy.

Keywords Electroencephalography (EEG) • Dementia with Lewy bodies (DLB) • Neuronal activity topography (NAT)

14.1 Introduction

In the human brain, a vast amount of biological information is continuously being transmitted from neuron to neuron. Electrical signals appear on the scalp because of the constant activity of this vast network, and these signals are called electroencephalograms (EEGs). The electroencephalograph is used to record the changes in the potential difference of the electrical signals between two points as brain wave data or EEG. While the change in potential difference is in the order of 50 μV and thus only one several hundredths of that of electrocardiograms, which are in the range of several tens to several hundreds of mV, it nevertheless contains abundant

M. Tanaka (✉) • T. Musha • Y. Kobayashi • H. Matsuzaki • Y. Kosugi
Brain Functions Lab., Inc., 1-508 Leading Venture Plaza, 75-1, Ono-cho, Tsurumi-ku, Yokohama 230-0046, Japan
e-mail: mtanaka@bfl.co.jp

K. Kosaka (ed.), *Dementia with Lewy Bodies*, DOI 10.1007/978-4-431-55948-1_14

information on brain activities. Thus, certain features of dementia are likely to be contained in EEG data.

The 2005 revised edition of the consensus clinical diagnostic criteria for dementia with Lewy bodies (DLB) [1] gives the presence of "prominent slow-wave activity on EEG with temporal lobe transient sharp waves" as the final (tenth) item under "Supportive features (commonly present, but not proven to have diagnostic specificity)." Slow-wave activity means the transition of the alpha-wave dominant rhythm in the vicinity of 10Hz, which appears normally in the occipital region in healthy adults, to slow alpha waves of about 8Hz, the irregular appearance of theta waves of 5–7Hz along with alpha waves, or the replacement of alpha with sustained theta or delta waves (0.5–4Hz).

However, slow-wave activity often occurs in Alzheimer's disease (AD) and other types of dementia as well. Furthermore, some studies have shown that slow-wave activities also occur in the background activities of healthy elderly subjects [2, 3]. Although one study [4] compared EEG between 14 patients with DLB-verified postmortem and 11 patients with AD-verified postmortem and found more evidence of slow-wave transient activity in the temporal lobe areas in the former group, another study [5] reported that it was not possible to distinguish EEG patterns between a group of 28 clinically diagnosed AD patients and a group of 34 clinically diagnosed DLB patients. Because of the difficulty of quantitatively demonstrating the difference between slow-wave activity due to aging or AD and that due to DLB, there have not been many efforts undertaken so far to employ EEG for DLB identification.

The present authors have been engaged in the development of a neuronal activity topography (NAT) analysis system as an EEG-based support system for the early identification of AD, which makes up between one third and one half of dementia patients. EEG was chosen because it has the merits that the equipment cost is not high, it does not cause radiation exposure and is noninvasive, it has no contraindications except in limited cases such as subjects using devices for deep brain stimulation (DBS) which delivers pulse signals to certain areas of the brain, and the examinations can be repeated with relative ease.

To obtain NAT, the miniscule differences in the brain activity of a subject in an awake, resting state with eyes closed are represented by two markers (sNAT and vNAT), which are obtained from EEG spectral analysis and used to represent the characteristics of certain disorders [6]. The EEG potentials of the subject when he/she is sitting, awake, resting, and with closed eyes are recorded for about 5 min using 21 (Fig. 14.1) or 19 electrodes attached to the scalp according to the International 10–20 system, then the EEG data is uploaded via the Internet and analyzed, and the results are given back to the user.

Conventionally, considerable time was required to quantitatively examine slow-wave activity by means of visual observation. Using NAT technology, however, it is possible to quantitatively check the features of large sets of data in a short time by comparing the patterns with representative patterns (templates) of certain disorders prepared in advance.

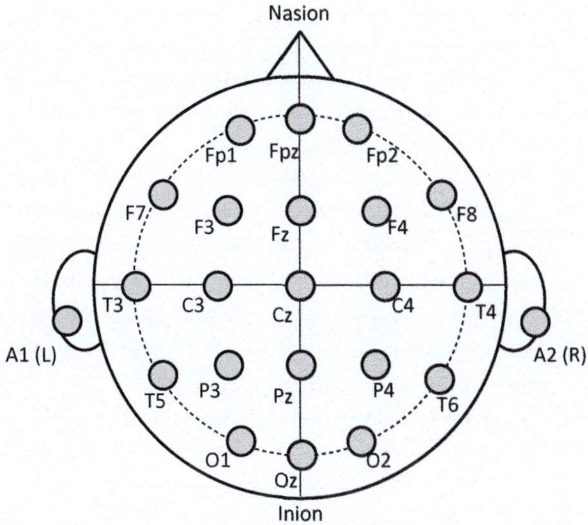

Fig. 14.1 Electrode positions in international 10–20 system

In this article, we shall first describe the EEG features of DLB patients in an awake, resting, and eyes-closed state that are visually recognizable and then discuss those features quantitatively obtained by NAT analysis.

14.2 EEG Visual Inspection

14.2.1 EEG of Healthy Aged Subject in Awake, Resting, and Eyes-Closed State

Figure 14.2 shows an example of the EEG data of a healthy aged subject with no cognitive function disorders. The EEG is that of a female subject, aged 70, who scored 29 on the Mini-Mental State Examination (MMSE). Alpha waves of about 12Hz appear prominently in the occipital region and display some waxing and waning. This is considered as a normal EEG. However, such clean EEG rhythms are not seen often among subjects aged 60 and over, who tend to display the slowing or diffusion of alpha waves, increase of theta waves, or slowing of waves in the temporal regions [2, 3].

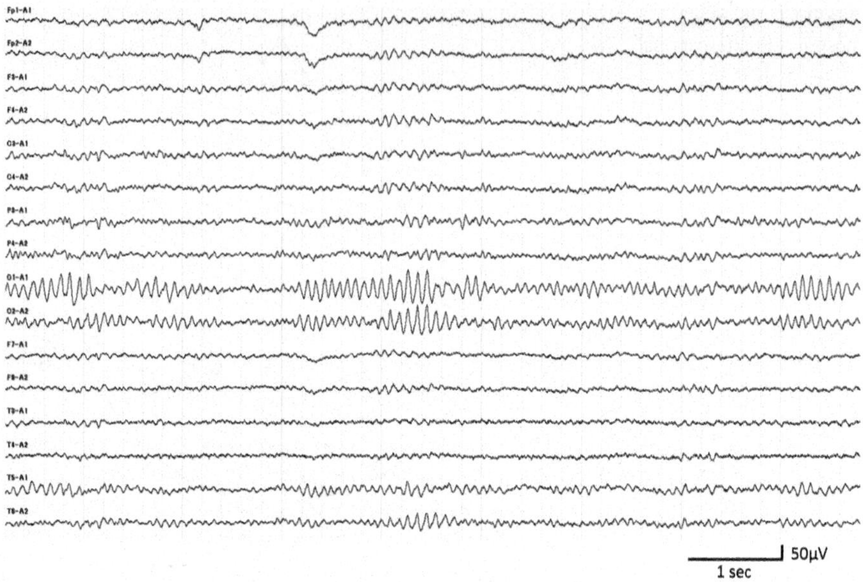

Fig. 14.2 Example of EEG of aged subject with normal cognitive functions in an awake, resting state with eyes closed (age 70, female, MMSE = 29. Alpha waves of about 12Hz appear dominantly in the occipital region and display waxing and waning)

14.2.2 EEG of DLB Patient in Awake, Resting, and Eyes-Closed State

Figure 14.3 shows an example of the EEG data of a DLB patient. The EEG is that of a female patient, aged 87, who scored 10 on MMSE. It displays a moderate slow abnormality with a predominance of theta waves and irregular, sustained alpha waves in the frontal region. The EEG is clearly different from that of Fig. 14.2, but it would be difficult for non-experts.

14.3 NAT (Neuronal Activity Topography)

To obtain NAT, two markers, sNAT and vNAT, which characterize the brain activity are defined from the power spectrum of the EEG potential recorded with electrodes and then analyzed [6]. This yields two types of information: (1) images of brain activities (i.e., the NAT images) and (2) a numerical index (i.e., likelihood) that indicates to what degree the obtained EEG is similar to those representing the average brain activity patterns specific to certain disorders (Fig. 14.4).

The details of sNAT and vNAT are given below.

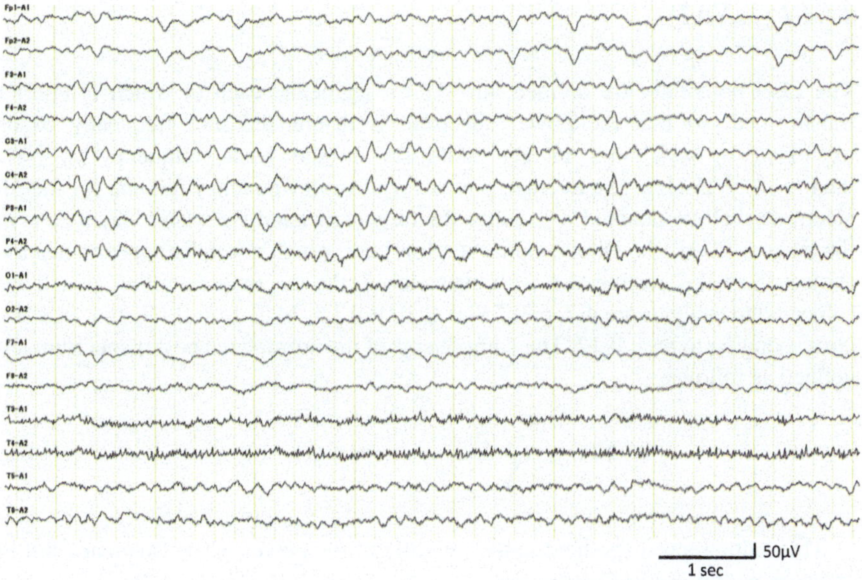

Fig. 14.3 Example of EEG of DLB patient in an awake, resting state with eyes closed (age 87, female, MMSE = 10. Moderate slow abnormality with theta waves predominating. Irregular sustained alpha waves are seen in the frontal region)

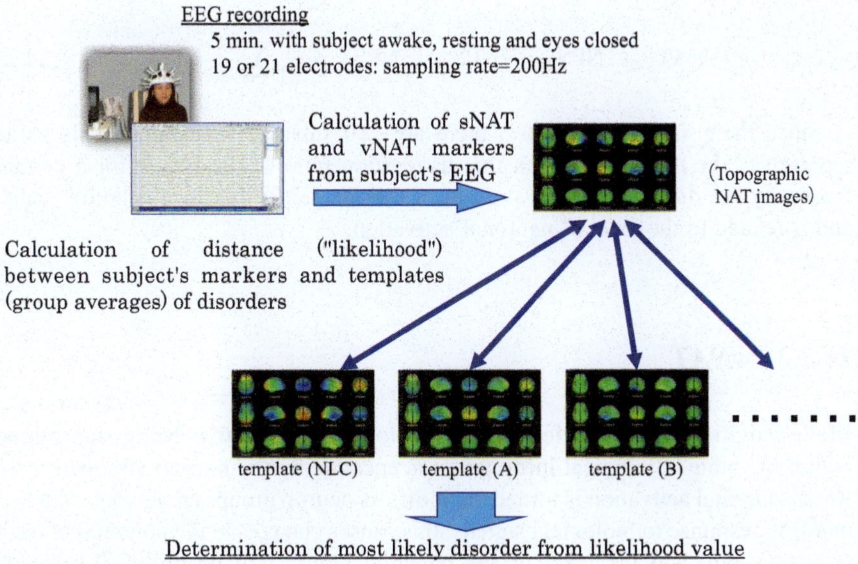

Fig. 14.4 NAT analysis flow

14.3.1 sNAT

The EEG potentials are divided into 0.64 s segments, each of which is Fourier transformed, so that the power spectrum is discretized into frequency bands expressed by mf_0, i.e., integer multiples of the basic frequency f_0 (=1/0.64 s = 1.5625 Hz). The average power for the mth frequency bin mf_0 for the jth electrode shall be denoted $S_{j,m}$. Since the frequency band we wish to analyze is in the range 4–20 Hz, i.e., theta, alpha, and low beta, which normally appear when the subject is awake, resting and with eyes closed, the ten frequency bins which are subjected to analysis are 4.7, 6.3, 7.8, 9.4, 10.9, 12.5, 14.1, 15.6, 17.2, and 18.8 Hz, corresponding to $m = 3$~12. The components of the normalized power spectrum are defined as follows:

$$\mathrm{NPS}_{j,m} \equiv \frac{S_{j,m}}{\sum_{n=3}^{12} S_{j,n}} \quad (m = 3 \sim 12) \tag{14.1}$$

This value represents the distribution ratio of the power of the frequency bin in question within the EEG spectrum.

To emphasize the variation of the distribution ratio of the EEG power for the frequency bin mf$_0$, we subtract the average value for all electrodes from the above and call it marker "sNAT." This marker consists of the ten submarkers, $\mathrm{sNAT}_{j,m}$, which are expressed as follows:

$$\mathrm{sNAT}_{j,m} \equiv \mathrm{NPS}_{j,m} - \overline{\mathrm{NPS}}_m, \quad \overline{\mathrm{NPS}}_m = \frac{1}{21}\sum_{j=1}^{21} \mathrm{NPS}_{j,m} \tag{14.2}$$

Since there are 21 electrodes, there are 210 submarkers in total. This value represents "the degree to which the distribution ratio of the power for a certain frequency bin differs from the average of that frequency bin for the entire scalp" and is related to the level of neuronal activation.

14.3.2 vNAT

Brain activities are a manifestation of biological information being transmitted within the brain. Biological information is encoded by the manner (frequency) in which neuronal activation is turned on or off. As neuron groups are locally switched on/off in response to biological signals, this causes changes in the potential of each frequency bin, and the level of the potential power will be different for each frequency bin. This causes the power levels of adjacent frequency bins to differ. In order to quantify this effect in a simple manner, the ratio of the power levels of two adjacent frequency bins is defined as:

$$p_{j,m} \equiv \frac{\mathrm{NPS}_{j,m+1}}{\mathrm{NPS}_{j,m}} \tag{14.3}$$

And $\mathrm{NPV}_{j,m}$ is defined, so that it will have the range 0–1, as follows:

$$\mathrm{NPV}_{j,m} \equiv \frac{4p_{j,m}}{\left(1+p_{j,m}\right)^2}; \quad m = 3 \sim 12 \tag{14.4}$$

As in the first marker, when the average value of all electrodes is subtracted from this to emphasize the variations, we obtain the second marker which we call vNAT. This marker consists of ten submarkers, $\mathrm{vNAT}_{j,m}$, defined as follows:

$$\mathrm{vNAT}_{j,m} \equiv \mathrm{NPV}_{j,m} - \overline{\mathrm{NPV}}_m, \quad \overline{\mathrm{NPV}}_m = \frac{1}{21}\sum_{j=1}^{21} \mathrm{NPV}_{j,m} \tag{14.5}$$

Since there are 21 electrodes, there are 210 submarkers in total. This value might be considered to be related to the synchronization of neuronal activation.

14.4 DLB in NAT

We investigate the features commonly found in the EEG patterns of DLB patients from the sNAT images obtained from NAT analysis and the differential likelihoods.

14.4.1 Subjects

Table 14.1 presents the data profiles of the normal control (NLC) group, AD patient group, and DLB patient group, which were used to obtain the templates. The NLC group consists of 52 subjects, who have scores of 26 or greater on MMSE, clinical dementia ratings (CDR) of 0, and no abnormalities in their magnetic resonance imaging (MRI) results or EEGs [6].

14.4.2 Topographic NAT Images

Figure 14.5 shows the average sNAT images of the template groups for NLC, AD, and DLB. The five images shown for each frequency bin consist of, from left to right, the image of the parietal region with the forehead in the upper part, that of the left temporal lobe where the forehead is to the left, that of the occipital region, that of the right temporal lobe where the forehead is to the right, and that of the frontal

Table 14.1 Template data profiles (NLC, AD, and DLB)

Template group	NLC	AD	DLB
Number	52	20	21
(Male/female)	(28/24)	(5/15)	(15/6)
Age (y)	65–85	71–95	59–90
(Mean ± SD)	71.9 ± 5.9	84.4 ± 6.3	77.7 ± 7.2
MMSE	29.1 ± 1.1	19.1 ± 3.5	22.4 ± 5.5
(Mean ± SD)			
Study	(T. Asada, 2010) [6]		(S. Orimo, 2014) [7]

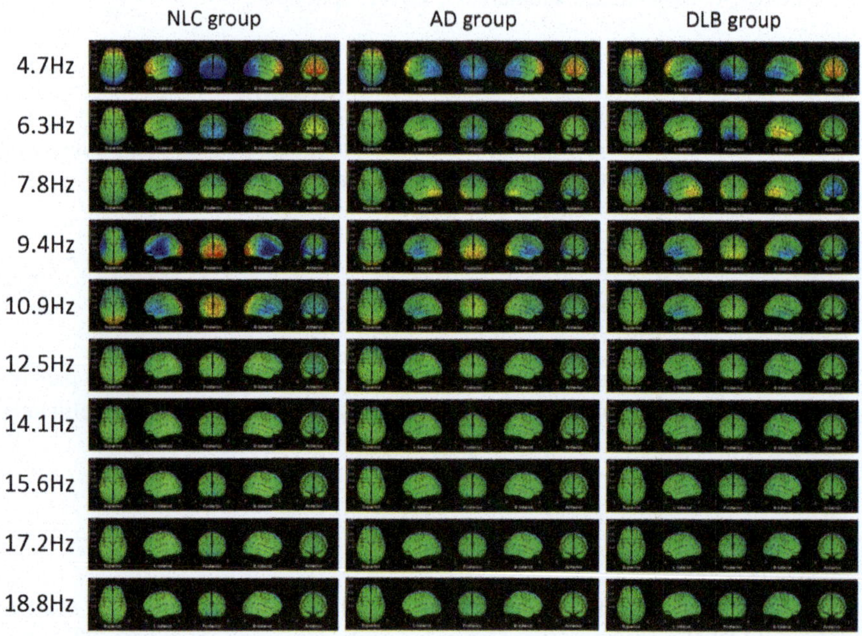

Fig. 14.5 sNAT images of template groups (NLC, AD, and DLB) (from *left*, NLC (normal control), AD group, and DLB group. *Green* represents average when power spectral distribution is normalized, *yellow* to *red* regions with relatively high power, and *light blue* to *blue* those with relatively low power)

region. As stated earlier, the sNAT image shows "the degree to which the distribution ratio of the power of that frequency bin for an electrode differs from the average level for all electrodes," and so the average level is shown in green sections with a relatively higher power distribution ratio in yellow shifting to red and those with lower power distribution ratio in light blue shifting to dark blue.

In the NLC group, the power distribution ratios of alpha waves from 9.4 to 10.9Hz in the occipital region and theta waves of 4.7Hz in the frontal region are relatively high, indicating that the dominant rhythm is in the vicinity of 10Hz. The

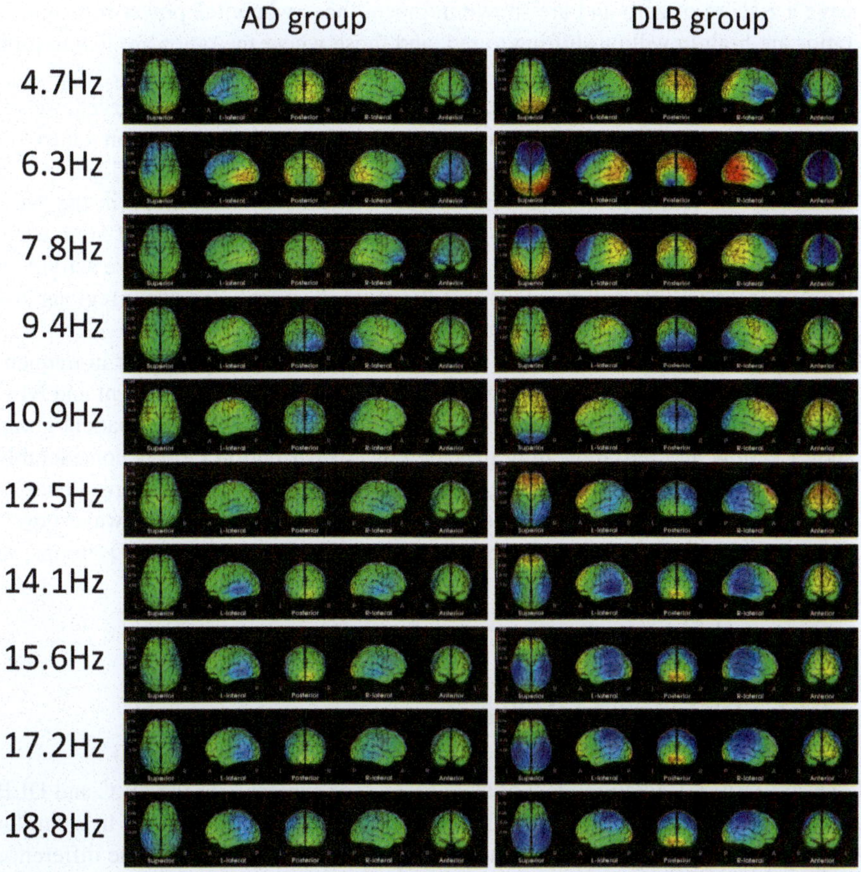

Fig. 14.6 NLC-normalized z-score images of sNAT of templates (from *left*, z-score images normalized with respect to NLC group of AD group and DLB group. Green represents z-score of around zero (roughly the same relative power to NLC group), *yellow* to *red* positive scores, and *light blue* to *blue* negative scores)

power distribution ratios of the AD patient group and NLC group are similar, although the former displays a weaker contrast in the color shadings. In the DLB patient group, the power distribution ratio of alpha waves in the occipital region is not so different from those for neighboring higher and lower frequencies, while those of 6.3 and 7.8Hz are higher at the temporal lobes. This group displays an even weaker color contrast than the AD group, indicating that the power distribution is flat overall.

To distinguish the features of the AD and DLB patient groups from those caused by aging in healthy aged subjects, NAT images showing z-scores normalized with respect to the NLC group were obtained and are shown in Fig. 14.6. Those sections where the power distribution ratios are at about the same level as the NLC group have a z-score of zero and are shown in green, those where the power distribution ratios are high in yellow shifting to red, and those where the ratios are low in light blue shifting to dark blue.

Focusing on the occipital region, where the dominant rhythm is observed, we see that in both the AD and DLB patient groups, the power distribution ratios for 9.4–12.5Hz in the occipital region are lower than those in the NLC group and those for 4.7–7.8Hz in the temporoparietal lobes higher than those in the NLC group. However, the DLB patient group displays a greater degree of slow-wave activity than the AD patient group. Thus, the characteristic of slow-wave activity in the AD and DLB patient groups is that it occurs in roughly the same regions in a similar pattern, but differs in magnitude.

Features that differ between the AD and DLB patient groups appear in frequencies of 10.9 and 12.5Hz in the frontal lobe. In this region, the AD patient and NLC groups display power distribution ratios that are similar, but the DLB patient group shows yellow and red, indicating that the power distribution ratio is considerably higher than in the NLC group. This can perhaps be explained by the prevalence of diffuse alpha among DLB patients, which results in a higher alpha-wave power distribution ratio in the frontal lobe as compared to the NLC and AD groups, in which diffuse alpha is not common.

14.4.3 Differential Likelihood

The similarities ("likelihoods") of state $sNAT^{X}$ of subject X to the NLC and DLB template states, respectively, $sNAT^{NLC}$ and $sNAT^{DLB}$, are computed. In a similar manner, the likelihoods are computed with respect to vNAT. Then, the difference between the respective likelihoods to the DLB and NLC templates, called the "differential likelihood," is obtained as follows:

$$\begin{aligned} &(\text{DLB} - \text{NLC})\ \text{differential likelihood} \\ &\quad = \text{likelihood of DLB} - \text{likelihood of NLC} \end{aligned} \tag{14.6}$$

If the differential likelihood of a subject is positive, then he or she is more likely to be closer to DLB than NLC. If negative, then the reverse holds.

Figure 14.7 shows a two-dimensional space diagram, where the abscissa and ordinate, respectively, represent the sNAT and vNAT components of the (DLB-NLC) differential likelihood. Three kinds of data set are plotted, i.e., a data set of the template NLC group, a data set of the template DLB patient group, and a data set of DLB patient group ("DLB-K"). DLB-K patient group characterized by (n = 17 (M = 8/F = 9), age = 79.1 ± 5.2 y, MMSE = 19.9 ± 6.7) was obtained from another study (Kosaka, 2014) at a different medical facility. The lower left part represents a region mostly occupied by the NLC group, while the upper right is mostly occupied by the DLB group. The broken line that defines the border between

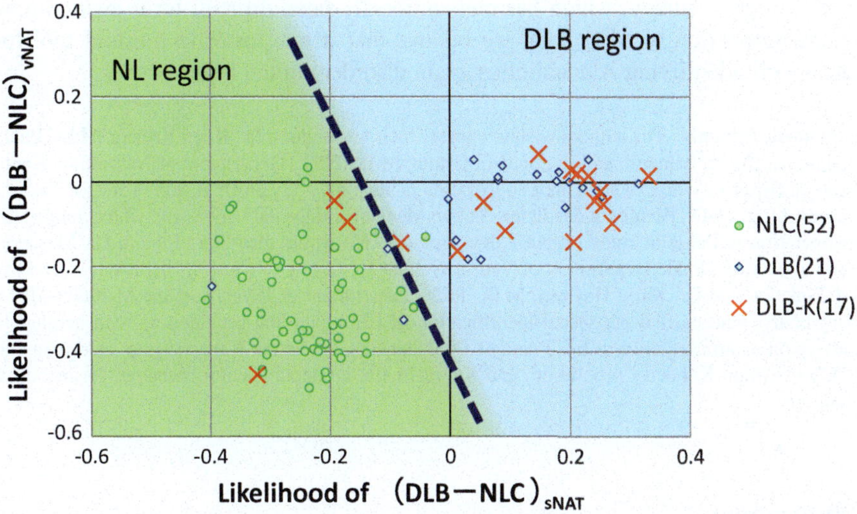

Fig. 14.7 (DLB-NLC) likelihood diagram of DLB and NLC groups (DLB-K group is a subject group from a medical institution that is different from the one from which DLB template was obtained. n = 17 (M = 8/F = 9), age = 79.1 ± 5.2y, and MMSE = 19.9 ± 6.7. Hit rate for DLB was about 82 % (14 of 17 patients). The *broken line* represents the border between the NL and DLB regions)

these two regions was determined from a discriminant analysis (canonical discriminant analysis which is an extension of Fisher's linear discriminant function) using the two templates. The hit rates for the templates were 98% (51 of 52 subjects) for the NLC group, 86 % (18 of 21 patients) for the DLB group, and 95 % overall. That for the DLB-K group was 82% (14 of 17 patients).

14.5 Conclusions

We were able to confirm the following two items as features of EEG patterns of DLB patients in an awake, resting state with their eyes closed:

(1) Slow-wave activity in the occipital region was observed in both the AD and DLB patient groups, but it was more pronounced in the latter.
(2) Diffuse alpha was also observed from NAT images and found to be more pronounced in the DLB group than in the AD group.

From the different distributional patterns of the differential likelihoods, determined from the difference between NAT patterns using the above features, the accuracy of identification of DLB and NL was about 95 %.

With NAT, it is possible to accumulate databases and increase the templates of various brain disorders. Since NAT allows one to separate DLB and NL subjects with a high accuracy, which has conventionally been difficult to do with simple visual inspection of EEG data, we believe that it may provide a useful tool for accurately identifying AD and other brain disorders in the future.

Acknowledgments The authors wish to express their gratitude to Dr. Kenji Kosaka, M.D., PhD., Clinic Ian Center Minami, and Dr. Satoshi Orimo, M.D., PhD., Department of Neurology, Kanto Central Hospital, who extended their cooperation in the joint study on DLB, and Professor Takashi Asada, M.D., PhD., Faculty of Medicine, Tokyo Medical and Dental University, who extended his cooperation in the joint study on NAT development. We would also like to thank Dr. Masanori Ishikawa, M.D., PhD., Department of Neuropsychiatry, Institute of Clinical Medicine, University of Tsukuba, and Dr. Karin Hayashi, M.D., PhD., Department of Psychosomatic Medicine, Toho University, who carried out visual identification of EEG data and provided us with invaluable advice on examining clinical EEG data of DLB patients. We thank Kazuo Ogino, chairman and CEO of Nihon Kohden Corporation, and Kaoru Imajo, its deputy senior manager, for technical support.

References

1. McKeith IG, Dickson DW, Lowe J, et al. Diagnosis and management of dementia with Lewy bodies: third report of the DLB consortium. Neurology. 2005;65(12):1863–72.
2. Silverman AJ, Busse EW, Barnes RH. Studies on the processes of aging: electroencephalographic findings in 400 elderly subjects. Electroencephalogr Clin Neurophysiol. 1955;7:67–74.
3. Nakano T, Mitasaka M, Ohtaka T, et al. Longitudinal changes in computerized EEG and mental function of the aged: a nine-year follow-up study. Int Psychogeriatr. 1992;4(1):9–23.
4. Briel RC, McKeith IG, Barker WA, et al. EEG findings in dementia with Lewy bodies and Alzheimer's disease. J Neurol Neurosurg Psychiatry. 1999;66(3):401–3.
5. Londos E, Passant U, Brun A, et al. Regional cerebral blood flow and EEG in clinically diagnosed dementia with Lewy bodies and Alzheimer's disease. Arch Gerontol Geriatr. 2003;36(3):231–45.
6. Musha T, Matsuzaki H, Kobayashi Y, et al. EEG markers for characterizing anomalous activities of cerebral neurons in NAT (neuronal activity topography) method. IEEE Trans Biomed Eng. 2013;60(8):2332–8.
7. Tanaka M, Orimo S, Kobayashi Y, et al. Discrimination of DLB, AD and NL in the NAT analysis (in Japanese). 55th annual meeting of the Japanese Society of Neurology; 2014. p. 72–7.

Chapter 15
Ventilatory Response to Hypercapnia in Dementia with Lewy Bodies

Katsuyoshi Mizukami

Abstract This chapter focuses on ventilatory response to hypercapnia (VRH) in patients with dementia with Lewy bodies (DLB). VRH is a rise in ventilation induced by increase in PCO_2. In our study, VRH was impaired in all examined DLB patients, while that of Alzheimer's disease (AD) and healthy elderly patients was normal. The mean VRH in DLB patients was significantly lower compared with Alzheimer's disease and healthy elderly patients. Impaired VRH can be observed also in the prodromal and mild stages of DLB. Hypercapnia primarily stimulates the central chemoreceptors, putatively located in the medulla oblongata. Thus, impaired VRH may be, in part, associated with the DLB lesions in the medulla oblongata. VRH is a promising diagnostic method for differentiating DLB from AD. Furthermore, it is important to bear in mind that DLB patients are susceptible to respiratory compromise and have risk of poor outcome due to respiratory complications.

Keywords DLB • Autonomic failure • Ventilatory response to hypercapnia

15.1 Introduction

Dementia with Lewy bodies (DLB) is a neurodegenerative disease characterized by progressive dementia with Parkinsonism, visual hallucinations, and cognitive fluctuations and is now thought to be the second most common form of dementia, after Alzheimer's disease (AD). Patients with DLB suffer from systematic autonomic dysfunction and have various autonomic symptoms, such as syncope, orthostatic hypotension, urinary incontinence, and constipation, at the early stages or even often before the onset of dementia [1–3]. In addition, the majority of patients show abnormal findings in the autonomic function assessments, such as a low uptake on ^{123}I-metaiodobenzylguanidine myocardial scintigraphy [4, 5] and impaired heart rate variability [6, 7].

K. Mizukami (✉)
Graduate School of Comprehensive Human Sciences, University of Tsukuba, 3-29-1 Otsuka, Bunkyo-ku, Tokyo 112-0012, Japan
e-mail: kmizukam@taiiku.tsukuba.ac.jp

K. Kosaka (ed.), *Dementia with Lewy Bodies*, DOI 10.1007/978-4-431-55948-1_15

Since our previous study disclosed the reduced impaired ventilatory response to hypercapnia in DLB [7], some articles have reported on the respiratory dysfunction of DLB patients. Sleep-disordered breathing is observed in over 70 % of DLB patients, and sleep-disordered breathing is observed most frequently in DLB patients among the major dementia diseases, such as Alzheimer's disease, vascular dementia, frontotemporal dementia, and DLB [8]. Another paper reported a higher prevalence of DLB patients with dysrhythmic breathing compared with patients with AD and patients without dementia [9].

This chapter focuses on ventilatory response to hypercapnia (VRH) in DLB patients.

15.2 Ventilatory Response to Hypercapnia

There are two kinds of ventilator response. One is ventilator response to hypoxia, which is a rise in ventilation induced by decrease in PO_2, and the other is ventilatory response to hypercapnia, which is a rise in ventilation induced by increase in PCO_2. Reduced ventilatory response leads to vulnerability to ventilatory failure during states of high demand (e.g., heart failure and pneumonia) and possible poor outcomes [10].

Elderly people are known to have diminished ventilatory response to hypoxia and hypercapnia [10, 11]. Kronenberg and Drage (1973) studied eight healthy young subjects and eight older subjects and noted a 50 % reduction in response to hypoxia and 40 % reduction in response to hypercapnia in the older subjects [11].

15.3 Ventilatory Response to Hypercapnia in DLB Patients

Mizukami et al. [7] reported reduced ventilatory response to hypercapnia in DLB patients. In this study, 15 patients with probable DLB (mean age 68.8 ± 7.3 years), 7 patients with AD (mean age 76.1 ± 8.6 years), and 12 healthy control subjects (mean age 69.3 ± 4.7 years) were examined. The mean scores of the Mini-Mental State Examination (MMSE) of the DLB, AD, and control subjects were 18.9 ± 5.8, 20.6 ± 5.1, and 29.3 ± 1.0, respectively. The mean duration of the illness of DLB and AD patients was 3.6 ± 2.0 years and 3.7 ± 2.2 years, respectively. In addition, 12 of 15 patients with DLB (80.0 %) showed a reduction in cerebral blood flow in the occipital lobe on single-photon emission computed tomography (SPECT), and 11 of 15 patients (73.3 %) showed low uptake on 123I-MIBG myocardial scintigraphy. All participants showed normal arterial blood gas analysis, %VC, and forced expiratory volume in 1 s (FEV1.0 %).

Ventilatory response to hypercapnia (VRH) was assessed using a dual control system for oxygen and carbon dioxide (Duograph KAY-100, CHEST Co., Tokyo). End-tidal oxygen partial pressure (PETO2) was kept constant at 180 Torr during the

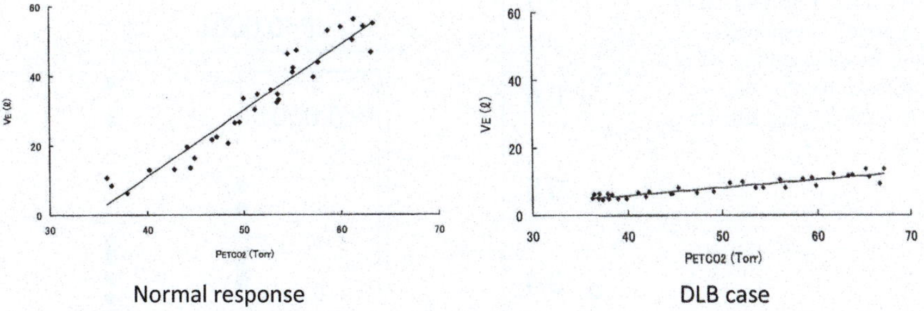

Fig. 15.1 Reduced respiratory response to hypercapnia

procedure. VRH was expressed as the slope of the regression line relating ventilation (L/min) to changes in end-tidal carbon dioxide partial pressure (PETCO2), corrected by body surface area (m^2) (ΔVE/PETCO2/BSA) (/min Torr/m^2) (Fig. 15.1).

The indices of VRH of the DLB patients, AD patients, and controls were 0.156 ± 0.10, 0.431 ± 0.04, and 0.466 ± 0.09, respectively (Fig. 15.2). VRH in DLB patients was significantly lower than that of AD patients ($p < 0.001$) and the controls ($p < 0.001$), while there was no statistical difference between the AD patients and controls (Table 15.1 and Fig. 15.2). All DLB patients demonstrated abnormally low VRH (normal range: male 0.34–1.20, female 0.39–0.95), while all of the AD or control subjects had normal VRH.

As shown in Table 15.1, there was no correlation between VRH and MMSE scores, disease duration, or Hoehn and Yahr stage. VRH was impaired even in very mild cases (i.e., cases 3 and 4).

This study suggested that VRH appears to be a promising diagnostic method for differentiating DLB from AD. In addition, decreased VRH may have clinical significance in DLB patients, who may be more susceptible to respiratory compromise.

15.4 Ventilatory Response to Hypercapnia in Patients During the Prodromal Stage of DLB

Our next study demonstrated that reduced VRH is observed during the prodromal stage of DLB [12]. Subjects were 167 patients (ranging from 50 to 83 years) primarily diagnosed with having mood disorders and hospitalized in our university hospital. According to the DLB criteria, diagnoses of probable and possible DLB were made. Several patients satisfying some but falling short of the DLB diagnosis criteria were defined as suspected DLB with supportive features. Twenty-three patients were diagnosed as either probable, possible, or suspected DLB (13.8 %). Low H/M ratio in 123I-metaiodobenzylguanidine (MIBG) myocardial

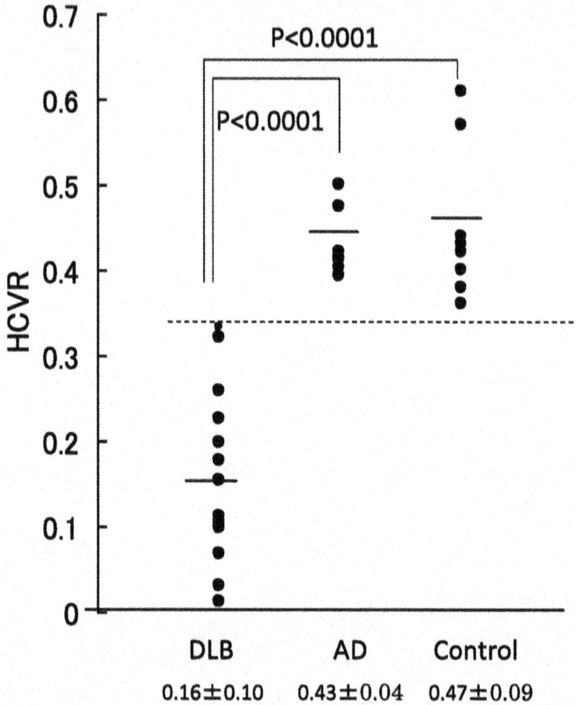

Fig. 15.2 Comparison of respiratory response to hypercapnia among DLB, AD, and healthy elderly subjects (Figure adapted from Ref. [7])

scintigraphy, a reduction in the cerebral blood flow in the occipital lobe revealed by brain perfusion SPECT, and reduced ventilatory response to hypercapnia in possible DLB and suspected DLB patients were 83.3 % and 50 %, 75 % and 88.9 %, and 83.3 % and 83.3 %, respectively. This study suggested that patients in the prodromal stage of DLB show highly positive findings of hypercapnic ventilation response.

Our next study examined the usefulness of VRH to predict depression converting DLB [13]. Participants were 35 consecutive patients with major depressive disorder and bradykinesia, first onset at 50 years or older. Longitudinal follow-up showed that all 18 patients with abnormal VRH developed DLB, whereas none of the 17 patients with normal VRH developed DLB within the study period. These results suggested the possibility that VRH may also be useful in the diagnosis of prodromal DLB.

15.5 Ventilatory Response in Other Neurodegenerative Diseases

Some neurodegenerative diseases, such as multiple system atrophy and Parkinson's disease (PD), show impaired ventilatory response. Chokroverty et al. (1978) reported that one of four patients with Shy-Drager syndrome had reduced ventilator

Table 15.1 Autonomic failures in DLB cases

	Sex	Age	Three core symptoms	MMSE	Barthel index	Duration from onset (years)	Yahr	Reduced occipital lobe perfusion in SPECT	Reduced MIBG H/M ratio	Ventilatory response to hypercapnia
1	M	70	Full	9	70	5	2	+	+	0.154
2	F	75	Full	21	70	8	3	+	+	0.322
3	F	56	VH(−)	27	100	1	2	+	+	0.176
4	F	77	Full	27	100	5	2	+	+	0.011
5	F	68	VH(−)	11	100	4	2	−	+	0.198
6	F	70	P(−)	21	95	1	0	−	−	0.067
7	M	73	Full	17	90	2	2	+	+	0.104
8	F	63	Full	18	80	5	2	−	+	0.257
9	F	55	Full	10	75	3	2	+	−	0.100
10	F	61	VH(−)	15	80	3	1	+	−	0.031
11	M	74	VH(−)	18	100	3	1	+	+	0.112
12	F	73	P(−)	18	100	5	0	+	−	0.097
13	M	74	Full	17	80	1	1	+	+	0.226
14	M	65	Full	25	100	5	1	+	+	0.332

Table adapted from Ref. [26]
VH visual hallucination, *P* Parkinsonism

response to hypercapnia [14]. In contrast, Tsuda et al. [15] showed normal ventilatory response to hypercapnia, but reduced ventilatory response to hypoxia in patients with multiple system atrophy. Two papers reported the results of ventilatory response in patients with Parkinson's disease. Onodera et al. [16] observed impaired ventilator response to hypoxia, but a normal response to hypercapnia in PD patients who were receiving dopaminergic medication. On the other hand, Seccombe et al. [17] reported that 7 of 15 patients with mild-to-moderate PD have a reduced ventilatory response to hypercapnia despite normal lung volume and flow.

15.6 Candidate Lesions for Ventilatory Response

It is well documented that hypercapnia primarily stimulates the central chemoreceptors near the ventral surface of the medulla oblongata, in which a muscarinic cholinergic mechanism is involved [18]. Involvement of cholinergic neurotransmitter systems is supported by the literature, demonstrating that mice lacking the acetylcholine esterase gene increases CO_2 chemosensitivity [19]. Other candidate brainstem areas for ventilatory response are the glutamatergic neurons of the retrotrapezoid nucleus [20, 21] and serotonergic neurons of the raphe nucleus [22, 23]. Since it is well documented that Lewy body pathology is remarkable in the ventrolateral medulla and the nucleus of raphe, in which chemoreceptors are thought to be located [24, 25], it is plausible that Lewy pathology in the medulla may be associated with impaired ventilatory response to hypercapnia in DLB.

15.7 Conclusion

Ventilatory response to hypercapnia may be a useful diagnostic method for DLB, although this warrants future multicenter study to confirm its usefulness. It is important to bear in mind that patients with DLB have impaired ventilatory response to hypercapnia, implying that patients with DLB may be susceptible to respiratory compromise and risk of poor outcome due to respiratory complications. The fact that the major cause of death in DLB patients is pneumonia [24] may, in part, be relevant to the impaired respiratory response to hypercapnia.

References

1. Horimoto Y, Matsumoto M, Akatsu H, et al. Autonomic dysfunctions in dementia with Lewy bodies. J Neurol. 2003;250:530–3.

2. Thaisetthawatkul P, Boeve BF, Benarroch EE, et al. Autonomic dysfunction in dementia with Lewy bodies. Neurology. 2004;62:1804–9.
3. Fujishiro H, Iseki E, Nakamura S, et al. Dementia with Lewy bodies: early diagnostic challenges. Psychogeriatrics. 2013;13:128–38.
4. Yoshita M, Taki J, Yokoyama K, et al. Value of 123I-MIBG radioactivity in the differential diagnosis of DLB from AD. Neurology. 2006;66:1850–4.
5. Yoshita M, Arai H, Arai H, et al. Diagnostic accuracy of 123I-meta-iodobenzylguanidine myocardial scintigraphy in dementia with Lewy bodies: a multicenter study. PLoS One. 2015;10(3):e0120540.
6. Allan LM, Ballard CG, Allen J, et al. Autonomic dysfunction in dementia. J Neurol Neurosurg Psychiatry. 2007;78:671–7.
7. Mizukami K, Homma T, Aonuma K, et al. Decreased ventilatory response to hypercapnia in dementia with Lewy bodies. Ann Neurol. 2009;65:614–7.
8. Guarnieri B, Adorni F, Musicco M, et al. Prevalence of sleep disturbances in mild cognitive impairment and dementing disorders: a multicenter Italian clinical cross-sectional study on 431 patients. Dement Geriatr Cogn Disord. 2012;33:50–8.
9. Hibi S, Yamaguchi Y, Umeda-Kameyama Y, et al. Respiratory dysrhythmia in dementia with Lewy bodies: a cross-sectional study. BMJ Open. 2013;3(9):e002870.
10. Sharma G, Goodwin J. Effect of aging on respiratory system physiology and immunology. Clin Interv Aging. 2006;1:253–60.
11. Kronenberg RS, Drage CW. Attenuation of the ventilatory and heart rate responses to hypoxia and hypercapnia with aging in normal men. J Clin Invest. 1973;52:1812–9.
12. Takahashi S, Mizukami K, Yasuno F, et al. Depression associated with dementia with Lewy bodies (DLB) and the effect of somatotherapy. Psychogeriatrics. 2009;9:56–61.
13. Takahashi S, Mizukami K, Arai T, et al. Ventilatory response to hypercapnia predeicts dementia with Lewy bodies in late-onset major depressive disorder. J Alzheimers Dis. 2016;50:751–58.
14. Chokroverty S, Sharp JT, Barron KD. Periodic respiration in erect posture in Shy-Drager syndrome. J Neurol Neurosurg Psychiatry. 1978;41:980–6.
15. Tsuda T, Onodera H, Okabe S, et al. Impaired chemosensitivity to hypoxia is a marker of multiple system atrophy. Ann Neurol. 2002;52:367–71.
16. Onodera H, Okabe S, Kikuchi Y, et al. Impaired chemosensitivity and perception of dyspnoea in Parkinson's disease. Lancet. 2000;356:739–40.
17. Seccombe LM, Giddings HL, Rogers PG, et al. Abnormal ventilatory control in Parkinson's disease--further evidence for non-motor dysfunction. Respir Physiol Neurobiol. 2011;179 (2–3):300–4.
18. Haji A, Takeda R, Okazaki M. Neuropharmacology of control of respiratory rhythm and pattern in mature mammals. Pharmacol Ther. 2000;86:277–304.
19. Boudinot E, Emery MJ, Mouisel E, et al. Increased ventilation and CO_2 chemosensitivity in acetylcholinesterase knockout mice. Respir Physiol Neurobiol. 2004;140:231–41.
20. Mulkey DK, Stornetta RL, Weston MC, et al. Respiratory control by ventral surface chemoreceptor neurons in rats. Nat Neurosci. 2004;7:1360–9.
21. Guyenet PG, Stornetta RL, Bayliss DA. Retrotrapezoid nucleus and central chemoreception. J Physiol. 2008;586:2043–8.
22. Richerson GB. Serotonin neurons as CO_2 sensors that maintain pH homeostasis. Nat Rev Neurosci. 2004;5:449–61.
23. Corcoran AE, Hodges MR, Wu Y, et al. Medullary serotonin neurons and central CO_2 chemoreception. Respir Physiol Neurobiol. 2009;168:49–58.
24. Hishikawa N, Hashizume Y, Yoshida M, et al. Clinical and neuropathological correlates of Lewy body disease. Acta Neuropathol. 2003;105(4):341–50.
25. Benarroch EE, Schmeichel AM, Dugger BN, et al. Dopamine cell loss in the periaqueductal gray in multiple system atrophy and Lewy body dementia. Neurology. 2009;73:106–12.
26. Mizukami K. Dementia with Lewy bodies and depressive state. Seishin Shinkeigaku Zasshi. 2012;114(3):289–96. [Article in Japanese].

Part V
Treatment

Chapter 16
Pharmacotherapy in Dementia with Lewy Bodies

Manabu Ikeda

Abstract Pharmacological management of dementia with Lewy bodies (DLB) remains challenging, because it is complicated by the risk of adverse reactions to medication. Treatments for one aspect of the disease may exacerbate other symptoms. In this chapter, I will introduce the results of pharmacological trials mainly investigating cognitive impairment and neuropsychiatric symptoms for DLB and Parkinson's disease and dementia (PDD), both separately and together. A recent meta-analysis indicated beneficial effects of donepezil and rivastigmine for cognitive and psychiatric symptoms, and these two drugs may be effective for improving cognition and reducing neurobehavioral disturbances over 1 year. Memantine can be used safely in patients with DLB and PDD, but its effects on symptoms may be variable. When using antipsychotics in DLB or PDD, the likely balance of risks vs. benefits requires very careful consideration. Agents that can modify underlying disease processes such as alpha-synuclein accumulation will be promising treatment candidates.

Keywords Dementia with Lewy bodies • Cholinesterase inhibitor • Donepezil • Rivastigmine • Memantine

16.1 Introduction

Dementia with Lewy bodies (DLB) is the second most common type of senile dementia following Alzheimer's disease (AD) [1]. The core clinical features of DLB are fluctuating cognition, visual hallucinations, and motor symptoms of parkinsonism as well as cognitive impairment characterized by deficits in attention, executive function, and visual perception [2]. Other features include neuropsychiatric symptoms such as delusions and depression, autonomic dysfunction, and sleep disorders such as REM sleep behavior disorder. In particular, fluctuating cognition, hallucinations, and delusions are challenging and stressful for both patients and

M. Ikeda, MD, PhD (✉)
Department of Psychiatry, Course of Integrated Medicine, Osaka University Graduate School of Medicine, 2-2, Yamadaoka, Suita-shi, Osaka 565-0871, Japan
e-mail: mikeda@psy.med.osaka-u.ac.jp

K. Kosaka (ed.), *Dementia with Lewy Bodies*, DOI 10.1007/978-4-431-55948-1_16

caregivers. The motor and autonomic features further reduce activities of daily living (ADL) and quality of life [3, 4]. Various therapeutic targets have been addressed pharmacologically. However, pharmacological management of DLB remains challenging, because it is complicated by the risk of adverse reactions to medication. Treatments for one aspect of the disease may exacerbate other symptoms. DLB patients can be exquisitely sensitive to antipsychotic agents for delusions and hallucinations and develop life-threatening sensitivity reactions, whereas antiparkinson medication given to improve motor symptoms can exacerbate neuropsychiatric symptoms. Because of these complex difficulties, very few randomized, placebo-controlled trials (RCTs) that are specific to DLB have been conducted [5], and most prescribing for DLB is "off-license." The distinction between DLB and Parkinson's disease and dementia (PDD) was introduced in the first consensus guidelines for the clinical and pathologic diagnosis of DLB in 1996 [2]. However, the clinical features of DLB and PDD have much in common. A recent Cochrane review considered the use of cholinesterase inhibitors (ChEIs) in both DLB and PDD [6]. In this review, I will introduce the results of pharmacological trials mainly investigating cognitive impairment and neuropsychiatric symptoms for DLB and PDD, both separately and together.

16.2 Previous Studies Using ChEIs in DLB and PDD

DLB is associated with a greater loss of cholinergic neurons in the nucleus basalis of Meynert and lower activity of choline acetyltransferase, the presynaptic synthetic enzyme for acetylcholine, than AD, but more postsynaptic muscarinic receptors in the cortex are preserved [7–9]. Loss of choline acetyltransferase activity is already prominent in the earliest stages of DLB [10]. Cholinergic depletion is not only correlated with cognitive impairment but also psychiatric symptoms such as hallucinations [11, 12]. Based on these pathological features, ChEIs may be effective for treating DLB [12, 13]. Retrospective data analysis of patients enrolled in tacrine trials who have since died and undergone an autopsy suggests that "responders" are more likely to have had DLB than AD [14]. A recent Cochrane review of DLB, PDD, and Parkinson's disease (PD) mild cognitive impairment studies concluded that ChEIs improve cognition, behavior, ADL, and mortality [15].

First, we will review open-label studies and placebo-controlled, double-blind studies using ChEIs in DLB and/or PDD. Second, we will introduce long-term, open-label, extension studies for DLB and PDD in detail.

16.2.1 Case Series and Open-Label Studies

16.2.1.1 Nine patients with DLB were treated with up to 10 mg donepezil daily for 12 weeks [16]. This treatment mostly improved hallucinations and sometimes improved cognition as measured by the Mini-Mental State Examination (MMSE) and overall function. Donepezil treatment was sometimes associated with worse parkinsonism.

16.2.1.2 Four patients with DLB and 12 with AD were treated with up to 5 mg donepezil daily for 24 weeks [17]. The tester was blinded to the disease classification of the patients. AD patients showed only a slight increase in cognitive scores, whereas the mean MMSE scores of DLB patients increased to a significantly greater degree. Across 6 months of treatment with donepezil, the Behavioral Symptoms in Alzheimer's Disease (BEHAVE-AD) scores tended to decline, and the decline was greater for DLB than for AD patients, but the difference did not reach statistical significance.

16.2.1.3 Eleven patients with DLB were treated with rivastigmine up to the maximum tolerated dose (mean 9.6 mg daily, range 3–12 mg) [18] in an open-label study. After 12 weeks of treatment, the mean Neuropsychiatric Inventory (NPI) scores fell by 73 % for delusions, 63 % for apathy, 45 % for agitation, and 27 % for hallucinations. Five of the patients (45 %) experienced very significant clinical improvements that had not been achieved with other treatments, including low-dose neuroleptics. The medication was well tolerated, and parkinsonian symptoms assessed by the unified Parkinson's disease rating scale (UPDRS) tended to improve.

16.2.1.4 A 20-week, open-label study was designed to assess the effects of donepezil treatment, followed by a 6-week withdrawal period and subsequent recommencement [19]. Eight patients with DLB and 11 with PDD were treated with up to 10 mg donepezil daily. The primary outcome measures were the MMSE, the total NPI, and the UPDRS III. Patients with DLB and PDD showed a significant improvement in cognition with treatment, loss of this improvement during withdrawal, and restoration of treatment gains during the 3-month recommencement period. Both groups also demonstrated favorable behavioral changes with treatment, and PDD patients in particular deteriorated significantly after withdrawal. The medication was well tolerated, and parkinsonian features were not significantly altered over the testing sessions.

16.2.1.5 A 24-week, multicenter, open-label study was designed to assess the safety and efficacy of galantamine in patients with DLB, and an interim analysis of the results was performed at 12 weeks [20]. Efficacy analyses were performed on data from 25 patients. Primary outcome measures were the NPI-12, the Cognitive Drug Research Computerized Assessment System (COGDRAS), and the Clinician's Global Impression of Change (CGIC) for global functioning. Marginally significant improvement was observed in scores on the NPI-12. Highly significant improvement was observed in scores on the NPI-4 subscale (delusions, hallucinations, apathy, and depression). Both positive and negative changes from baseline were observed in the attention and visuospatial orientation subsets of COGDRAS testing. Scores on the CGIC improved significantly. Improvements were also found in secondary efficacy variables, including cognitive, functional, ADL, sleep, and confusion assessments. Motor scores, as measured by the UPDRS motor subscale, showed mild improvement, which demonstrates that galantamine has no adverse effect on parkinsonian symptoms.

16.2.1.6 A 12-week, multicenter, open-label study was designed to determine the feasibility of conducting a randomized clinical trial of 5 mg/day donepezil in patients with mild-to-moderate DLB [21]. Twelve patients with probable DLB were evaluated at weeks 4, 8, and 12 using the modified NPI with an extra domain to additionally evaluate fluctuation in cognitive functions (NPI-11), the Japanese version of Alzheimer's Disease Assessment Scale-cognitive subscale (ADAS-J-cog), and the UPDRS. The NPI-11 scores were significantly improved at weeks 8 and 12 compared with baseline. Despite a significant improvement in ADAS-J-cog at week 4, no more improvement was noted thereafter. Deterioration was not noted in UPDRS scores.

16.2.2 Randomized Placebo-Controlled Studies

16.2.2.1 A multinational RCT consisting of 20 weeks of treatment followed by 3 weeks of rest was designed to examine the efficacy, tolerability, and safety of rivastigmine, given twice a daily, at doses up to 12 mg/day in patients with DLB [22]. One hundred twenty patients with DLB were evaluated at baseline and at weeks 12, 20, and 23. Primary outcome measures were NPI-4 and a combined score indicating the speed of response to selected tests from the cognitive drug research computerized cognitive assessment system. Secondary efficacy measures were the clinical global change-plus (CGC-plus), the total score of the NPI-10, and other cognitive tasks. NPI-4 and NPI-10 scores were significantly improved at week 20 compared with baseline. The difference between rivastigmine and placebo for analyses of the last observation was significant at week 20. Twice as many (63 % vs. 30 %) patients on rivastigmine vs. placebo showed at least a 30 % improvement from baseline on the NPI-4 at week 20. For the computerized cognitive assessment system speed score, the difference between rivastigmine and placebo was significant at weeks 12 and 20. No significant difference between rivastigmine and placebo was seen in the mean CGC-plus score and the mean MMSE score. After drug discontinuation, differences between rivastigmine and placebo tended to disappear. Deterioration was not noted in the UPDRS motor subscale for rivastigmine compared with baseline and placebo.

16.2.2.2 We examined the efficacy and safety of donepezil given once daily at 3, 5, or 10 mg for 12 weeks in 140 patients with DLB in a multicenter, exploratory RCT (Fig. 16.1a, b) [23]. An open-label long-term extension study was then conducted in patients who had completed the double-blind study to examine the safety and efficacy of donepezil at 5 mg for 52 weeks [24]. The double-blind study showed that donepezil at 5 and 10 mg/day significantly improved cognitive impairment (MMSE score). The responder rate (MMSE change $\geq$3) was significantly higher in all donepezil groups compared to placebo. Scores for NPI-2 (hallucinations and cognitive fluctuation) and NPI-4 were significantly more improved at the

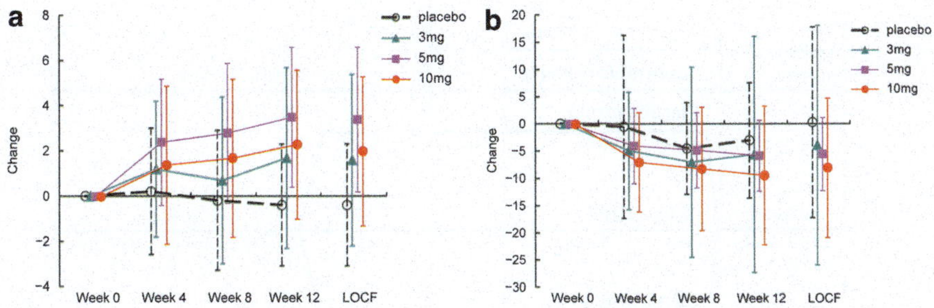

Fig. 16.1 Mean changes from baseline in the (**a**) Mini-Mental State Examination and (**b**) Neuropsychiatric Inventory (NPI-10) in the exploratory RCT of donepezil in DLB [23]

final evaluation (last observation carried forward, LOCF) in the 5-mg (except NPI-4) and 10-mg groups than in the placebo group. The distributions of the Clinician's Interview-Based Impression of Change plus Caregiver Input (CIBIC-plus) at LOCF in all active groups were significantly superior to that of placebo. Significant improvement was found in the Zarit Caregiver Burden Interview (ZBI) at 10 mg/day. Deterioration was not noted in the UPDRS III score in any active groups at the final evaluation.

16.2.2.3 Recently, we conducted a phase 3 study, integrating an RCT [25] and an open-label long-term extension study [26] (Fig. 16.2a, b). Patients with DLB ($n = 142$) were randomly assigned to placebo or 5 mg or 10 mg donepezil that was administered once daily for 12 weeks. Co-primary endpoints were changes in cognitive function assessed using MMSE and behavioral and neuropsychiatric symptoms using the NPI-2. The predefined superiority of donepezil to the placebo was not confirmed in either active group in the primary analysis. MMSE significantly improved compared to placebo in the 10-mg group, whereas the change in MMSE in the 5-mg group was not significant. This result may be due to a relatively higher number of earlier discontinuations. Thirty-one patients discontinued treatment, with more discontinuations in the 5-mg group than in the 10-mg group. In the 5-mg group, eight patients (17.0 %) discontinued by week 4 when the blood concentrations of 5 mg donepezil reached the steady state, whereas only one (3.0 %) had discontinued in the previous study [23]. Although NPI-2 improved compared to baseline in active groups, the differences from placebo were not significant. The placebo group also showed improvement. Evaluation of psychiatric symptoms may be affected by advanced education and instructions for caregivers. Although the incidence of parkinsonism was slightly higher in the 10-mg group, the change in the UPDRS III score was minimal without a significant difference from the placebo group.

16.2.2.4 A double-blind, randomized, placebo-controlled, crossover study was designed to examine the safety and efficacy of donepezil [27]. Fourteen patients with PD and cognitive impairment received donepezil (5 or 10 mg/day) or matching placebo during two sequential periods lasting 10 weeks each. The primary outcome measures were the MMSE score, the CIBIC-plus score, and the motor subscale of

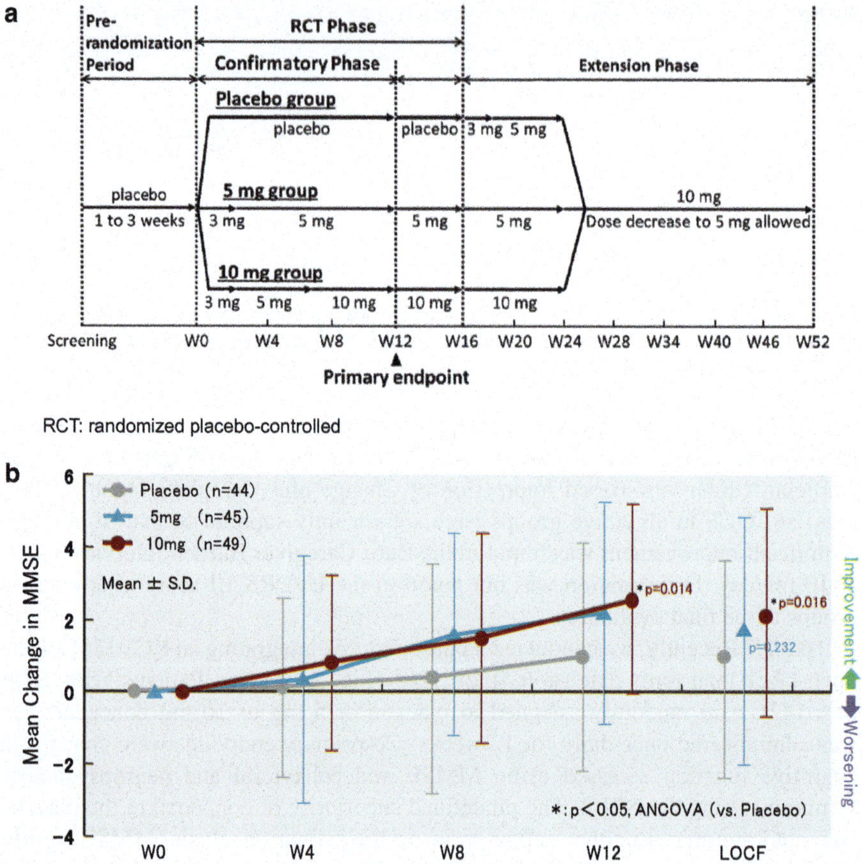

Fig. 16.2 (**a**) Study flow and (**b**) mean changes from baseline in the Mini-Mental State Examination in the phase 3 RCT of donepezil in DLB [25]

the UPDRS. After 10 weeks of treatment, the mean MMSE score was increased by 2.1 (SD 2.7) points on donepezil and 0.3 (SD 3.2) points on placebo, and the CIBIC-plus score was 3.3 (SD 0.9) on donepezil and 4.1 (SD 0.8) on placebo. Statistical analysis of the repeated measurements and crossover study design showed significant effects of donepezil compared with placebo for MMSE ($p = 0.013$) and CIBIC-plus ($p = 0.034$). Parkinsonism did not increase during donepezil treatment.

16.2.2.5 An RCT was designed to examine the safety and efficacy of donepezil [28]. Nine PD patients with dementia or cognitive impairment received placebo, and seven patients received donepezil (2.5–10 mg/day) for a mean (SD) duration of 15.2 (3.4) weeks. The primary outcome measures were derived from a neuropsychological battery that assessed global cognitive status as well as memory, attention, psychomotor speed, and visuospatial and executive functions. The study was completed by 10 out of 16 (62.5 %) subjects. Patients on donepezil showed selective and significant improvement on the memory subscale of the Dementia Rating

Scale (DRS). A trend toward improvement in a measure of psychomotor speed and attention was also observed. No group differences were seen in the MMSE score, DRS total score, psychiatric status, motor function, or ADL as measured at baseline or the end-point.

16.2.2.6 Patients in whom mild-to-moderate dementia developed at least 2 years after they received a clinical diagnosis of PD were randomly assigned to receive placebo or 3–12 mg rivastigmine per day for 24 weeks [29]. A total of 541 patients with PDD were randomly assigned to treatment with rivastigmine or placebo in a ratio of 2:1. The primary outcome measures were the scores for the ADAS-cog and Alzheimer's Disease Cooperative Study-Clinician's Global Impression of Change (ADCS-CGIC). The outcomes were better among patients treated with rivastigmine than among those who received placebo; however, the differences between these two groups were moderate and similar to those reported in trials of rivastigmine for AD. Rivastigmine-treated patients had a mean improvement of 2.1 points in the score on the 70-point ADAS-cog from a baseline score of 23.8, compared with a 0.7-point worsening in the placebo group from a baseline score of 24.3 ($p < 0.001$). Clinically meaningful improvements in the scores for the ADCS-CGIC were observed in 19.8 % of patients in the rivastigmine group and 14.5 % of those in the placebo group, and clinically meaningful worsening was observed in 13.0 % and 23.1 %, respectively (mean scores at 24 weeks, 3.8 and 4.3, respectively; $p = 0.007$). Significantly better outcomes were seen with rivastigmine with respect to all secondary outcome measures such as ADCS-ADL, NPI-10, MMSE, the Clinical Dementia Scale (CDR), power of attention tests, etc. Deterioration was not noted in the UPDRS III score in any active groups at the final evaluation.

16.2.2.7 A double-blind, randomized, placebo-controlled, crossover study was designed to examine the safety and efficacy of donepezil [30]. Twenty-two patients with PDD were randomized to receive either donepezil (5 or 10 mg/day) (during 10 weeks) followed by identical placebo (during 10 weeks) or placebo followed by donepezil, with an open-label washout period of 6 weeks between the two periods. The primary outcome measure was the ADAS-cog. A 1.9-point trend toward better scores on the ADAS-cog on treatment was observed compared with placebo, but the difference was not statistically significant. The secondary cognitive measures showed a statistically significant 2-point benefit on the MMSE and no change on the Mattis Dementia Rating Scale. The CGIC showed a significant 0.37-point improvement with donepezil. No improvement was observed on the Brief Psychiatric Rating Scale (BPRS). No worsening of PD symptoms was observed as measured by the total or motor sections of the UPDRS.

16.2.2.8 A 24-week, multinational RCT was designed to examine the efficacy and safety of donepezil given once daily in patients with PDD [31]. Five hundred fifty patients with PDD were randomized to donepezil (5 or 10 mg) or placebo and were evaluated at baseline and at weeks 12 and 24. Co-outcome measures were the ADAS-cog and the CIBIC-plus. ADAS-cog mean changes from baseline to week 24 (end-point) were not significant for donepezil in the intent-to-treat population by the predefined statistical model. Alternative ADAS-cog analysis in which the treatment-by-country interaction term was removed from the model revealed a significant, dose-dependent benefit with donepezil. The 10-mg group, but not the 5-mg group, had significantly better CIBIC-plus scores compared with placebo. Secondary outcome measures—MMSE, Delis–Kaplan Executive Function System, and Brief Test of Attention that represents cognitive functions particularly relevant to PDD—showed a significant benefit for both donepezil doses. No significant differences in ADL or behavior were observed. Adverse events (AEs) were more common with donepezil but mostly mild/moderate in severity.

16.2.3 Long-Term Safety Studies in DLB

16.2.3.1 Twenty-nine patients with DLB were recruited from a placebo-controlled trial of rivastigmine [22] and treated for up to 96 weeks [32]. All patients were recruited after a 3-week open-label washout phase. Of the 29 patients, nine discontinued treatment during the course of the trial: four discontinued because of side effects, four were nonresponders, and one died from an unrelated cause. Improvement from baseline was seen in cognitive function as measured by the MMSE and neuropsychiatric symptoms as measured by the NPI over the first 24 weeks of treatment. By 96 weeks, neither the MMSE scores nor the NPI scores were significantly worse than at baseline. UPDRS total and subscale scores were not significantly increased from baseline in weeks 36–96, showing no detectable deterioration in parkinsonism over the treatment period.

16.2.3.2 A 52-week, multicenter, open-label extension study was designed to investigate the safety and efficacy of long-term administration of donepezil in patients with DLB (Fig. 16.3) [24]. Up to 8 weeks after the completion of the preceding RCT [23], 108 patients started treatment with 3 mg donepezil daily for 2 weeks, followed by 5 mg daily for the remaining 50 weeks. Ninety patients (83.3 %) completed 24 weeks of treatment, and 81 patients (75 %) completed 52 weeks. The overall discontinuation rate of this study was 25 % ($n = 27$), and 18 patients discontinued treatment due to AEs. Three patients underwent a dose reduction from 5 to 3 mg/day due to occurrence of AEs. Cognitive function, behavioral and psychiatric symptoms, cognitive fluctuations, and caregiver burden were assessed using the MMSE, the NPI, Cognitive Fluctuation Inventory, and the ZBI, respectively. Cognitive function and dementia-related behavioral symptoms including cognitive fluctuations improved after the start of donepezil treatment, and improvement was maintained for 52 weeks, although a relationship between the washout period and attenuation of the treatment effect was suggested. Reduction in caregiver burden that was observed in the preceding RCT returned to the baseline level at 52 weeks. However, of note, burden on caregivers did not increase throughout the cumulative observational period. Delayed AE onset induced by long-term administration of donepezil was unlikely to appear. The long-term study showed that donepezil at 5 mg/day was well tolerated and sustained improvement in cognitive impairment and psychiatric symptoms over 52 weeks, or up to 64 weeks if the preceding treatment period is included.

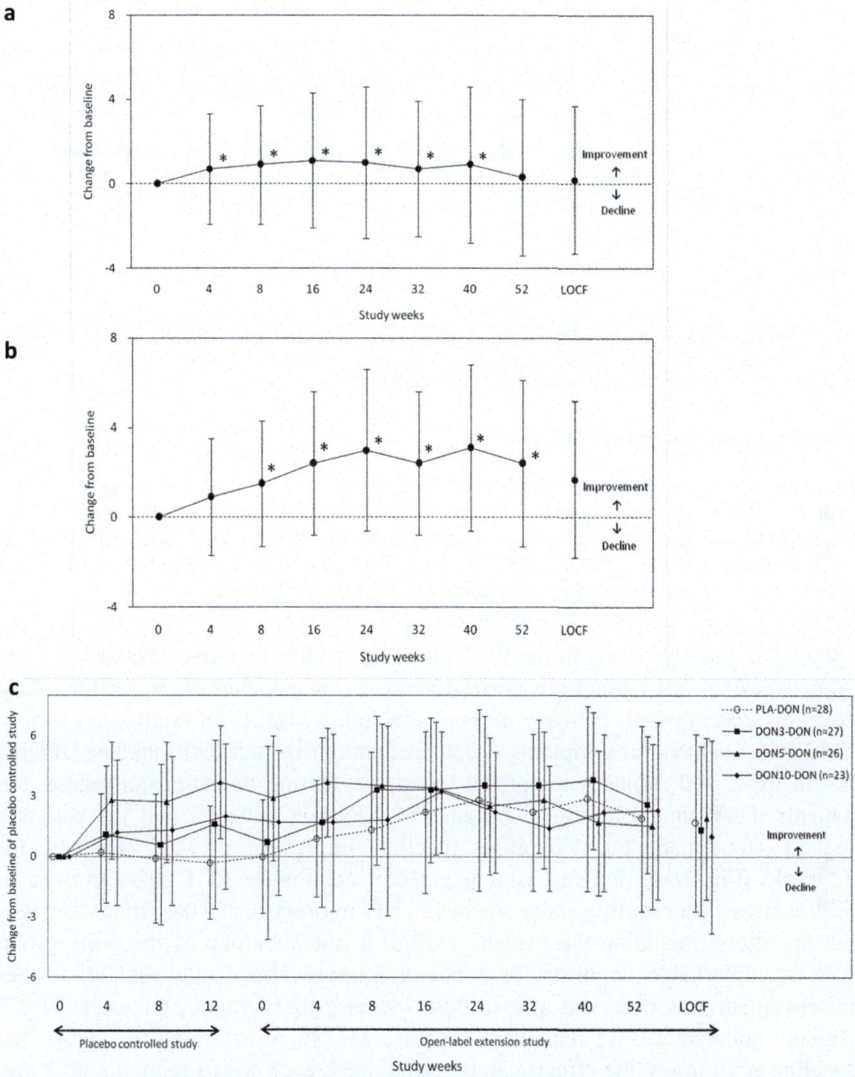

Fig. 16.3 Mean change in MMSE score [24]. (**a**) Overall mean change during the treatment period ($n = 103$). (**b**) Mean change in the placebo group of the preceding RCT ($n = 27$). (**c**) Mean cumulative changes by treatment group in the preceding RCT throughout both the preceding RCT and this extension study. Notes: * indicates $P < 0.05$. P values were calculated compared to baseline using paired t-tests in (**a**) and (**b**). No statistical test was performed in (**c**). Vertical bars indicate standard deviations. *LOCF* last observation carried forward

16.2.3.3 The long-term efficacy and safety of 10 mg donepezil in patients with dementia with DLB were investigated in a 52-week phase 3 trial. This study consisted of a 16-week RCT [25] and a 36-week open-label extension phase [26]. Of 142 DLB patients enrolled in the RCT phase, 110 entered the extension

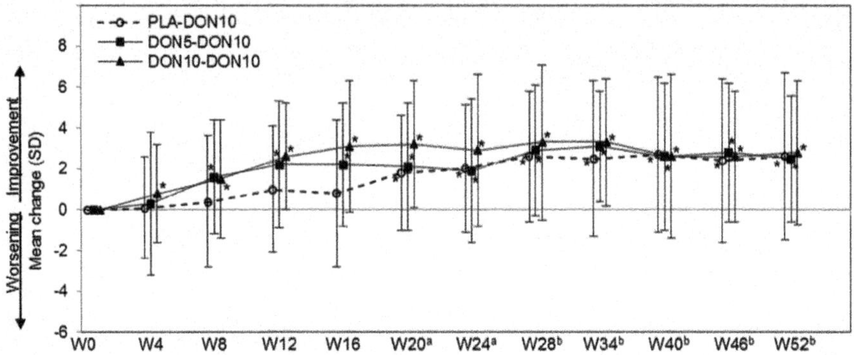

MMSE: mini-mental state examination, FAS: full analysis set

* P <0.05 (paired t-test versus Week 0)

Fig. 16.4 Mean changes in the Mini-Mental State Examination by treatment group throughout both the placebo-controlled phase and open-label extension phase [26]. Placebo → 10 mg (PLA-DON10) started treatment with 3 mg at week 16, and the dose was increased to 5 mg at week 18. Placebo → 10 mg (PLA-DON10) and donepezil 5 mg → 10 mg (DON5-DON10) started treatment with 10 mg at week 24 (dose decreased to 5 mg was allowed)

phase. The placebo group of the RCT phase initiated active treatment at week 16. After week 24, all patients received 10 mg. Dose reduction to 5 mg for safety concerns was allowed. Efficacy measures included MMSE for cognitive function and NPI for behavioral symptoms. Safety evaluations included AEs and the UPDRS III. In total, 100 subjects completed the study. During the extension phase, ten patients discontinued treatment because of AEs (six patients) and the patient's request (four patients). Cognitive function improvement was sustained for 52 weeks (Fig. 16.4). Patients who received placebo in the RCT phase showed an improvement after starting active treatment. NPI improved in all the groups throughout the study, including the placebo period. In the subgroup of the 5-mg group without remarkable cognitive or behavioral improvement at week 24, further improvement was observed after a dose increase to 10 mg. After week 24, 21 patients underwent dose reduction. Because MMSE scores remained above the baseline at all times, the effects can be maintained, even with a reduction to 5 mg. The incidence of any AEs did not increase over time. Thus, the possibility of delayed onset of AEs with long-term treatment seems low. Most of the treatment-related AEs were mild or moderate, and only parkinsonism had an incidence of 5 % or more.

16.2.4 Comments

Case studies and open trials of ChEIs in DLB or PDD have consistently shown improvements in neuropsychiatric symptoms. Donepezil [16, 17 19, 21], rivastigmine [18], and galantamine [20] reduced various psychotic symptoms such as hallucinations, delusions, apathy, etc.

No head-to-head trials have been performed to compare the efficacy of ChEIs in DLB and PDD, but donepezil and rivastigmine have a wide evidence base. As mentioned above, six RCTs for donepezil, two for DLB [23, 25], and four for PDD [27, 28, 30, 31] have been performed, and two RCTs for rivastigmine, one for DLB [22], and one for PDD [29] have also been performed. A recent meta-analysis [33] indicated beneficial effects of donepezil and rivastigmine for cognitive and psychiatric symptoms. Rivastigmine, but not donepezil, was associated with a greater risk of AEs.

Results from our two long-term studies suggest that improvement in cognitive impairment by donepezil at 5 and 10 mg is sustainable for at least 1 year in patients with DLB. In an open-label long-term study of donepezil in patients with mild-to-moderate AD, the improvement in MMSE was maintained until 24 weeks after administration started and then gradually waned and deteriorated [34]. Considering this result in the context of a similar or faster progression in cognitive impairment in DLB than in AD [35, 36], the duration during which the cognitive improvement induced by donepezil persists in patients with DLB may surpass that in patients with AD. Rivastigmine is also effective in improving cognition and reducing neurobehavioral disturbances over 96 weeks [32]. The major limitation of these three long-term studies is their open-label, single-arm design. However, due to the progressive nature of DLB in which mortality is accelerated, allocating patients to a placebo is not appropriate for long periods of time.

Theoretically, ChEIs can exacerbate parkinsonism. However, this was rare and rarely bothersome enough to warrant the discontinuation of medication. Although severe autonomic dysfunctions such as symptomatic bradycardia and QT prolongation were not remarkable, such fragile patients were usually excluded from these trials. We should confirm the AEs induced by ChEIs in DLB or PDD in a real clinical setting.

16.3 Previous Studies Using Memantine in DLB and PDD

Memantine, which is a selective, noncompetitive blocker of NMDA receptors, has been used to treat AD and vascular dementia. The mechanism of action is related to the modulation of glutamatergic transmission, which mediates cortico-cortical and cortico-subcortical interactions in the brain. Changes in markers of glutamatergic activity have been identified in patients with DLB [37]. Evidence for striatal glutamatergic overactivity has been reported in animal models of parkinsonism [38]. Given that Alzheimer-type pathology such as amyloid deposits and neurofibrillary tangles is common in DLB and PDD, the observation that therapy with memantine is effective in these patients is not surprising.

16.3.1 Case Series and Open-Label Studies

16.3.1.1 Three patients with DLB experienced worsening delusions and visual hallucinations as a result of memantine therapy [39]. Significant resolution occurred once treatment was discontinued.

16.3.1.2 To determine the effect of memantine for the treatment of DLB, the authors reviewed the charts of 11 subjects with DLB that were prospectively evaluated and treated with memantine (with or without ChEIs) for varying lengths of time [40]. Nine of eleven DLB subjects on memantine were also on ChEIs. Seven of 11 were stable or improved with memantine, and the remaining four worsened or responded adversely when exposed to the drug. AEs included increased hallucinations and sedation. No adverse effects on motor function were observed.

16.3.1.3 An open, controlled, 16-week study was performed to evaluate the efficacy and safety of memantine in patients with DLB or PDD [41]. The study included 23 patients who were divided into two groups: 14 patients received memantine at a dose of 20 mg/day, and nine patients constituted the control group. Patients did not receive ChEIs for at least 2 months prior to inclusion in the study. Efficacy was evaluated using a battery of quantitative neuropsychological tests (MMSE, Mattis Dementia Scale, clock-drawing test), clinical scales for assessment of fluctuations in mental states (the clinician assessment of fluctuation (CAF) scale, the one-day fluctuation assessment scale (ODFAS)), scales for assessment of behavioral and psychotic disorders, and the general clinical impression scale. Motor impairments were evaluated using UPDRS III. The results demonstrated that memantine had positive effects on the patients' general status and cognitive functions (increases on the MMSE by 1.5 points), mainly because of improvements in attention and control functions. Reductions in the severity of fluctuations in mental state, aggressiveness, lack of spontaneity, and disinhibition were also observed. The severity of psychotic and motor disorders did not change significantly. Tolerance of memantine was good, and only two patients withdrew from the study because of episodes of confusion during the dose titration period.

16.3.2 Randomized Placebo-Controlled Studies

16.3.2.1 A 22-week RCT was designed to examine the safety and tolerability of memantine (20 mg/day), in 25 patients suffering from PDD [42]. Global, cognitive, and behavioral outcome measures were administered at baseline, at end of study drug treatment (week 16), and at drug termination (week 22). The primary outcome measure was global cognitive impairment with emphasis on subcortical functions as assessed by the DRS. Secondary outcome measures were the NPI, MMSE, and CIBIC-Plus to assess global change by an independent assessor. Memantine was well tolerated by participants at 20 mg/day dosing. No participant withdrew due to memantine-related AEs. Statistically significant differences between groups on the

DRS total and the NPI total as well as the MMSE were not observed. At week 16, a trend toward improvement in global functioning in mean CIBIC-Plus scores in the memantine (60 %) versus the placebo group (43 %) was observed. Six weeks after drug withdrawal, a significantly greater proportion (70 %) of memantine-treated participants deteriorated globally compared with those treated with placebo (29 %). These findings suggest that continued treatment with memantine may be needed to maintain a global level of functioning over time. No worsening of motor symptoms as measured by the motor sections of the UPDRS III was seen.

16.3.2.2 A 24-week, multinational RCT was designed to examine the efficacy and safety of memantine (20 mg/day) in patients with PDD or DLB [43]. Stable treatment with ChEIs was allowed before (at least 6 months before enrollment) and during the trial. The primary outcome measure was CGIC, which ranged from 1 to 7 points; a low score indicates a better outcome. Analysis was performed by intention to treat based on the LOCF. Seventy-two patients with PDD or DLB were randomly assigned and started treatment: 34 with memantine and 38 with placebo; 56 (78 %) completed the study. All withdrawals were due to AEs, but the proportion of withdrawals was similar in both groups. At week 24, the patients in the memantine group had better CGIC scores than those taking placebo. No differences were observed in the mean CGIC LOCF between the memantine- and placebo-treated patients with DLB. The mean score in the PDD group was 4.3 in the placebo group and 2.9 in the memantine group, suggesting a more pronounced global response in patients with PDD. With the exception of improved speed on attentional tasks in the memantine group, no significant differences were found between the groups in secondary outcome measures. Patients with DLB or PDD may benefit from treatment with memantine, which was well tolerated.

16.3.2.3 A 24-week, multinational RCT was designed to examine the efficacy and safety of memantine (20 mg/day) in patients with mild-to-moderate PDD or DLB [44]. Patients were randomly assigned to placebo or memantine (20 mg per day) and did not receive ChEIs for at least 6 weeks prior to enrolling in the study. No primary outcome measure was defined. Safety analyses were done for all patients who took at least one dose of memantine or placebo, and efficacy analyses were done for all patients who had at least one valid post-baseline assessment. Of the 199 patients randomly assigned to treatment, 34 with DLB and 62 with PDD were given memantine, and 41 with DLB and 58 with PDD were given placebo; 159 (80 %) patients completed the study: 80 in the memantine group and 79 in the placebo group. At week 24, patients with DLB who received memantine showed greater improvement according to ADCS-CGIC scores compared to those who received placebo. No significant differences were noted between the two treatments in patients with PDD or in the total population. NPI scores showed significantly greater improvement in the memantine group than in the placebo group in patients with DLB, but not in those with PDD or in the total patient population. No significant differences were found between the two treatment groups in any of the study populations in most of the cognitive test scores, ADCS-ADL scores, and the ZBI scores. The incidence of AEs and number of discontinuations due to AEs were similar in the two groups. Memantine seems to improve global clinical status and behavioral symptoms of patients with mild-to-moderate DLB.

16.3.3 Long-Term Safety Studies

A 30-week extension trial [45] was performed that was a continuation of the RCT to study memantine in DLB and PDD [43]. The objective was to evaluate the presence of recurrence of symptoms upon drug withdrawal. Furthermore, another aim was to explore washout dynamics to inform clinical practice. The trial comprised a 4-week washout period and a 26-week open-label treatment period. Outcome measures were the presence of recurrence of symptoms upon drug withdrawal, CGIC, and modified motor UPDRS. Recurrence of symptoms occurred more frequently ($p = 0.04$) in patients receiving memantine (58 %) than in patients receiving placebo (25 %). A significant global deterioration ($p = 0.0003$) was observed during washout within the memantine group as measured by CGIC. The patients seemed to recover during the open-label treatment, but these findings were not significant.

16.3.4 Comments

Data from case series and open trials of memantine in DLB and PDD are contradictory [39–41]. Among the subjects in the same trial, some improved and others worsened or responded adversely [40]. Results from three RCTs have also been contradictory. Relatively small RCTs of memantine in PDD showed no efficacy in the primary outcome measure (DRS for global cognitive impairment) [42]. In large RCT for DLB or PDD, patients in the active group had better CGIC (primary outcome measure) scores than those taking placebo [43]. In the largest RCT in patients with DLB or PDD, ADCS-CGIC and NPI scores showed significantly greater improvement in the memantine group than in the placebo group in patients with DLB, but not in those with PDD or in the total patient population [44]. A long-term extension study showed that any possible memantine-associated benefits may be rapidly lost after drug withdrawal [45]. The incidence of AEs and the number of discontinuations due to AEs were similar in the active group and the placebo group among these RCTs. Memantine can be used safely in patients with DLB and PDD, but its effects on symptoms may be variable.

16.4 Previous Studies Using Antipsychotics in DLB and PDD

Psychotic symptoms in DLB or PDD patients are particularly difficult to treat due to the extreme sensitivity of these patients to anticholinergic and antidopaminergic medications [46]. These patients are particularly sensitive to developing extrapyramidal symptoms (EPS) and also to the potentially fatal complication of neuroleptic sensitivity, which affects ~50 % of DLB patients [47]. Furthermore, meta-analyses of pooled data from RCTs indicate that the use of antipsychotics in older individuals with dementia is associated with an increased risk of cardiovascular disease and mortality [48]. Therefore, a need exists for antipsychotic drugs with less propensity to induce EPS and reduced affinity for dopamine and acetylcholine receptors [46]. Although clozapine is useful in treating PD psychosis [49], very few studies have been conducted in patients with DLB or PDD. Two patients with DLB were intolerant of clozapine, showing no extrapyramidal side effects, but an increase in confusion and behavioral symptoms [50]. Olanzapine appears to be poorly tolerated in a considerable number of patients, even at low dosages (2.5 mg/day) [51], although low-dose olanzapine (5 mg/day) may reduce psychosis in patients with DLB without worsening parkinsonism [52]. Worsening of motor function and psychiatric symptoms was reported in 80 % of individuals with PDD, even those given low-dose olanzapine [53]. Risperidone has been associated with a high risk of neuroleptic malignant syndrome [47, 54, 55]. An RCT showed a higher withdrawal rate (65 %) and worsening psychiatric symptoms on the NPI and global impression on CGIC [56]. Despite an attractive in vitro profile (a partial dopamine agonist), aripiprazole can induce serious extrapyramidal side effects such as parkinsonism and tardive dyskinesia [57]. Quetiapine reduces psychiatric manifestations of DLB without causing neuroleptic sensitivity or increasing EPS [58–60]. An RCT of quetiapine in DLB ($n = 23$), PDD ($n = 9$), and AD with parkinsonian features ($n = 8$) showed good tolerance and no worsening parkinsonism, although no significant differences in the primary outcome measure of efficacy (BPRS) was observed [61]. Hence, quetiapine may be an attractive candidate for the treatment of psychoses in DLB at this point. The use of antipsychotics in DLB or PDD requires very careful consideration of the likely balance of risks vs. benefits [62].

16.5 Conclusion

The interplay among cognitive, psychiatric, motor, and autonomic symptoms of DLB makes the management of these symptoms complex and challenging. In particular, the pharmacological management of DLB is usually polypharmacy due to multiple pharmacological treatment targets and is complicated by the risk of adverse reactions to medication [63]. Improved treatment for target symptoms may be associated with worsening of symptoms in other domains. No treatments are currently licensed for DLB except donepezil for DLB in Japan or for PDD except rivastigmine in several countries including the USA.

As described above, high-level evidence is still rare in the pharmacological intervention for DLB and PDD. Compared with AD, it is difficult to enroll a large number of patients into clinical trials, especially RCTs, for DLB owing to its faster progression, wide variety of symptoms including severe BPSD, greater caregiver burden, and easily induced severe adverse events. In the previous two RCTs of donepezil, the number of patients enrolled by each center was generally small (none by 5 and only 1 patient by 14 out of 48 centers at phase 2 and none by 14 and only 1 by 15 out of 72 centers at phase 3) [23, 25]. Similar recruitment difficulties impeded an RCT of rivastigmine for DLB [22]. It might be inevitable that patients are recruited from various specialty departments, such as neurology, psychiatry, geriatrics, and so on, of multinational centers for future RCTs in DLB and that those studies take a long time for enrollment. Therefore, it is very important to confirm the adequacy of using the consensus criteria in those studies by comparing patient characteristics among trials conducted at different times and subjects enrolled from different types of specialty centers [64].

A very recent meta-analysis indicated improvements with donepezil and rivastigmine for cognition, psychotic symptoms, and ADL (without worsening motor symptoms or parkinsonism) but with AEs in DLB and PDD [33]. Moreover, based on the analysis of pooled datasets from phase 2 and 3 trials, we conclude that DLB can be treated effectively and safely without relevant worsening of EPS, but careful attention must be paid to symptom progression when drugs are administered to patients with relatively severe parkinsonism [65]. Memantine seems to be relatively well tolerated in DLB and PDD, but the efficacy is controversial. Moreover, the results may be driven by data from PDD rather than DLB subjects and may only be present with concurrent ChEI treatment [63, 66]. Treatments for parkinsonism, depression, and autonomic dysfunctions in DLB and PDD have been omitted for lack of space. Please refer to recent comprehensive review articles [33, 63]. No disease-modifying therapies exist, although ChEIs offer the greatest hope for symptomatic improvement without significant compromise of motor function. Agents that can modify underlying disease processes such as alpha-synuclein accumulation will be promising treatment candidates.

References

1. McKeith I, Mintzer J, Aarsland D, et al. International Psychogeriatric Association Expert Meeting on DLB: dementia with Lewy bodies. Lancet Neurol. 2004;3:19–28.
2. McKeith IG, Galasko D, Kosaka K, et al. Consensus guidelines for the clinical and pathologic diagnosis of dementia with Lewy bodies (DLB): report of the consortium on DLB international workshop. Neurology. 1996;47:1113–24.
3. Allan L, McKeith I, Ballard C, et al. The prevalence of autonomic symptoms in dementia and their association with physical activity, activities of daily living and quality of life. Dement Geriatr Cogn Disord. 2006;22:230–7.
4. McKeith IG, Rowan E, Askew K, et al. More severe functional impairment in dementia with lewy bodies than Alzheimer disease is related to extrapyramidal motor dysfunction. Am J Geriatr Psychiatry. 2006;14:582–8.
5. Boot BP, McDade EM, McGinnis SM, et al. Treatment of dementia with Lewy bodies. Curr Treat Options Neurol. 2013;15:738–64.
6. Rolinski M, Fox C, Maidment I, et al. Cholinesterase inhibitors for dementia with Lewy bodies, Parkinson's disease dementia and cognitive impairment in Parkinson's disease. Cochrane Database Syst Rev. 2012. CD006504.
7. Lippa CF, Smith TW, Perry E. Dementia with Lewy bodies: choline acetyltransferase parallels nucleus basalis pathology. J Neural Transm. 1999;106:525–35.

8. Perry EK, Haroutunian V, Davis KL, et al. Neocortical cholinergic activities differentiate Lewy body dementia from classical Alzheimer's disease. Neuroreport. 1994;5:747–9.
9. Perry EK, Irving D, Kerwin JM, et al. Cholinergic transmitter and neurotrophic activities in Lewy body dementia: similarity to Parkinson's and distinction from Alzheimer disease. Alzheimer Dis Assoc Disord. 1993;7:69–79.
10. Tiraboschi P, Hansen LA, Alford M, et al. Early and widespread cholinergic losses differentiate dementia with Lewy bodies from Alzheimer disease. Arch Gen Psychiatry. 2002;59:946–51.
11. Ballard C, Piggott M, Johnson M, et al. Delusions associated with elevated muscarinic binding in dementia with Lewy bodies. Ann Neurol. 2000;48:868–76.
12. McKeith IG, Dickson DW, Lowe J, et al. Diagnosis and management of dementia with Lewy bodies: third report of the DLB Consortium. Neurology. 2005;65:1863–72.
13. O'Brien JT, Burns A, BAP Dementia Consensus Group. Clinical practice with anti-dementia drugs: a revised (second) consensus statement from the British Association for Psychopharmacology. J Psychopharmacol. 2011;25:997–1019.
14. Levy R, Eagger S, Griffiths M, et al. Lewy bodies and response to tacrine in Alzheimer's disease. Lancet. 1994;15;343(8890):176.
15. Rolinski M, Fox C, Maidment I, et al. Cholinesterase inhibitors for dementia with Lewy bodies, Parkinson's disease dementia and cognitive impairment in Parkinson's disease (review). Cochrane Database Syst Rev. 2012;3:CD0066504.
16. Shea C, MacKnight C, Rockwood K. Donepezil for treatment of dementia with Lewy bodies: a case series of nine patients. Int Psychogeriatr. 1998;10:229–38.
17. Samuel W, Caligiuri M, Galasko D, et al. Better cognitive and psychopathologic response to donepezil in patients prospectively diagnosed as dementia with Lewy bodies: a preliminary study. Int J Geriatr Psychiatry. 2000;15:794–902.
18. McKeith IG, Grace JB, Walker Z, et al. Rivastigmine in the treatment of dementia with Lewy bodies: preliminary findings from an open trial. Int J Geriatr Psychiatry. 2000;15:387–92.
19. Minett TS, Thomas A, Wilkinson LM, et al. What happens when donepezil is suddenly withdrawn? An open label trial in dementia with Lewy bodies and Parkinson's disease with dementia. Int J Geriatr Psychiatry. 2003;18:988–93.
20. Edwards KR, Hershey L, Wray L, et al. Efficacy and safety of galantamine in patients with dementia with Lewy bodies: a 12-week interim analysis. Dement Geriatr Cogn Disord. 2004;17 Suppl 1:40–8.
21. Mori S, Mori E, Iseki E, et al. Efficacy and safety of donepezil in patients with dementia with Lewy bodies: preliminary findings from an open-label study. Psychiatry Clin Neurosci. 2006;60:190–5.
22. McKeith I, Del Ser T, Spano P, et al. Efficacy of rivastigmine in dementia with Lewy bodies: a randomised, double-blind, placebo-controlled international study. Lancet. 2000;356:2031–6.
23. Mori E, Ikeda M, Kosaka K, et al. Donepezil for dementia with Lewy bodies: a randomized, placebo-controlled trial. Ann Neurol. 2012;72:41–52.
24. Ikeda M, Mori E, Kosaka K, Donepezil-DLB Study Investigators, et al. Long-term safety and efficacy of donepezil in patients with dementia with Lewy bodies: results from a 52-week, open-label, multicenter extension study. Dement Geriatr Cogn Disord. 2013;36:229–41.
25. Ikeda M, Mori E, Matsuo K, et al. Donepezil for dementia with Lewy bodies: a randomized placebo-controlled, confirmatory phase III trial. Alzheimers Res Ther. 2015. doi:10.1186/s13195-014-0083-0.
26. Mori E, Ikeda M, Nagai R, et al. Long-term donepezil use for dementia with Lewy bodies: results from an open-label extension of phase III trial. Alzheimers Res Ther. 2015. doi:10.1186/s13195-014-0081-2.
27. Aarsland D, Laake K, Larsen JP, et al. Donepezil for cognitive impairment in Parkinson's disease: a randomised controlled study. J Neurol Neurosurg Psychiatry. 2002;72:708–12.
28. Leroi I, Brandt J, Reich SG, et al. Randomized placebo-controlled trial of donepezil in cognitive impairment in Parkinson's disease. Int J Geriatr Psychiatry. 2004;19:1–8.

29. Emre M, Aarsland D, Albanese A, et al. Rivastigmine for dementia associated with Parkinson's disease. N Engl J Med. 2004;351:2509–18.
30. Ravina B, Putt M, Siderowf A, et al. Donepezil for dementia in Parkinson's disease: a randomised, double blind, placebo controlled, crossover study. J Neurol Neurosurg Psychiatry. 2005;76:934–9.
31. Dubois B, Tolosa E, Katzenschlager R, et al. Donepezil in Parkinson's disease dementia: a randomized, double-blind efficacy and safety study. Mov Disord. 2012;27:1230–8.
32. Grace J, Daniel S, Stevens T, et al. Long-term use of rivastigmine in patients with dementia with Lewy bodies: an open-label trial. Int Psychogeriatr. 2001;13:199–205.
33. Stinton C, McKeith I, Taylor JP, et al. Pharmacological management of Lewy body dementia: a systematic review and meta-analysis. Am J Psychiatry. 2015;172:731–42.
34. Tohgi H, Homma A, Imai Y, et al. Long-term safety and efficacy of acetylcholinesterase inhibitor E2020 in patients with Alzheimer-type dementia: 52-week open label study. Clin Eval. 2000;28:97–126.
35. Ballard C, O'Brien J, Morris CM, et al. The progression of cognitive impairment in dementia with Lewy bodies, vascular dementia and Alzheimer's disease. Int J Geriatr Psychiatry. 2001;16:499–503.
36. Olichney JM, Galasko D, Salmon DP, et al. Cognitive decline is faster in Lewy body variant than in Alzheimer's disease. Neurology. 1998;51:351–7.
37. Dalfó E, Albasanz JL, Martín M, et al. Abnormal metabotropic glutamate receptor expression and signaling in the cerebral cortex in diffuse lewy body disease is associated with irregular α-synuclein/phospholipase C ($PLC\beta_1$) interactions. Brain Pathol. 2004;14:388–9.
38. Starr MS. Glutamate/dopamine D1/D2 balance in the basal ganglia and its relevance to Parkinson's disease. Synapse. 1995;19:264–93.
39. Ridha BH, Josephs KA, Rossor NM. Delusions and hallucinations in dementia with Lewy bodies: worsening with memantine. Neurology. 2005;65:481–2.
40. Sabbagh MN, Hake AM, Ahmed S, et al. The use of memantine in dementia with Lewy bodies. J Alzheimers Dis. 2005;7:285–9.
41. Levin OS, Batukaeva LA, Smolentseva IG, et al. Efficacy and safety of memantine in Lewy body dementia. Neurosci Behav Physiol. 2009;39:597–604.
42. Leroi I, Overshott R, Byrne EJ, et al. Randomized controlled trial of memantine in dementia associated with Parkinson's disease. Mov Disord. 2009;24:1217–21.
43. Aarsland D, Ballard C, Walker Z, et al. Memantine in patients with Parkinson's disease dementia or dementia with Lewy bodies: a double-blind, placebo-controlled, multicentre trial. Lancet Neurol. 2009;8:613–18.
44. Emre M, Tsolaki M, Bonuccelli U, 11018 Study Investigators, et al. Memantine for patients with Parkinson's disease dementia or dementia with Lewy bodies: a randomised, double-blind, placebo-controlled trial. Lancet Neurol. 2010;9:969–77.
45. Johansson C, Ballard C, Hansson O, et al. Efficacy of memantine in PDD and DLB: an extension study including washout and open-label treatment. Int J Geriatr Psychiatry. 2011;26:206–13.
46. Baskys A. Lewy body dementia: the litmus test for neuroleptic sensitivity and extrapyramidal symptoms. J Clin Psychiatry. 2004;65 Suppl 11:16–22.
47. Ballard C, Grace J, McKeith I, et al. Neuroleptic sensitivity in dementia with Lewy bodies and Alzheimer's disease [letter]. Lancet. 1998;351:1032–3.
48. Schneider LS, Dagerman KS, Insel P. Risk of death with atypical antipsychotic drug treatment for dementia: meta-analysis of randomized placebo-controlled trials. JAMA. 2005;294:1934–43.
49. Olanow CW, Watts RL, Koller WC. An algorithm (decision tree) for the management of Parkinson's disease (2001): treatment guidelines. Neurology. 2001;56(11 Suppl 5):S1–S88.
50. Burke WJ, Pfeiffer RF, McComb RD. Neuroleptic sensitivity to clozapine in dementia with Lewy bodies. J Neuropsychiatry Clin Neurosci. 1998;10:227–9.

51. Walker Z, Grace J, Overshot R, et al. Olanzapine in dementia with Lewy bodies: a clinical study. Int J Geriatr Psychiatry. 1999;14:459–66.
52. Cummings JL, Street J, Masterman D, et al. Efficacy of olanzapine in the treatment of psychosis in dementia with Lewy bodies. Dement Geriatr Cogn Disord. 2002;13:67–73.
53. Marsh L, Lyketsos C, Reich SG. Olanzapine for the treatment of psychosis in patients with Parkinson's disease and dementia. Psychosomatics. 2001;42:477–81.
54. Sechi G, Agnetti V, Masuri R, et al. Risperidone, neuroleptic malignant syndrome and probable dementia with Lewy bodies. Prog Neuropsychopharmacol Biol Psychiatry. 2000;24:1043–51.
55. Morikawa M, Kishimoto T. Probable dementia with Lewy bodies and risperidone-induced delirium [letter]. Can J Psychiatry. 2002;47:976.
56. Culo S, Mulsant BH, Rosen J, et al. Treating neuropsychiatric symptoms in dementia with Lewy bodies: a randomized controlled-trial. Alzheimer Dis Assoc Disord. 2010;24:360–4.
57. Boylan LS, Hirsch S. Motor worsening and tardive dyskinesia with aripiprazole in Lewy body dementia. BMJ Case Rep. 2009;2009. pii: bcr06.2008.0205. doi:10.1136/bcr.06.2008.0205.
58. Takahashi H, Yoshida K, Sugita T, et al. Quetiapine treatment of psychotic symptoms and aggressive behavior in patients with dementia with Lewy bodies: a case series. Prog Neuropsychopharmacol Biol Psychiatry. 2003;27:549–53.
59. Fernandez HH, Trieschmann ME, Burke MA, et al. Quetiapine for psychosis in Parkinson's disease versus dementia with Lewy bodies. J Clin Psychiatry. 2002;63:513–15.
60. Davis P, Baskys A. Quetiapine effectively reduces psychotic symptoms in patients with Lewy Body dementia: an advantage of the unique pharmacological profile? Brain Aging. 2002;2:49–53.
61. Kurlan R, Cummings J, Raman R, et al. Quetiapine for agitation or psychosis in patients with dementia and parkinsonism. Neurology. 2007;68:1356–63.
62. Barber R, Boddy B. Lewy body disease. In: Ritchie CW, Ames D, Masters CL, Cummings J, editors. Therapeutic strategies in dementia. Oxford: Clinical Publishing; 2007. p. 301–17.
63. Boot MP. Comprehensive treatment of dementia with Lewy bodies. Alzheimers Res Ther. 2015. doi:10.1186/s13195-015-0128-z.
64. Ikeda M, Mori E, Iseki E, et al. Adequacy of using consensus guidelines for diagnosis of dementia with Lewy bodies in clinical trials for drug development. Dement Geriatr Cogn Disord. 2016;41:55–67.
65. Mori E, Ikeda M, Nakagawa M, et al. Effects of donepezil on extrapyramidal symptoms in patients with dementia with Lewy bodies: a secondary pooled analysis of two randomized-controlled and two open-label long-term extension studies. Dement Geriatr Cogn Disord. 2015;40:186–98.
66. Aarsland D, Ballard C, Rongve A, et al. Clinical trials of dementia with Lewy bodies and Parkinson's disease dementia. Curr Neurol Neurosci Rep. 2012;12:492–501.

Chapter 17
Traditional Chinese Medicine for Treatment of Dementia

Koh Iwasaki and Shin Takayama

Abstract Dementia has been considered as a disease since the seventeenth century in traditional Asian medicine. In the nineteenth century, Wan Qingren described about dementia in a scientific manner at first time in the world. Recently, a traditional herbal medicine yokukansan (YKS) is paid attention to ameliorate behavioral and psychological symptoms of dementia (BPSD) without deterioration of extrapyramidal symptoms. YKS improves BPSD and ADL of demented people. Also, it ameliorates hallucination of dementia with Lewy bodies (DLB). Pharmacological mechanism of YKS is mainly owing to *Uncaria* and contained alkaloids related to serotonergic and glutamatergic functions.

Keywords DLB • BPSD • Traditional Asian medicine • Yokukansan

17.1 Dementia in Traditional Chinese Medicine

Dementia with Lewy bodies (DLB) is the second most common cause of dementia. In Japan, a clinical trial to treat DLB using traditional Asian medicine was recently started.

In China and Japan, the historical term for dementia was 痴呆 (chiho in Japanese, Chidai in Chinese). The term Chidai was originally proposed by the traditional Chinese doctor Zhang Jingyue (張景岳) in his famous text entitled *Jingyue guanshu* (景岳全書) in 1624. Zhang Jingyue argued that the man became Chidai when he exhibited severe mental stress, despair, lost ambition, and being overly worrisome or fearful. Patients with Chidai lose adequate cognition or discernment and exhibit meaningless speech, abnormal behavior, and autonomic

K. Iwasaki (✉)
Ishinomaki-Ogatsu Municipal Clinic, 9-16 Kotakihama-Ohama, Ogatsu Ward, Ishinomaki City, Miyagi, Japan

Tohoku University, Sendai, Japan
e-mail: iwasaki.koh67@gmail.com

S. Takayama
Department of Kampo Medicine, Tohoku University Hospital, 1-1 Seiryo-Machi, Aoba Ward, Sendai City, Miyagi 980-8574, Japan

K. Kosaka (ed.), *Dementia with Lewy Bodies*, DOI 10.1007/978-4-431-55948-1_17

nervous system dysfunction. Despite this loss in cognitive function, the body condition remains otherwise healthy. Zhang Jingyue considered dementia as an acquired disease.

In the nineteenth century, Wan Qingren (王清任) expanded this idea in his text entitled *Yilingaicuo* (医林改錯) in 1830. He stated that memory disturbance in children resulted from poor brain development; however, poor memory in the elderly resulted from brain atrophy. According to the text, the brain function in Chidai people weakens, and the brain atrophies and collapses, ultimately, resulting in death. Wan Qingren published these observations approximately 70 years before Alois Alzheimer reported his first case in Europe. Wan Qingnin was the first in the world to describe dementia in a scientific manner.

17.2 Yokukansan, a Traditional Asian Herbal Medicine

17.2.1 Characteristics

抑肝散, known as yokukansan (YKS) in Japanese and Yi-Gan San in Chinese, is a traditional Asian herbal medicine [1]. It was originally described in the 保嬰撮要 [2] (Bâo yïng cuö yào, *Synopsis for Protecting the Infant*), which was authored by 薛鎧 (Xue Kai) and 薛己 (Xue Ji, a son of Xue Kai) during the Ming dynasty in China in 1555 or 1556 as a remedy for restlessness and agitation in children [3]. YKS comprises a mixture of dried herbs as follows: 4 g of *Atractylodes lanceae rhizoma* (蒼朮), 4 g of *Poria* (茯苓), 3 g of *Cnidii rhizoma* (川芎), 3 g of *Angelicae radix* (当帰), 2 g of *Bupleuri radix* (柴胡), 1.5 g of *Glycyrrhizae radix* (甘草), and 3 g of *Uncariae uncus cum ramulus* (釣藤鈎) [4]. These herbs are registered in the Pharmacopoeia of Japan ver. 15. Patients consume 2.5 g of YKS powder (1.08 g of the extract) three times daily. YKS has been approved by the Japanese Ministry of Health, Labour and Welfare, and prescriptions are covered by the National Health Insurance plan.

17.2.2 Clinical Evidence

In 2005, we reported that YKS improved behavioral and psychological symptoms of dementia (BPSD), such as hallucination, delusion, agitation, and aggression [4] (Figs. 17.1 and 17.2). More than 130 studies have since reported the effects and mechanisms of YKS on psychosomatic and neurological symptoms (searched on PubMed on 8 March 2015). In 2009, Mizukami et al. published an expansive crossover trial investigating the effects of YKS on BPSD [5]. A meta-analysis has also been performed examining the effect of YKS on BPSD [6].

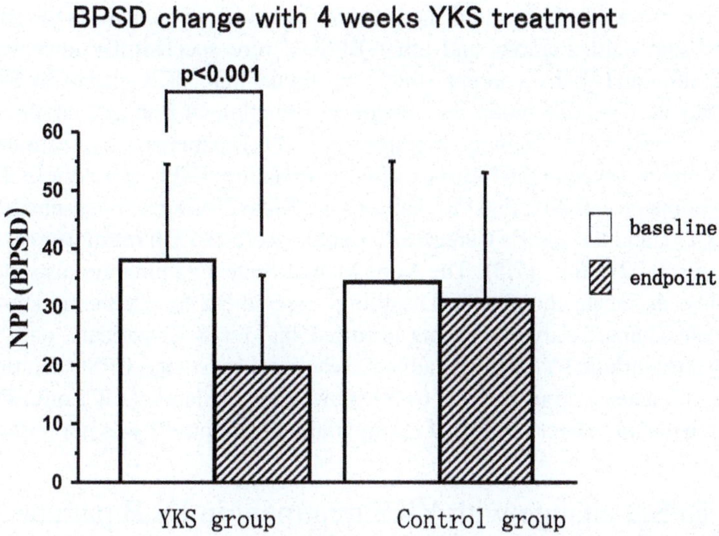

Fig. 17.1 Change in NPI score. NPI significantly improved in the YGS group ($n = 27$, from 37.9 ± 16.1 to 19.5 ± 15.6, mean $\pm$ SD; $p < 0.001$) but did not change significantly in the control group ($n = 25$). In the NPI subscales, significant improvements were shown in hallucinations, agitation/aggression, irritability/lability, and aberrant motor activity. No treatment-emergent adverse event was seen in either group during the observation period

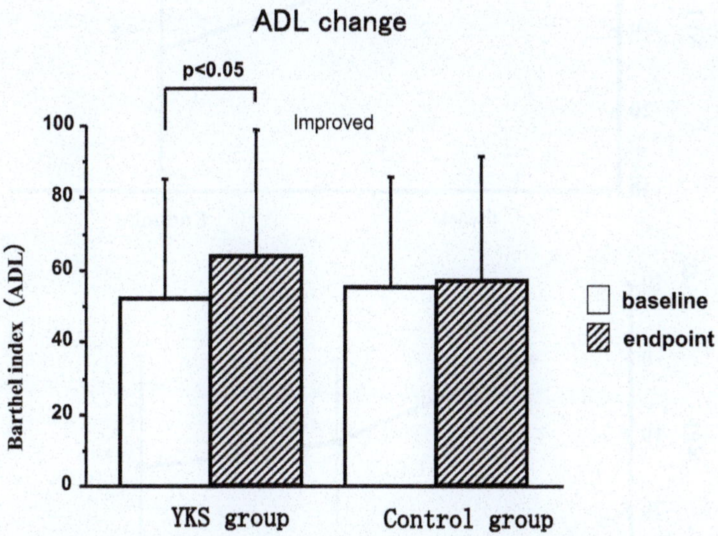

Fig. 17.2 Barthel index. Barthel index scores significantly improved in the YGS group (from 56.4 ± 34.2 to 62.9 ± 35.2; $p < 0.05$) but did not change significantly in the control group

On the other hand, we published a case series of 15 patients with DLB and reported that hallucinations and other BPSDs were successfully improved with YKS treatment [7]. In a larger study, we found that YKS improved BPSD in DLB patients without worsening cognitive function and improved the burden score in caregivers [8]. Namely, in a study of 63 DLB patients, significant improvements were observed in the Neuropsychiatric Inventory (NPI) score (mean decrease of 12.5 points, $p < 0.001$; Figs. 17.3 and 17.4), Behave-AD insomnia subscale score ($p = 0.011$), and the Zarit's Caregiver's Burden score (J-ZBI; mean decrease of 3.5 points, $p = 0.024$; Fig. 17.5). The Mini-Mental State Examination also increased 1.1 points as mean, though the Disability Assessment for Dementia showed no significant change. Adverse events occurred in 11 (18 %) patients, and 3 (5 %) patients discontinued YKS due to adverse reactions, spasticity, BPSD deterioration, edema, and nausea. Four patients (6 %) showed hypokalemia (<3.5 mEq/L) at the study conclusion. Deterioration of extrapyramidal symptoms was not observed.

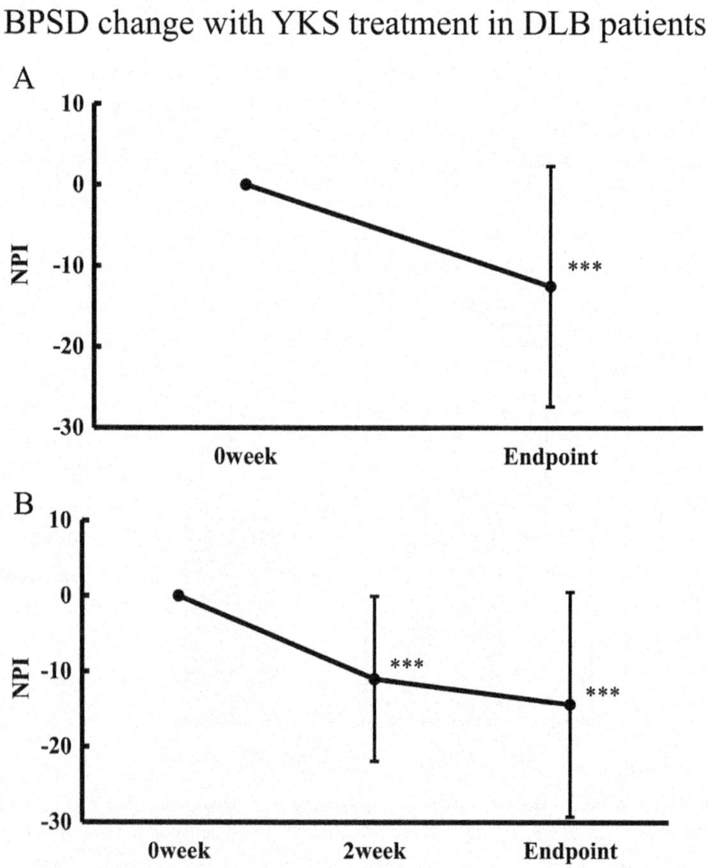

Fig. 17.3 BPSD change with YKS treatment in DLB patients. ***$p < 0.001$. Abbreviation: *NPI* neuropsychiatric inventory

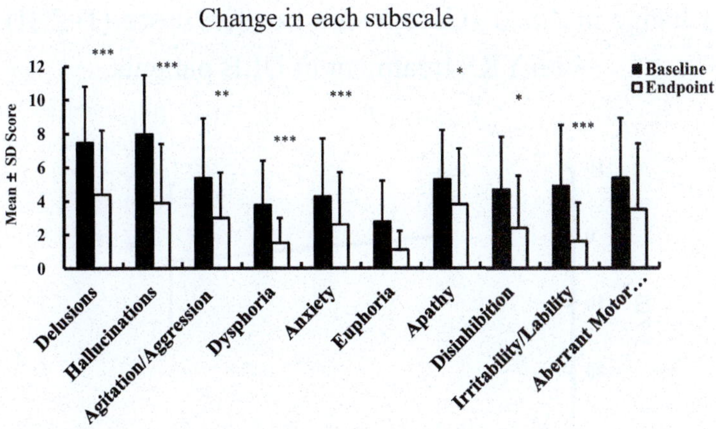

Fig. 17.4 Change in each subscale. $^{***}p < .001$, $^{**}p < .01$, $^{*}p < .05$

17.2.3 Pharmacological Mechanisms

In a 2009 report, Sekiguchi et al. demonstrated that YKS treatment ameliorated aggressive behavior in mice administered with beta-amyloid protein [9]. They also demonstrated that YKS did not suppress motor activity, nor did it induce catalepsy. Takeda et al. reported that YKS attenuated abnormal glutamate release in rats receiving a diet deficient in zinc [10], and in another study, they reported that YKS significantly suppressed the increase in extracellular glutamate and aspartate in the hippocampus of zinc-deficient rats after KCl stimulation [11]. In 2008, Egashira et al. reported that YKS inhibited the 2,5-dimethoxy-4-iodoamphetamine-induced head-twitch response and decreased expression of 5-hydroxytryptamine 2A receptors in the prefrontal cortex [12]. Terawaki et al. reported a partial agonistic effect of YKS on human recombinant serotonin 1A receptors expressed in the membranes of Chinese hamster ovary cells [13]. These reports collectively suggest the involvement of serotonergic and glutamatergic functions in the underlying mechanism of YKS. Tabuchi et al. reported that YKS ameliorated cognitive disturbances in APP transgenic mice, which are an animal model of Alzheimer's disease [14]. Shimada et al. in 2001 reported that an aqueous extract of the hooks and stems of *Uncaria sinensis* (Oliv.) *Havil., Uncariae uncus cum ramulus*, a herb included in YKS, protected against glutamate-induced neuronal death in cultured cerebellar granule cells [15]. They suggested that oxindole alkaloids, such as isorhynchophylline, isocorynoxeine, and rhynchophylline, and indole alkaloids, such as hirsuteine and hirsutine, were the active components in *Uncaria* [16]. These compounds may cause the clinical effects of YKS. Similarly, in 2012, Nishi et al. reported that at least some of the effects of YKS may be due to an alkaloid found in the hooks of *Uncaria* known as geissoschizine methyl ether (GM), which acted as a partial agonist at the 5-HT1A receptor [17]. This assessment was supported by their concurrent finding that treatment with GM reduced

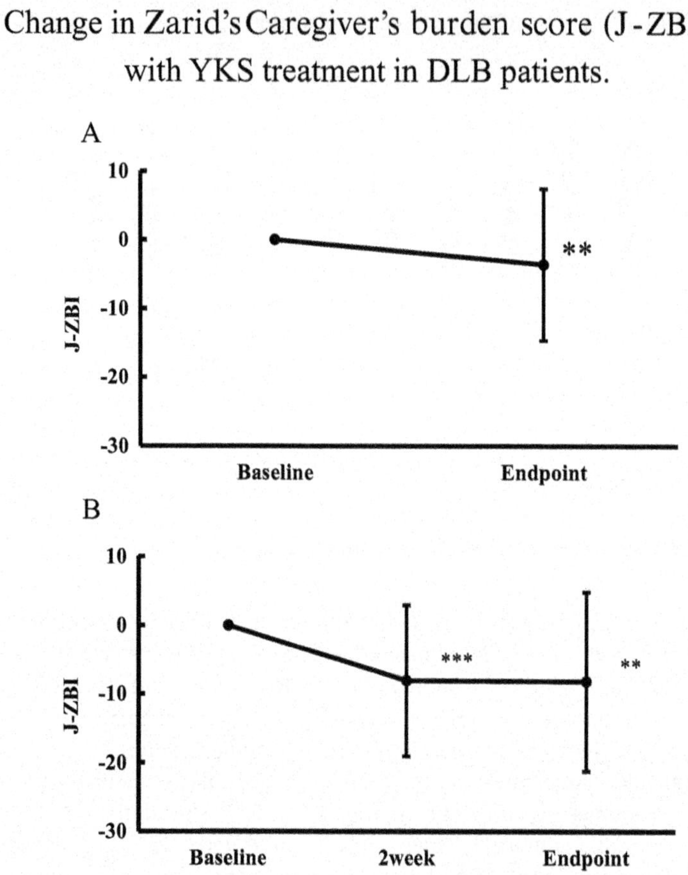

Fig. 17.5 Change in Zarit's Caregiver's burden score (J-ZBI) with YKS treatment in DLB patients. $***p < .001$, $**p < .01$. Abbreviation: *J-ZBI* Zarit burden interview-Japanese edition

aggression and increased social behavior in socially isolated mice, while treatment with YKS lacking *Uncaria* hooks did not.

17.2.4 Adverse Effects

YKS contains *Glycyrrhizae radix*; therefore, care must be taken to avoid derangements in the potassium concentration. *Glycyrrhizae radix* may cause hypokalemia (low serum potassium) [18].

References

1. Ikarashi Y, Iizuka S, Imamura S, et al. Effects of yokukansan, a traditional Japanese medicine, on memory disturbance and behavioral and psychological symptoms of dementia in thiamine-deficient rats. Biol Pharm Bull. 1701;2009:32(10).
2. https://www.tumblr.com/search/herbal%20psychopharmacology
3. Miyaoka T, Horiguchi J. Clinical potential of Yi-Gan San (yokukansan) for the treatment of psychiatric disorders. Curr Psychiatry Rev. 2009;5(4):271–5.
4. Iwasaki K, Satoh-Nakagawa T, Maruyama M, et al. A randomized, observer-blind, controlled trial of the traditional Chinese medicine Yi-Gan San for improvement of behavioral and psychological symptoms and activities of daily living in dementia patients. J Clin Psychiatry. 2005;66:248–52.
5. Mizukami K, Asada T, Kinoshita T, et al. A randomized cross-over study of a traditional Japanese medicine (kampo), yokukansan, in the treatment of the behavioral and psychological symptoms of dementia. Int J Neuropsychopharmacol. 2009;12:191–9.
6. Matsuda Y, Kishi T, Shibayama H, et al. Yokukansan in the treatment of behavioral and psychological symptoms of dementia: a systematic review and meta-analysis of randomized controlled trials. Hum Psychopharmacol. 2013;28(1):80–6.
7. Iwasaki K, Maruyama M, Tomita N, et al. Effects of the traditional Chinese herbal medicine Yi-Gan San for cholinesterase inhibitor-resistant visual hallucinations and neuropsychiatric symptoms in patients with dementia with Lewy bodies. J Clin Psychiatry. 2005;66:1612–3.
8. Iwasaki K, Kosaka K, Mori H, et al. Improvement in delusions and hallucinations in patients with dementia with Lewy bodies upon administration of yokukansan, a traditional Japanese medicine. Psychogeriatrics. 2012;12(4):235–41.
9. Sekiguchi K, Yamaguchi T, Tabuchi M, et al. Effects of yokukansan, a traditional Japanese medicine, on aggressiveness induced by intracerebroventricular injection of amyloid beta protein into mice. Phytother Res. 2009;23(8):1175–81.
10. Takeda A, Tamano H, Itoh H, et al. Attenuation of abnormal glutamate release in zinc deficiency by zinc and Yokukansan. Neurochem Int. 2008;53:230–5.
11. Takeda A, Itoh H, Tamano H, et al. Suppressive effect of Yokukansan on excessive release of glutamate and aspartate in the hippocampus of zinc-deficient rats. Nutr Neurosci. 2008;11:41–6.
12. Egashira N, Iwasaki K, Ishibashi A, et al. Repeated administration of Yokukansan inhibits DOI-induced head-twitch response and decreases expression of 5-hydroxytryptamine (5-HT) 2A receptors in the prefrontal cortex. Prog Neuropsychopharmacol Biol Psychiatry. 2008;32:1516–20.
13. Terawaki K, Ikarashi Y, Sekiguchi K, et al. Partial agonistic effect of yokukansan on human recombinant serotonin 1A receptors expressed in the membranes of Chinese hamster ovary cells. J Ethnopharmacol. 2010;127(2):306–12.
14. Tabuchi M, Yamaguchi T, Iizuka S, et al. Ameliorative effects of yokukansan, a traditional Japanese medicine, on learning and non-cognitive disturbances in the Tg2576 mouse model of Alzheimer's disease. J Ethnopharmacol. 2009;122(1):157–62.
15. Shimada Y, Goto H, Kogure T, et al. Protective effect of phenolic compounds isolated from the hooks and stems of *Uncaria sinensis* on glutamate-induced neuronal death. Am J Chin Med. 2001;29:173–80.
16. Shimada Y, Goto H, Itoh T, et al. Evaluation of the protective effects of alkaloids isolated from the hooks and stems of *Uncaria sinensis* on glutamate-induced neuronal death in cultured cerebellar granule cells from rats. J Pharm Pharmacol. 1999;51:715–22.
17. Nishi A, Yamaguchi T, Sekiguchi K, et al. Geissoschizine methyl ether, an alkaloid in Uncaria hook, is a potent serotonin (1A) receptor agonist and candidate for amelioration of aggressiveness and sociality by yokukansan. Neuroscience. 2012;207:124–36.
18. Crean AM, Abdel-Rahman SE, Greenwood JP. A sweet tooth as the root cause of cardiac arrest. Can J Cardiol. 2009;25(10):357–8.

The manufacturer's authorised representative in the EU is Springer Nature Customer Service Centre GmbH, Europaplatz 3, 69115 Heidelberg, Germany. If you have any concerns regarding our products, please contact ProductSafety@springernature.com

Printed and bound by CPI Group (UK) Ltd, Croydon, CR0 4YY
22/09/2026
02220946-0004